ippincott's

DRUGS TO KNOW for the
NCLEX-RN®

Wolters Kluwer | Lippincott Williams & Wilkins
Health

Philadelphia · Baltimore · New York · London
Buenos Aires · Hong Kong · Sydney · Tokyo

STAFF

Acquisitions Editor
Bill Lamsback

Clinical Director
Joan M. Robinson, RN, MSN

Product Director
David Moreau

Product Manager
Rosanne Hallowell

Editor
Shana Harrington

Copy Editor
Heather Ditch

Editorial Assistants
Karen J. Kirk, Jeri O'Shea,
Linda K. Ruhf

Art Director
Elaine Kasmer

Cover Designer
Melissa Walter

Vendor Manager
Cynthia Rudy

Manufacturing Manager
Beth J. Welsh

Production and Indexing Services
S4Carlisle Publishing Services

LDKNRN020714

Library of Congress Cataloging-in-Publication Data
Lippincott's drugs to know for the NCLEX-RN. — 1st ed.
    p. ; cm.
    Drugs to know for the NCLEX-RN
    Includes bibliographical references and index.
I. Lippincott Williams & Wilkins. II.
    Title: Drugs to know for the NCLEX-RN.
    [DNLM: 1. Pharmaceutical
    Preparations — Handbooks.
    2. Drug Therapy — nursing — Handbooks.
    3. Pharmacological
    Phenomena — Handbooks. QV 39]
615.103—dc23
    ISBN 978-1-4511-7198-3 (alk. paper)
    2012001227

CCS0614

Contents

Appendices

How to use this book: Studying for NCLEX® medication-related questions

Lippincott's Drugs to Know for the NCLEX-RN® is designed as a quick and easy review to use when studying for the NCLEX-RN. Overall, the NCLEX-RN examination assesses the nurse's knowledge and skills that are crucial for meeting the client's needs, with the goal of promoting, maintaining, and restoring the client's health. One significant category included in the NCLEX-RN examination is pharmacological and parenteral therapies, which assesses the nurse's skill and knowledge in administering medications and parenteral therapies.

This versatile book provides a straightforward way to enhance your study for the pharmacological category of the NCLEX-RN. Covering more than 300 key medications, it is organized alphabetically by drug class and then by drugs within each class. Each individual drug is described on its own page in a consistent format, including the drug's pronunciation, trade and brand names, and a focus on key points covered by the NCLEX-RN: Indications, Action, Adverse Reactions, Nursing Considerations, and Patient Teaching. Patient safety is also addressed (pay particular attention to the five appendices for this information). If you encounter an unfamiliar abbreviation in the drug entries, refer to the Guide to abbreviations on page vii. Because all of the text has been reviewed by a clinical expert, you can be sure that the information provided is up-to-date and clinically accurate.

The NCLEX-RN exam questions require the nurse to demonstrate the principles of clinical decision making and critical thinking as they apply to nursing practice. Specifically, as described by the NCLEX exam makers themselves, the pharmacology-related questions assess the nurse's ability to

- identify a contraindication to the administration of a medication to the client.
- identify actual and potential incompatibilities of prescribed client medications.
- identify symptoms/evidence of an allergic reaction (for example, to medications).
- assess the client for actual or potential side effects and adverse effects of medications.
- provide information to the client on common side effects, adverse effects, and potential interactions of medications, and when to notify the primary health care provider.
- educate the client on medication self-administration procedures.
- educate the client about medications.
- prepare and administer medications, using rights of medication administration.

- review pertinent data prior to medication administration (for example, vital signs, lab results, allergies, and potential interactions).
- use clinical decision making and critical thinking when addressing expected effects and outcomes of medications.

  With *Lippincott's Drugs to Know for the NCLEX-RN*®, you can review with confidence for that last step to licensure, the NCLEX-RN. Please note, however, that this book is intended to serve as a study aid only. Because of the abbreviated information contained within, it shouldn't be used as a guide to clinical practice.

Guide to abbreviations

ACE	angiotensin-converting enzyme	I.V.	intravenous
ADH	antidiuretic hormone	lb	pound
ADHD	attention deficit hyperactivity disorder	MAO	monoamine oxidase
		MS	multiple sclerosis
AIDS	acquired immunodeficiency syndrome	NMDA	N-methyl-D-aspartate
		NNRI	non-nucleoside reverse transcriptase inhibitor
ARB	angiotensin receptor blocker	NSAID	nonsteroidal anti-inflammatory drug
AV	atrioventricular	ODT	orally dissolving tablet
BPH	benign prostatic hypertrophy	OTC	over-the-counter
BSA	body surface area	oz	ounce
BUN	blood urea nitrogen	PABA	para-aminobenzoic acid
CBC	complete blood count	PCA	patient-controlled analgesia
CNS	central nervous system	PE	pulmonary embolism
COPD	chronic obstructive pulmonary disease	P.O.	by mouth
		P.R.	by rectum
CV	cardiovascular	PT	prothrombin time
D_5W	dextrose 5% in water	PTT	partial thromboplastin time
ECG	electrocardiogram	PVC	premature ventricular contraction
EEG	electroencephalogram		
EENT	eyes, ears, nose, throat	RAAS	renin–angiotensin–aldosterone system
GABA	gamma-aminobutyric acid		
GFR	glomerular filtration rate	RBC	red blood cell
GGT	gamma-glutamyltransferase	SA	sinoatrial
GI	gastrointestinal	S.L.	sublingual
GU	genitourinary	SSNRI	selective serotonin and norepinephrine reuptake inhibitor
G6PD	glucose-6-phosphate dehydrogenase		
H_1	histamine$_1$	SSRI	selective serotonin reuptake inhibitor
H_2	histamine$_2$	T_3	triiodothyronine
HIV	human immunodeficiency virus	T_4	thyroxine
		UTI	urinary tract infection
HMG-CoA	3-hydroxy-3-methylglutaryl coenzyme A	WBC	white blood cell
I.M.	intramuscular		

Alpha blockers

clonidine hydrochloride
doxazosin mesylate
guanfacine hydrochloride
prazosin hydrochloride
terazosin hydrochloride

INDICATIONS

➤ Hypertension; mild to moderate urinary obstruction in men with BPH

ACTION

Selective alpha blockers decrease vascular resistance and increase vein capacity, thereby lowering blood pressure and causing orthostatic and exercise hypotension, mild to moderate miosis, interference with ejaculation, and pink, warm skin. They also relax nonvascular smooth muscle, especially in the prostate capsule, which reduces urinary problems in men with BPH. Because alpha$_1$ blockers don't block alpha$_2$ receptors, they don't cause transmitter overflow.

Nonselective alpha blockers antagonize both alpha$_1$ and alpha$_2$ receptors. Generally, alpha blockade results in tachycardia, palpitations, and increased renin secretion because of abnormally large amounts of norepinephrine (from transmitter overflow) released from adrenergic nerve endings as a result of the blockade of alpha$_1$ and alpha$_2$ receptors. Norepinephrine's effects are counterproductive to the major uses of nonselective alpha blockers.

ADVERSE REACTIONS

Alpha blockers may cause severe orthostatic hypotension and syncope, especially with the first few doses. The most common adverse effects are dizziness, headache, drowsiness, somnolence, and malaise. These drugs also may cause tachycardia, palpitations, fluid retention (from excess renin secretion), and aggravation of respiratory tract infection.

CONTRAINDICATIONS AND CAUTIONS

• Contraindicated in patients with MI, coronary insufficiency, or angina or with hypersensitivity to these drugs or any of their components. Also contraindicated in combination therapy with phosphodiesterase type 5 inhibitors (sildenafil, tadalafil, vardenafil).
• In elderly patients, hypotensive effects may be more pronounced.

clonidine hydrochloride
KLOE-ni-deen

Catapres, Catapres-TTS, Duraclon, Jenloga

Pharmacologic class: Centrally acting alpha agonist

INDICATIONS
➤ Essential and renal hypertension

ACTION
Unknown. Thought to stimulate alpha$_2$ receptors and inhibit the central vasomotor centers, decreasing sympathetic outflow to the heart, kidneys, and peripheral vasculature, and lowering peripheral vascular resistance, blood pressure, and heart rate.

ADVERSE REACTIONS
CNS: drowsiness, dizziness, sedation, weakness
CV: bradycardia, severe rebound hypertension
GI: constipation, dry mouth, nausea
Skin: pruritus, dermatitis with transdermal patch

NURSING CONSIDERATIONS
• Monitor blood pressure and pulse rate frequently.
• Elderly patients may be more sensitive than younger ones to drug's hypotensive effects.
• Noticeable antihypertensive effects of transdermal clonidine may take 2 to 3 days.
• Don't confuse clonidine with quinidine or clomiphene; or Catapres with Cetapred or Combipres.
• Closely monitor blood pressure if administered with beta blockers: may cause life-threatening hypertension.

PATIENT TEACHING
• Advise patient that stopping drug abruptly may cause severe rebound high blood pressure. Tell him dosage must be reduced gradually over 2 to 4 days, as instructed by prescriber.
• Tell patient to take the last dose immediately before bedtime.
• Reassure patient that the transdermal patch usually remains attached despite showering and other routine daily activities. Also tell him to place patch at a different site each week.

doxazosin mesylate
dox-AY-zo-sin

Cardura, Cardura XL

Pharmacologic class: Alpha blocker

INDICATIONS
➤ Essential hypertension
➤ BPH

ACTION
Acts on the peripheral vasculature to reduce peripheral vascular resistance and produce vasodilation. Drug also decreases smooth muscle tone in the prostate and bladder neck.

ADVERSE REACTIONS
CNS: dizziness, asthenia, headache
CV: orthostatic hypotension, arrhythmias
Hematologic: leukopenia, neutropenia

NURSING CONSIDERATIONS
• Monitor blood pressure closely.
• If syncope occurs, place patient in a recumbent position and treat supportively.
• Don't confuse doxazosin with doxapram, doxorubicin, or doxepin.
• Don't confuse Cardura with Coumadin, K-Dur, Cardene, or Cordarone.
• Give extended-release tablet with breakfast.
• Don't give evening dose the night before switching to extended-release from immediate-release formula.

PATIENT TEACHING
• Instruct the patient to swallow extended-release tablets whole: don't chew, divide, cut, or crush.
• Advise the patient that he is susceptible to a first-dose effect (marked low blood pressure on standing up with dizziness or fainting). This is most common after first dose but also can occur during dosage adjustment or interruption of therapy.
• Advise patient to rise slowly from sitting or lying position.
• Advise patient to avoid driving and other hazardous activities until drug's effects are known.

guanfacine hydrochloride
GWAHN-fa-seen

Intuniv, Tenex

Pharmacologic class: Centrally acting antiadrenergic

INDICATIONS
➤ Hypertension
➤ Pediatric hypertension
➤ Attention deficit hyperactivity disorder

ACTION
Reduces sympathetic outflow from the vasomotor center to the heart and blood vessels, resulting in a decrease in peripheral vascular resistance and a reduction in heart rate.

ADVERSE REACTIONS
CNS: dizziness, somnolence
CV: bradycardia
GI: constipation, dry mouth

NURSING CONSIDERATIONS
• Monitor blood pressure frequently.
• Rebound hypertension may occur and, if it occurs, will be noticeable within 2 to 4 days after therapy ends.
• Don't confuse guanfacine with guanidine, guaifenesin, or guanabenz. Don't confuse Tenex with Xanax, Entex, or Ten-K.
• Don't give extended-release tablet with high-fat meal; give with water, milk, or other liquid.
• Don't crush, break, or allow patient to chew extended-release tablets.
• Use cautiously in patients with severe coronary insufficiency, recent MI, cerebrovascular disease, or chronic renal or hepatic insufficiency.
• Closely monitor blood pressure if administered with tricyclic antidepressants: may inhibit antihypertensive effects.

PATIENT TEACHING
• Advise patient to avoid activities that require alertness before drug's effects are known; drowsiness may occur.
• Warn patient that he may have a lower tolerance to alcohol and other CNS depressants during therapy.
• Caution patient that drug may decrease saliva and contribute to dental caries, periodontal disease, oral candidiasis, and discomfort. Advise patient to have routine dental exams.

prazosin hydrochloride
PRA-zo-sin

Minipress

Pharmacologic class: Alpha blocker

INDICATIONS
➤ Mild to moderate hypertension

ACTION
Unknown. Thought to act by blocking alpha-adrenergic receptors.

ADVERSE REACTIONS
CNS: dizziness, first-dose syncope, headache, drowsiness
CV: orthostatic hypotension, palpitations
GI: vomiting, diarrhea, abdominal cramps, nausea

NURSING CONSIDERATIONS
• Monitor patient's blood pressure and pulse rate frequently.
• Elderly patients may be more sensitive to drug's hypotensive effects.
• Be alert for first-dose syncope if first dose is more than 1 mg.
• Be aware that concurrent use of diuretics may increase the frequency of syncope.

PATIENT TEACHING
• Warn patient that dizziness may occur with first dose. If he experiences dizziness, tell him to sit or lie down. Reassure him that this effect disappears with continued dosing.
• Caution patient to avoid driving or performing hazardous tasks for the first 24 hours after starting this drug or increasing the dose.
• Tell patient not to suddenly stop taking drug, but to notify prescriber if unpleasant adverse reactions occur.
• Advise patient to minimize low blood pressure and dizziness upon standing by rising slowly and avoiding sudden position changes.

terazosin hydrochloride

ter-AY-zoe-sin

Hytrin

Pharmacologic class: Alpha blocker

INDICATIONS
➤ Hypertension
➤ Symptomatic BPH

ACTION
Improves urine flow in patients with BPH by blocking alpha-adrenergic receptors in the bladder neck and prostate, relieving urethral pressure. Drug also reduces peripheral vascular resistance and blood pressure via arterial and venous dilation.

ADVERSE REACTIONS
CNS: headache, dizziness, asthenia, first-dose syncope
CV: peripheral edema, palpitations, orthostatic hypotension
GI: nausea
Hematologic: thrombocytopenia

NURSING CONSIDERATIONS
• Monitor blood pressure frequently.
• Be aware that concurrent use with other antihypertensives may cause excessive hypotension.

PATIENT TEACHING
• Tell patient not to stop drug suddenly, but to notify prescriber if adverse reactions occur.
• Warn patient to avoid hazardous activities that require mental alertness, such as driving or operating heavy machinery, for 12 hours after first dose.
• Tell patient that light-headedness can occur, especially during the first few days of therapy. Advise him to rise slowly to minimize this effect and to report signs and symptoms to prescriber.

Alzheimer's disease drugs

donepezil hydrochloride
memantine hydrochloride
rivastigmine tartrate

INDICATIONS
➤ Treatment of mild to moderate dementia of the Alzheimer's type

ACTION
Current theories attribute signs and symptoms of Alzheimer's disease to a deficiency of cholinergic neurotransmission. It's suggested that these drugs improve cholinergic function by increasing acetylcholine through reversible inhibition of its hydrolysis by cholinesterase. Memantine is an NMDA receptor antagonist. Persistent activation of the NMDA receptors is thought to contribute to symptoms of Alzheimer's disease. There is no evidence that any of the drugs alter the course of the underlying disease process.

ADVERSE REACTIONS
Weight loss, diarrhea, anorexia, nausea, vomiting, dizziness, headache, bradyarrhythmias; hypertension and constipation (memantine).

CONTRAINDICATIONS AND CAUTIONS
• Contraindicated in patients hypersensitive to any of the drug components.
• May exaggerate neuromuscular blocking effects of succinylcholine-type and similar neuromuscular blocking agents used during anesthesia.
• Use cautiously with concomitant drugs that slow heart rate. There is an increased risk for heart block.
• Use cautiously with NSAIDs because the drug increases gastric acid secretion. There is increased risk of developing ulcers and active or occult GI bleeding.
• Use cautiously in patients with moderate hepatic or renal impairment. The drugs are not recommended in severe hepatic impairment or severe renal impairment (creatinine clearance less than 9 ml/minute).
• Use cautiously in patients with a history of asthma or COPD.

donepezil hydrochloride
doe-NEP-ah-zill

Aricept, Aricept ODT

Pharmacologic class: Cholinesterase inhibitor

INDICATIONS
➤ Mild to moderate Alzheimer's dementia
➤ Moderate to severe Alzheimer's disease

ACTION
Thought to increase acetylcholine level by inhibiting cholinesterase enzyme, which causes acetylcholine hydrolysis.

ADVERSE REACTIONS
CNS: headache, insomnia, seizures
CV: bradycardia, heart block
EENT: cataract, blurred vision, eye irritation, sore throat
GI: nausea, diarrhea, vomiting, GI bleeding

NURSING CONSIDERATIONS
• Allow ODT to dissolve on tongue; then follow with water.
• Give drug at bedtime, without regard for food.
• Monitor patient for evidence of active or occult GI bleeding.
• Monitor patient for bradycardia because of potential for vagotonic effects.
• Don't confuse Aricept with Ascriptin.

PATIENT TEACHING
• Stress that drug doesn't alter underlying degenerative disease but can temporarily stabilize or relieve symptoms. Effectiveness depends on taking drug at regular intervals.
• Advise patient and caregiver to report immediately significant adverse effects or changes in overall health status and to inform health care team that patient is taking drug before he receives anesthesia.
• Tell patient to avoid OTC cold or sleep remedies because of risk of increased anticholinergic effects.

memantine hydrochloride

meh-MAN-teen

Namenda, Namenda XR

Pharmacologic class: NMDA receptor antagonist

INDICATIONS
➤ Moderate to severe Alzheimer's dementia

ACTION
Antagonizes NMDA receptors, the persistent activation of which seems to increase Alzheimer symptoms.

ADVERSE REACTIONS
CNS: stroke, aggressiveness, agitation, confusion, depression, dizziness, headache, insomnia, somnolence, syncope, transient ischemic attack, vertigo
CV: heart failure, edema, hypertension
GI: anorexia, constipation, diarrhea, nausea, vomiting
GU: incontinence, urinary frequency, UTI

NURSING CONSIDERATIONS
• Patients may take capsules intact or capsules may be opened, sprinkled on applesauce, and then swallowed. Don't allow patients to divide, chew, or crush capsules.
• In elderly patients, even those with a normal creatinine level, use of this drug may impair renal function. Don't give drug to patients with severe renal impairment.
• Monitor patient carefully for adverse reactions as he may not be able to recognize changes or communicate effectively.

PATIENT TEACHING
• Explain that drug doesn't cure Alzheimer's disease but may aid patient in maintaining function for a longer period of time.
• Tell patient or caregiver to report adverse effects.
• Urge patient to avoid alcohol, which may reduce drug's effectiveness.

rivastigmine tartrate
riv-ah-STIG-meen

Exelon, Exelon Patch

Pharmacologic class: Cholinesterase inhibitor

INDICATIONS
➤ Mild to moderate Alzheimer's dementia
➤ Mild to moderate dementia associated with Parkinson's disease

ACTION
Thought to increase acetylcholine level by inhibiting cholinesterase enzyme, which causes acetylcholine hydrolysis.

ADVERSE REACTIONS
CNS: headache, dizziness
CV: bradycardia
GI: nausea, vomiting, diarrhea, anorexia, abdominal pain

NURSING CONSIDERATIONS
• Monitor patient for severe nausea, vomiting, and diarrhea, which may lead to dehydration and weight loss.
• Monitor patient for evidence of active or occult GI bleeding.
• For P.O.: Give drug with food in the morning and evening. Solution may be taken directly or mixed with small glass of water, cold fruit juice, or soda.
• For transdermal: Apply patch once daily to clean, dry, hairless skin on the upper or lower back, upper arm, or chest, in a place not rubbed by tight clothing. Change the site daily, and don't use the same site within 14 days.

PATIENT TEACHING
• Tell caregiver to give drug with food in the morning and evening.
• Advise patient that memory improvement may be subtle and that drug more likely slows future memory loss.
• Teach patient or caregiver the recommended sites for patch placement and the frequency of changing the site. Stress the importance of not using the same site within 14 days.

Aminoglycosides

amikacin sulfate
gentamicin sulfate
tobramycin sulfate

INDICATIONS

➤ Septicemia; postoperative, pulmonary, intra-abdominal, and urinary tract infections; skin, soft tissue, bone, and joint infections; aerobic gram-negative bacillary meningitis not susceptible to other antibiotics; serious staphylococcal, *Pseudomonas aeruginosa*, and *Klebsiella* infections; enterococcal infections; nosocomial pneumonia; anaerobic infections involving *Bacteroides fragilis*; tuberculosis; initial empiric therapy in febrile, leukopenic patients

ACTION

Aminoglycosides are bactericidal. They bind directly and irreversibly to 30S ribosomal subunits, inhibiting bacterial protein synthesis. They're active against many aerobic gram-negative and some aerobic gram-positive organisms and can be used in combination with other antibiotics for short courses of therapy.

ADVERSE REACTIONS

Ototoxicity and nephrotoxicity are the most serious complications. Neuromuscular blockade also may occur. Oral forms most commonly cause diarrhea, nausea, and vomiting. Parenteral drugs may cause vein irritation, phlebitis, and sterile abscess.

CONTRAINDICATIONS AND CAUTIONS

• Contraindicated in patients hypersensitive to these drugs.
• Use cautiously in patients with a neuromuscular disorder and in those taking neuromuscular blockades.
• Use at lower dosages in patients with renal impairment.
• In pregnant women, can cause fetal harm. In breast-feeding women, safety hasn't been established.
• In neonates and premature infants, the half-life of aminoglycosides is prolonged because of immature renal systems. In infants and children, dosage adjustment may be needed.
• Elderly patients have an increased risk of nephrotoxicity and commonly need a lower dose and longer intervals; they're also susceptible to ototoxicity and superinfection.

amikacin sulfate

am-i-KAY-sin

Pharmacologic class: Aminoglycoside

INDICATIONS

➤ Serious infections caused by sensitive strains of *Pseudomonas aeruginosa*, *Escherichia coli*, *Proteus*, *Klebsiella*, or *Staphylococcus*
➤ Uncomplicated UTI caused by organisms not susceptible to less toxic drugs

ACTION

Inhibits protein synthesis by binding directly to the 30S ribosomal subunit; bactericidal.

ADVERSE REACTIONS

CNS: neuromuscular blockade
EENT: ototoxicity
GU: azotemia, nephrotoxicity, increase in urinary excretion of casts
Musculoskeletal: arthralgia
Respiratory: apnea

NURSING CONSIDERATIONS

• Be aware that I.V. loop diuretics such as furosemide may increase ototoxicity.
• Obtain specimen for culture and sensitivity tests before giving first dose. Begin therapy while awaiting results.
• Obtain blood for peak level 1 hour after I.M. injection and 30 minutes to 1 hour after I.V. infusion ends; for trough levels, draw blood just before next dose.
• Monitor renal function, including urine output, specific gravity, urinalysis, BUN and creatinine levels, and creatinine clearance. Report any evidence of declining renal function.
• Watch for signs and symptoms of superinfection (especially of upper respiratory tract), such as continued fever, chills, and increased pulse rate.
• Don't confuse amikacin with anakinra.

PATIENT TEACHING

• Instruct patient to promptly report adverse reactions to prescriber.
• Encourage patient to maintain adequate fluid intake.

gentamicin sulfate (injection)

jen-ta-MYE-sin

Pharmacologic class: Aminoglycoside

INDICATIONS

➤ Serious infections caused by sensitive strains of *Pseudomonas aeruginosa*, *Escherichia coli*, *Proteus*, *Klebsiella*, *Serratia*, or *Staphylococcus*

ACTION

Inhibits protein synthesis by binding directly to the 30S ribosomal subunit; bactericidal.

ADVERSE REACTIONS

CNS: encephalopathy, seizures, fever, headache, lethargy, confusion, dizziness, numbness, peripheral neuropathy, vertigo, ataxia, tingling
CV: hypotension
EENT: ototoxicity, tinnitus
GU: nephrotoxicity
Hematologic: agranulocytosis, leukopenia, thrombocytopenia, anemia
Respiratory: apnea
Other: anaphylaxis

NURSING CONSIDERATIONS

• Be aware that I.V. loop diuretics such as furosemide may increase ototoxicity.
• Obtain specimen for culture and sensitivity tests before giving first dose. Begin therapy while awaiting results.
• Obtain blood for peak level 1 hour after I.M. injection and 30 minutes to 1 hour after I.V. infusion ends; for trough levels, draw blood just before next dose.
• Monitor renal function, including urine output, specific gravity, urinalysis, BUN and creatinine levels, and creatinine clearance. Report any evidence of declining renal function.
• Watch for signs and symptoms of superinfection (especially of upper respiratory tract), such as continued fever, chills, and increased pulse rate.

PATIENT TEACHING

• Instruct patient to promptly report adverse reactions, such as dizziness, vertigo, unsteady gait, ringing in the ears, hearing loss, numbness, tingling, or muscle twitching.
• Encourage patient to drink plenty of fluids.
• Warn patient to avoid hazardous activities if adverse CNS reactions occur.

tobramycin sulfate
toe-bra-MYE-sinTOBI

Pharmacologic class: Aminoglycoside

INDICATIONS
➤ Serious infection by sensitive strains of *Escherichia coli*, *Proteus*, *Klebsiella*, *Enterobacter*, *Serratia*, *Morganella morganii*, *Staphylococcus aureus*, *Citrobacter*, *Pseudomonas*, or *Providencia*

ACTION
Generally bactericidal. Inhibits protein synthesis by binding directly to the 30S ribosomal subunit.

ADVERSE REACTIONS
CNS: seizures, headache, lethargy, confusion, disorientation, fever
EENT: ototoxicity, hoarseness, pharyngitis
GU: nephrotoxicity
Hematologic: leukopenia, thrombocytopenia, agranulocytosis
Respiratory: bronchospasm

NURSING CONSIDERATIONS
• Be aware that I.V. loop diuretics such as furosemide may increase ototoxicity.
• Obtain specimen for culture and sensitivity tests before giving first dose. Begin therapy while awaiting results.
• Obtain blood for peak level 1 hour after I.M. injection and 30 minutes to 1 hour after I.V. infusion ends; for trough levels, draw blood just before next dose.
• Monitor renal function, including urine output, specific gravity, urinalysis, BUN and creatinine levels, and creatinine clearance. Report any evidence of declining renal function.
• Watch for signs and symptoms of superinfection (especially of upper respiratory tract), such as continued fever, chills, and increased pulse rate.
• Don't confuse tobramycin with Trobicin.

PATIENT TEACHING
• Caution patient not to perform hazardous activities if adverse CNS reactions occur.
• Encourage patient to maintain adequate fluid intake.
• Teach patient how to use and maintain nebulizer. Tell patient using several inhaled therapies to use this drug last.
• Instruct patient not to use if the inhalation solution is cloudy or contains particles or if it has been stored at room temperature for longer than 28 days.

Angiotensin-converting enzyme inhibitors

benazepril hydrochloride
captopril
enalapril maleate
fosinopril sodium
lisinopril
quinapril hydrochloride
ramipril
trandolapril

INDICATIONS
➤ Hypertension, heart failure, left ventricular dysfunction, MI (ramipril, lisinopril), and diabetic nephropathy (captopril)

ACTION
ACE inhibitors prevent conversion of angiotensin I to angiotensin II, a potent vasoconstrictor. Besides decreasing vasoconstriction and thus reducing peripheral arterial resistance, inhibiting angiotensin II decreases adrenocortical secretion of aldosterone. This reduces sodium and water retention and extracellular fluid volume.

ACE inhibition also causes increased levels of bradykinin, which results in vasodilation. This decreases heart rate and systemic vascular resistance.

ADVERSE REACTIONS
The most common adverse effects of therapeutic doses are angioedema of the face and limbs, dry cough, dysgeusia, fatigue, headache, hyperkalemia, hypotension, proteinuria, rash, and tachycardia. Severe hypotension may occur at toxic drug levels.

CONTRAINDICATIONS AND CAUTIONS
• Contraindicated in patients hypersensitive to these drugs.
• Use cautiously in patients with impaired renal function or serious autoimmune disease and in those taking other drugs known to decrease WBC count or immune response.
• Women of childbearing potential taking ACE inhibitors should report pregnancy immediately to prescriber. High risks of fetal morbidity and mortality are linked to ACE inhibitors, especially in the second and third trimesters. Some ACE inhibitors appear in breast milk. To avoid adverse effects in infants, instruct patient to stop breast-feeding during therapy. In children, safety and effectiveness haven't been established; give drug only if potential benefits outweigh risks. Elderly patients may need lower doses because of impaired drug clearance.

benazepril hydrochloride
ben-A-za-pril

Lotensin

Pharmacologic class: ACE inhibitor

INDICATIONS
➤ Hypertension

ACTION
Inhibits ACE, preventing conversion of angiotensin I to angiotensin II, a potent vasoconstrictor. Less angiotensin II decreases peripheral arterial resistance, decreasing aldosterone secretion, which reduces sodium and water retention and lowers blood pressure.

ADVERSE REACTIONS
CNS: headache, dizziness, drowsiness, fatigue, somnolence
CV: symptomatic hypotension
GU: impotence
Metabolic: hyperkalemia
Musculoskeletal: arthralgia, arthritis, myalgia
Respiratory: dry, persistent, nonproductive cough
Other: hypersensitivity reactions, angioedema

NURSING CONSIDERATIONS
• Measure blood pressure when drug level is at peak (2 to 6 hours after administration) and at trough (just before a dose) to verify adequate blood pressure control.
• Don't confuse benazepril with Benadryl or Lotensin with Loniten or lovastatin.

PATIENT TEACHING
• Instruct patient to avoid salt substitutes containing potassium. May cause hyperkalemia.
• Inform patient that light-headedness can occur. Tell him to rise slowly to minimize this effect.
• Warn patient to use caution in hot weather and during exercise. Inadequate fluid intake, vomiting, diarrhea, and excessive perspiration can lead to light-headedness and fainting.
• Advise patient to report signs of infection, such as fever and sore throat. Tell him to call prescriber if he develops easy bruising or bleeding; swelling of tongue, lips, face, eyes, mucous membranes, or extremities; difficulty swallowing or breathing; or hoarseness.

captopril
KAP-toe-pril

Capoten

Pharmacologic class: ACE inhibitor

INDICATIONS
➤ Hypertension
➤ Heart failure
➤ Left ventricular dysfunction after acute MI

ACTION
Inhibits ACE, preventing conversion of angiotensin I to angiotensin II, a potent vasoconstrictor. Less angiotensin II decreases peripheral arterial resistance, decreasing aldosterone secretion, which reduces sodium and water retention and lowers blood pressure.

ADVERSE REACTIONS
CNS: dizziness, fainting, headache
CV: tachycardia, hypotension
Hematologic: leukopenia, agranulocytosis, thrombocytopenia, pancytopenia, anemia
Metabolic: hyperkalemia
Respiratory: dry, persistent, nonproductive cough, dyspnea
Skin: urticarial rash, maculopapular rash
Other: angioedema

NURSING CONSIDERATIONS
• Give 1 hour before meals to enhance drug absorption.
• Antacids may decrease captopril effect. Separate dosage times.
• Monitor patient's blood pressure and pulse rate frequently.
• Assess patient for signs of angioedema.
• Don't confuse captopril with Capitrol.

PATIENT TEACHING
• Instruct patient to avoid salt substitutes containing potassium. May cause hyperkalemia.
• Inform patient that light-headedness can occur. Tell him to rise slowly to minimize this effect.
• Tell patient to use caution in hot weather and during exercise. Lack of fluids, vomiting, diarrhea, and excessive perspiration can lead to light-headedness and syncope.
• Advise patient to report signs and symptoms of infection, such as fever and sore throat.

enalapril maleate

eh-NAH-leh-prel

Vasotec

Pharmacologic class: ACE inhibitor

INDICATIONS
➤ Hypertension
➤ Symptomatic heart failure
➤ Asymptomatic left ventricular dysfunction

ACTION
May inhibit ACE, preventing conversion of angiotensin I to angiotensin II, a potent vasoconstrictor. Less angiotensin II decreases peripheral arterial resistance, decreasing aldosterone secretion, reducing sodium and water retention, and lowering blood pressure.

ADVERSE REACTIONS
CNS: asthenia, headache, dizziness, fatigue, vertigo, syncope
CV: hypotension, chest pain
GU: decreased renal function (in patients with bilateral renal artery stenosis or heart failure)
Respiratory: dry, persistent, tickling, nonproductive cough, dyspnea
Other: angioedema

NURSING CONSIDERATIONS
• Closely monitor blood pressure response to drug.
• Monitor potassium intake and potassium level.
• Don't confuse enalapril with Anafranil or Eldepryl.

PATIENT TEACHING
• Instruct patient to avoid salt substitutes containing potassium. May cause hyperkalemia.
• Inform patient that light-headedness can occur. Tell him to rise slowly to minimize this effect.
• Tell patient to use caution in hot weather and during exercise. Lack of fluids, vomiting, diarrhea, and excessive perspiration can lead to light-headedness and syncope.
• Advise patient to report signs and symptoms of infection, such as fever and sore throat.

fosinopril sodium
foh-SIN-oh-pril

Monopril

Pharmacologic class: ACE inhibitor

INDICATIONS
➤ Hypertension
➤ Heart failure

ACTION
Inhibits ACE, preventing conversion of angiotensin I to angiotensin II, a potent vasoconstrictor. Less angiotensin II decreases peripheral arterial resistance, thus decreasing aldosterone secretion, which reduces sodium and water retention and lowers blood pressure.

ADVERSE REACTIONS
CNS: dizziness, stroke, headache, fatigue, syncope, paresthesia
CV: palpitations, hypotension, orthostatic hypotension
GI: pancreatitis, nausea, vomiting, diarrhea
Hepatic: hepatitis
Metabolic: hyperkalemia
Respiratory: dry, persistent, tickling, nonproductive cough; bronchospasm
Other: angioedema, decreased libido, gout

NURSING CONSIDERATIONS
• Monitor blood pressure for drug effect.
• Antacids may decrease fosinopril effect. Separate dosage times.
• Monitor potassium intake and potassium level.
• Assess renal and hepatic function.
• Don't confuse fosinopril with lisinopril. Don't confuse Monopril with Monurol.

PATIENT TEACHING
• Instruct patient to avoid salt substitutes containing potassium. May cause hyperkalemia.
• Inform patient that light-headedness can occur. Tell him to rise slowly to minimize this effect.
• Tell patient to use caution in hot weather and during exercise. Lack of fluids, vomiting, diarrhea, and excessive perspiration can lead to light-headedness and syncope.
• Advise patient to report signs and symptoms of infection, such as fever and sore throat.

lisinopril
lye-SIN-oh-pril

Prinivil, Zestril

Pharmacologic class: ACE inhibitor

INDICATIONS
➤ Hypertension
➤ Adjunct treatment for heart failure
➤ Hemodynamically stable patients within 24 hours of acute MI to improve survival

ACTION
Causes decreased production of angiotensin II and suppression of the renin–angiotensin–aldosterone system.

ADVERSE REACTIONS
CNS: dizziness, headache, fatigue, paresthesia
CV: orthostatic hypotension, hypotension, chest pain
EENT: nasal congestion
GI: diarrhea, nausea, dyspepsia
Metabolic: hyperkalemia
Respiratory: dyspnea; dry, persistent, tickling, nonproductive cough
Other: angioedema

NURSING CONSIDERATIONS
• Monitor blood pressure frequently. If drug doesn't adequately control blood pressure, diuretics may be added.
• Don't confuse lisinopril with fosinopril or Lioresal. Don't confuse Zestril with Zostrix, Zetia, Zebeta, or Zyrtec. Don't confuse Prinivil with Proventil or Prilosec.

PATIENT TEACHING
• Instruct patient to avoid salt substitutes containing potassium. May cause hyperkalemia.
• Inform patient that light-headedness can occur. Tell him to rise slowly to minimize this effect.
• Tell patient to use caution in hot weather and during exercise. Lack of fluids, vomiting, diarrhea, and excessive perspiration can lead to light-headedness and syncope.
• Advise patient to report signs and symptoms of infection, such as fever and sore throat.

quinapril hydrochloride
KWIN-ah-pril

Accupril

Pharmacologic class: ACE inhibitor

INDICATIONS
➤ Hypertension
➤ Heart failure

ACTION
Prevents conversion of angiotensin I to angiotensin II, a potent vaso-constrictor. Less angiotensin II decreases peripheral arterial resistance, decreasing aldosterone secretion, which reduces sodium and water retention and lowers blood pressure.

ADVERSE REACTIONS
CNS: headache, dizziness, fatigue, depression
CV: hypertensive crisis, hypotension, chest pain
GI: abdominal pain, vomiting, nausea, diarrhea
Metabolic: hyperkalemia
Respiratory: dry, persistent, tickling, nonproductive cough; dyspnea

NURSING CONSIDERATIONS
• Give drug 1 hour before or 2 hours after meals, or with a light meal.
• Don't give drug with a high-fat meal.
• Assess renal and hepatic function.
• Monitor blood pressure for effectiveness of therapy.
• Monitor potassium level.
• Avoid using with tetracycline. May decrease absorption.

PATIENT TEACHING
• Instruct patient to avoid salt substitutes containing potassium. May cause hyperkalemia.
• Inform patient that light-headedness can occur. Tell him to rise slowly to minimize this effect.
• Tell patient to use caution in hot weather and during exercise. Lack of fluids, vomiting, diarrhea, and excessive perspiration can lead to light-headedness and syncope.
• Advise patient to report signs and symptoms of infection, such as fever and sore throat.
• Tell patient to avoid taking with a high-fat meal because this may decrease absorption of drug.

ramipril
ra-MI-pril

Altace

Pharmacologic class: ACE inhibitor

INDICATIONS
➤ Hypertension
➤ Heart failure after an MI

ACTION
Prevents conversion of angiotensin I to angiotensin II, a potent vasoconstrictor. Less angiotensin II decreases peripheral arterial resistance, decreasing aldosterone secretion, which reduces sodium and water retention and lowers blood pressure.

ADVERSE REACTIONS
CV: hypotension, heart failure, MI, postural hypotension
GI: nausea, vomiting, diarrhea
Metabolic: hyperkalemia
Respiratory: dyspnea; dry, persistent, tickling, nonproductive cough

NURSING CONSIDERATIONS
• If necessary, open capsule and sprinkle contents on a small amount of applesauce or mix with 4 oz of water or apple juice. Give to patient immediately.
• Monitor blood pressure regularly for drug effectiveness.
• Monitor potassium level.

PATIENT TEACHING
• Tell patient that if he has difficulty swallowing capsules, he can open drug and sprinkle contents on a small amount of applesauce.
• Instruct patient to avoid salt substitutes containing potassium. May cause hyperkalemia.
• Inform patient that light-headedness can occur. Tell him to rise slowly to minimize this effect.
• Tell patient to use caution in hot weather and during exercise. Lack of fluids, vomiting, diarrhea, and excessive perspiration can lead to light-headedness and syncope.
• Advise patient to report signs and symptoms of infection, such as fever and sore throat.

trandolapril
tran-DOLE-ah-pril

Mavik

Pharmacologic class: ACE inhibitor

INDICATIONS
➤ Hypertension
➤ Heart failure or ventricular dysfunction after MI

ACTION
Thought to inhibit ACE, reducing angiotensin II formation, which decreases peripheral arterial resistance, decreases aldosterone secretion, reduces sodium and water retention, and lowers blood pressure.

ADVERSE REACTIONS
CNS: dizziness, headache, fatigue, syncope, stroke
CV: hypotension, bradycardia, chest pain, intermittent claudication
GI: pancreatitis, dyspepsia, diarrhea
Hematologic: neutropenia, leukopenia
Metabolic: hyperkalemia
Respiratory: persistent, nonproductive cough; dyspnea

NURSING CONSIDERATIONS
• Don't give antacid 1 hour before or up to 2 hours after dose.
• Monitor potassium level closely.
• Watch for hypotension. Excessive hypotension can occur when drug is given with diuretics.
• Assess patient's renal function.

PATIENT TEACHING
• Instruct patient to report yellowing of skin or eyes.
• Instruct patient to avoid salt substitutes containing potassium. May cause hyperkalemia.
• Inform patient that light-headedness can occur. Tell him to rise slowly to minimize this effect.
• Tell patient to use caution in hot weather and during exercise. Lack of fluids, vomiting, diarrhea, and excessive perspiration can lead to light-headedness and syncope.
• Advise patient to report signs and symptoms of infection, such as fever and sore throat.

Angiotensin II receptor blockers

irbesartan
losartan potassium
olmesartan medoxomil
valsartan

INDICATIONS
➤ Hypertension; nephropathy in type 2 diabetics (losartan and irbe-sartan); heart failure (valsartan); hypertension with left ventricular hypertrophy (losartan)

ACTION
ARBs act by interfering with the RAAS. They selectively block the binding of angiotensin II to the angiotensin II receptor. This prevents vasoconstricting and aldosterone-secreting effects of angiotensin II (a potent vasoconstrictor), resulting in a blood pressure decrease.

ADVERSE REACTIONS
ARBs commonly cause orthostatic changes in heart rate, headache, hypotension, nausea, and vomiting.

CONTRAINDICATIONS AND CAUTIONS
• Contraindicated in patients hypersensitive to these drugs and in those with hypotension.
• Use cautiously in patients with hepatic or renal dysfunction.
• In pregnant women, use cautiously when potential benefits to the mother outweigh risks to the fetus. Check each drug because some are safe only in the first trimester. In breast-feeding women, use cautiously; some ARBs appear in breast milk. Elderly patients are more susceptible to adverse reactions and may need lower maintenance doses; monitor these patients closely.
• May increase the risk of cancer; however, the benefits continue to outweigh the risk.

irbesartan
er-bah-SAR-tan

Avapro

Pharmacologic class: Angiotensin II receptor antagonist

INDICATIONS
➤ Hypertension
➤ Nephropathy in patients with type 2 diabetes

ACTION
Produces antihypertensive effect by competitive antagonist activity at the angiotensin II receptor.

ADVERSE REACTIONS
CNS: fatigue, anxiety, dizziness, headache
CV: chest pain, edema, tachycardia
GI: diarrhea, dyspepsia, abdominal pain, nausea, vomiting
Respiratory: upper respiratory tract infection, cough
Skin: rash

NURSING CONSIDERATIONS
• Drug may be given with a diuretic or other antihypertensive, if needed, for control of hypertension.
• Symptomatic hypotension may occur in volume- or sodium-depleted patients (vigorous diuretic use or dialysis). Correct the cause of volume depletion before administration or before a lower dose is used.
• If hypotension occurs, place patient in a supine position and give an I.V. infusion of normal saline solution, if needed. When blood pressure has stabilized after a transient hypotensive episode, drug may be continued.
• Dizziness and orthostatic hypotension may occur more frequently in patients with type 2 diabetes and renal disease.

PATIENT TEACHING
• Warn woman of childbearing age of consequences of drug exposure to fetus. Tell her to call prescriber immediately if pregnancy is suspected.

losartan potassium
low-SAR-tan

Cozaar

Pharmacologic class: Angiotensin II receptor antagonist

INDICATIONS
➤ Hypertension
➤ Nephropathy in type 2 diabetic patients
➤ Stroke prevention in patients with hypertension and left ventricular hypertrophy

ACTION
Inhibits vasoconstrictive and aldosterone-secreting action of angiotensin II by blocking angiotensin II receptor on the surface of vascular smooth muscle and other tissue cells.

ADVERSE REACTIONS
Patients with hypertension or left ventricular hypertrophy:
CNS: dizziness, asthenia, fatigue, headache, insomnia
CV: edema, chest pain
Respiratory: cough, upper respiratory infection
Other: angioedema

Patients with nephropathy:
CNS: asthenia, fatigue
CV: chest pain, hypotension, orthostatic hypotension
GI: diarrhea, dyspepsia, gastritis
GU: UTI
Metabolic: hyperkalemia, hypoglycemia, weight gain
Musculoskeletal: back pain
Respiratory: cough, bronchitis
Other: flulike syndrome, angioedema

NURSING CONSIDERATIONS
• Monitor patient's blood pressure closely to evaluate effectiveness of therapy.
• Monitor patients who are also taking diuretics for hypotension.
• Monitor creatinine and BUN levels.
• Don't confuse Cozaar with Zocor.

PATIENT TEACHING
• Instruct patient to avoid salt substitutes containing potassium. May cause hyperkalemia.

olmesartan medoxomil
ol-ma-SAR-tan

Benicar

Pharmacologic class: Angiotensin II receptor antagonist

INDICATIONS
➤ Pediatric hypertension
➤ Hypertension

ACTION
Blocks vasoconstrictor and aldosterone-secreting effects of angiotensin II by selectively blocking the binding of angiotensin II to the angiotensin I, or AT_1, receptor in the vascular smooth muscle.

ADVERSE REACTIONS
CNS: headache
EENT: pharyngitis, rhinitis, sinusitis
GI: diarrhea
GU: hematuria
Metabolic: hyperglycemia, hypertriglyceridemia
Musculoskeletal: back pain
Respiratory: bronchitis, upper respiratory tract infection
Other: flulike symptoms, accidental injury

NURSING CONSIDERATIONS
• Closely monitor patients with heart failure for oliguria, azotemia, and acute renal failure.
• Monitor patient's blood pressure closely to evaluate effectiveness of therapy.
• Monitor patients who are also taking diuretics for hypotension.
• Monitor creatinine and BUN levels.
• Drug may be made into suspension by pharmacist if patient is unable to swallow pills. Shake suspension well before use.

PATIENT TEACHING
• Tell patient to take drug exactly as prescribed and not to stop taking it, even if he feels better.
• Tell patient to take drug without regard to meals.
• Tell patient to report to health care provider any adverse reactions promptly, especially light-headedness and fainting.

valsartan
val-SAR-tan

Diovan

Pharmacologic class: Angiotensin II receptor antagonist

INDICATIONS
➤ Hypertension
➤ New York Heart Association class II to IV heart failure
➤ To reduce CV death in stable post-MI patients with left ventricular failure or dysfunction

ACTION
Blocks the binding of angiotensin II to receptor sites in vascular smooth muscle and the adrenal gland, which inhibits the pressor effects of the renin–angiotensin–aldosterone system.

ADVERSE REACTIONS
CNS: dizziness, headache, insomnia, fatigue, vertigo
CV: edema, hypotension, orthostatic hypotension, syncope
GI: abdominal pain, diarrhea, nausea, dyspepsia
GU: renal impairment
Hematologic: neutropenia
Metabolic: hyperkalemia
Respiratory: upper respiratory tract infection, cough
Other: angioedema, viral infection

NURSING CONSIDERATIONS
• Watch for hypotension. Excessive hypotension can occur when drug is given with high doses of diuretics.
• Correct volume and sodium depletions before starting drug.

PATIENT TEACHING
• Tell women of childbearing age to notify prescriber if pregnancy occurs. Drug will need to be stopped.
• Advise patient that drug may be taken without regard for food.

Antacids

aluminum hydroxide
calcium carbonate

INDICATIONS
➤ Hyperacidity; hyperphosphatemia (aluminum hydroxide); hypomagnesemia (magnesium oxide); postmenopausal hypocalcemia (calcium carbonate)

ACTION
Antacids reduce the total acid load in the GI tract and elevate gastric pH to reduce pepsin activity. They also strengthen the gastric mucosal barrier and increase esophageal sphincter tone.

ADVERSE REACTIONS
Antacids containing aluminum may cause aluminum intoxication, constipation, hypophosphatemia, intestinal obstruction, and osteomalacia. Antacids containing magnesium may cause diarrhea or hypermagnesemia (in renal failure). Calcium carbonate, magaldrate, magnesium oxide, and sodium bicarbonate may cause constipation, milk-alkali syndrome, or rebound hyperacidity.

CONTRAINDICATIONS AND CAUTIONS
• Calcium carbonate and magnesium oxide are contraindicated in patients with severe renal disease. Sodium bicarbonate is contraindicated in patients with hypertension, renal disease, or edema; patients who are vomiting; patients receiving diuretics or continuous GI suction; and patients on sodium-restricted diets.
• In patients with mild renal impairment, give magnesium oxide cautiously.
• Give aluminum preparations and calcium carbonate cautiously in elderly patients; in those receiving antidiarrheals, antispasmodics, or anticholinergics; and in those with dehydration, fluid restriction, chronic renal disease, or suspected intestinal absorption problems.
• Pregnant women should consult their prescriber before using antacids. Breastfeeding women may take antacids. In infants, serious adverse effects are more likely from changes in fluid and electrolyte balance; monitor them closely. Elderly patients have an increased risk of adverse reactions; monitor them closely; also, give these patients aluminum preparations, calcium carbonate, and magnesium oxide cautiously.

aluminum hydroxide
a-LOO-mi-num

AlternaGEL, Alu-Cap, Alu-Tab, Amphojel, Dialume

Pharmacologic class: Aluminum salt

INDICATIONS
➤ Acid indigestion

ACTION
Neutralizes acid in GI tract, elevates gastric pH to reduce pepsin activity, strengthens gastric mucosal barrier, and increases esophageal sphincter tone.

ADVERSE REACTIONS
CNS: encephalopathy
GI: constipation, intestinal obstruction
Metabolic: hypophosphatemia
Musculoskeletal: osteomalacia

NURSING CONSIDERATIONS
• May decrease the effect of tetracycline absorption. Give antacid 1 to 2 hours before tetracycline.
• May decrease quinolone effect. Give antacid at least 6 hours before or 2 hours after quinolone.
• Enteric-coated drug may be released prematurely in stomach. Separate doses by at least 1 hour.
• Use cautiously in patients with chronic renal disease.
• Shake suspension well.
• May interfere with imaging techniques using sodium pertechnetate Tc-99m or technetium-99m sulfur colloid.
• Watch for aluminum toxicity in patients with severe renal impairment (dialysis encephalopathy, osteomalacia). Aluminum isn't well removed by dialysis.

PATIENT TEACHING
• Instruct patient to shake suspension well and to follow with a small amount of milk or water to facilitate passage.
• Urge patient to notify prescriber about signs and symptoms of GI bleeding, such as tarry stools or coffee-ground vomitus.

calcium carbonate

KAL-see-um

Alka-Mints, Cal-Carb Forte, Calci-Chew, Calci-Mix, Calel-D, Cal-Gest, Caltrate, Chooz, Dicarbosil, Equilet, Maalox Antacid Caplets, Nephro-Calci, Oscal, Oysco, Oyst-Cal, Rolaids, Surpass, Titralac, Trial, Tums

Pharmacologic class: Calcium salt

INDICATIONS

➤ Acid indigestion, calcium supplement

ACTION

Reduces total acid load in GI tract, elevates gastric pH to reduce pepsin activity, strengthens gastric mucosal barrier, and increases esophageal sphincter tone.

ADVERSE REACTIONS

CNS: headache, irritability, weakness
GI: nausea, constipation, flatulence, rebound hyperacidity

NURSING CONSIDERATIONS

• Shake suspension well before administration.
• Record amount and consistency of stools. Manage constipation with laxatives or stool softeners.
• Monitor calcium level, especially in patients with mild renal impairment.
• Watch for evidence of hypercalcemia (nausea, vomiting, headache, confusion, and anorexia).

PATIENT TEACHING

• Advise patient not to take calcium carbonate indiscriminately or to switch antacids without prescriber's advice.
• Tell patient who takes chewable tablets to chew thoroughly before swallowing and to follow with a glass of water.
• Tell patient who uses suspension form to shake well and take with a small amount of water to facilitate passage.
• Urge patient to notify prescriber about signs and symptoms of GI bleeding, such as tarry stools or coffee-ground vomitus.

Antianemics

epoetin alfa
ferrous fumarate
ferrous sulfate
folic acid

INDICATIONS
➤Anemia associated with chronic renal failure (epoetin alfa); zidovudine therapy in patients with HIV and cancer patients on chemotherapy (epoetin alfa); reduce the need for allogenic blood transfusions in surgical patients (epoetin alfa); iron deficiency (ferrous fumarate, ferrous sulfate); RDA (folic acid); megaloblastic or macrocytic anemia from folic acid or other nutritional deficiency (folic acid)

ACTION
Epoetin stimulates RBC production in the bone marrow. Ferrous fumarate and ferrous sulfate provide elemental iron, an essential component in the formation of hemoglobin. Folic acid stimulates normal erythropoiesis and nucleoprotein synthesis.

ADVERSE REACTIONS
Antianemic agents may cause fatigue, headache, weakness, nausea, vomiting, diarrhea, constipation, rash, and urticaria.

CONTRAINDICATIONS AND CAUTIONS
• Contraindicated in patients hypersensitive to any of the drug components.
• Epoetin alfa shouldn't be used in patients with breast, non–small-cell lung, head and neck, lymphoid, and cervical cancers, or for the treatment of cancers with curative potential.

epoetin alfa (erythropoietin)

e-poe-E-tin

Epogen, Procrit

Pharmacologic class: Recombinant human erythropoietin

INDICATIONS

➤ Anemia caused by chronic renal failure, zidovudine therapy in HIV-infected patients, or chemotherapy

➤ Reduce need for allogenic blood transfusion in anemic patients scheduled to have elective, noncardiac, nonvascular surgery

ACTION

Mimics effects of erythropoietin. Functions as a growth factor and as a differentiating factor, enhancing RBC production.

ADVERSE REACTIONS

CNS: asthenia, dizziness, fatigue, headache, paresthesia, seizures
CV: edema, hypertension, increased clotting of arteriovenous grafts
GI: diarrhea, nausea, vomiting
Metabolic: hyperkalemia, hyperphosphatemia, hyperuricemia
Musculoskeletal: arthralgia
Respiratory: cough, shortness of breath, upper respiratory infection

NURSING CONSIDERATIONS

- Store solution in refrigerator and protect from light.
- Don't shake or dilute.
- Don't use if solution is discolored or has particulate matter.
- To prevent deep vein thrombosis, consider prophylaxis.
- Don't confuse Epogen with Neupogen.

PATIENT TEACHING

- Inform patient that pain or discomfort in limbs and pelvis, and coldness and sweating may occur after injection (usually within 2 hours). Symptoms may last for 12 hours and then disappear.
- Advise women that they may resume menstruating after therapy and to consider the need for contraception.

ferrous fumarate

FAIR-us

Feostat, Hemocyte, Ircon, Nephro-Fer

Pharmacologic class: Hematinic

INDICATIONS
➤ Iron deficiency
➤ As a supplement during pregnancy

ACTION
Provides elemental iron, an essential component in the formation of hemoglobin.

ADVERSE REACTIONS
GI: nausea, vomiting, constipation, diarrhea, black stools, GI irritation. Other: temporarily stained teeth from suspension and drops.

NURSING CONSIDERATIONS
• Between-meal doses are preferable. Drug can be given with some foods, although absorption may be decreased.
• Give tablets with juice (preferably orange juice) or water but not with milk or antacids.
• Don't crush tablets.
• May yield false-positive guaiac test results. May decrease uptake of technetium-99m and interfere with skeletal imaging.
• Be aware that oral iron may turn stools black. Although this is harmless, it could mask presence of melena.
• Monitor hemoglobin level, hematocrit, and reticulocyte count during therapy.

PATIENT TEACHING
• Tell parents to keep all iron-containing products out of the reach of children and to immediately call prescriber or poison control center if an accidental overdose occurs.
• Tell patient to take suspension with straw and place drops at back of throat to avoid staining teeth.
• Advise patient not to substitute one iron salt for another; the amount of elemental iron may vary.
• Advise patient to report constipation and change in stool color or consistency.

ferrous sulfate
FAIR-us

Feosol, Fer-Gen-Sol, Fer-In-Sol, FeroSul

Pharmacologic class: Hematinic

INDICATIONS
➤ Iron deficiency

ACTION
Provides elemental iron, an essential component in the formation of hemoglobin.

ADVERSE REACTIONS
GI: nausea, constipation, black stools
Other: temporarily stained teeth from liquid forms

NURSING CONSIDERATIONS
• Between-meal doses are preferable. Drug can be given with some foods, although absorption may be decreased.
• Give tablets with juice (preferably orange juice) or water but not with milk or antacids.
• Don't crush tablets.
• May yield false-positive guaiac test results. May decrease uptake of technetium-99m and interfere with skeletal imaging.
• Be aware that oral iron may turn stools black. Although this is harmless, it could mask presence of melena.
• Monitor hemoglobin level, hematocrit, and reticulocyte count during therapy.
• Don't confuse different iron salts; elemental content may vary.
• *Cereals, cheese, coffee, eggs, milk, tea, whole-grain breads, yogurt:* May decrease iron absorption. Discourage use together.

PATIENT TEACHING
• Instruct patient not to crush or chew extended-release form.
• Advise patient not to substitute one iron salt for another; the amount of elemental iron may vary.
• Advise patient to report constipation and change in stool color or consistency.

folic acid (vitamin B$_9$)
FOE-lik

Pharmacologic class: Folic acid derivative

INDICATIONS
➤ RDA
➤ Megaloblastic or macrocytic anemia from folic acid or other nutritional deficiency, hepatic disease, alcoholism, intestinal obstruction, or excessive hemolysis

ACTION
Stimulates normal erythropoiesis and nucleoprotein synthesis.

ADVERSE REACTIONS
CNS: altered sleep pattern, general malaise, difficulty concentrating, confusion, impaired judgment, irritability, hyperactivity
GI: anorexia, nausea, flatulence, bitter taste
Respiratory: bronchospasm

NURSING CONSIDERATIONS
• The U.S. Public Health Service recommends use of folic acid during pregnancy to decrease fetal neural tube defects. Patients with history of fetal neural tube defects in pregnancy should increase folic acid intake for 1 month before and 3 months after conception.
• Patients with small-bowel resections and intestinal malabsorption may need parenteral administration.
• Don't confuse folic acid with folinic acid.
• Protect injectate from light and heat; store at room temperature.

PATIENT TEACHING
• Teach patient about proper nutrition to prevent recurrence of anemia.
• Stress importance of follow-up visits and laboratory studies.
• Teach patient about foods that contain folic acid: liver, oranges, whole wheat, broccoli, and Brussels sprouts.

Antiarrhythmics

amiodarone hydrochloride
flecainide acetate
lidocaine hydrochloride
procainamide hydrochloride
propafenone hydrochloride
quinidine gluconate/quinidine sulfate

INDICATIONS
➤ Atrial and ventricular arrhythmias

ACTION
Class I drugs reduce the inward current carried by sodium ions, which stabilizes neuronal cardiac membranes. Class IA drugs depress phase 0, prolong the action potential, and stabilize cardiac membranes. Class IB drugs depress phase 0, shorten the action potential, and stabilize cardiac membranes. Class IC drugs block the transport of sodium ions, which decreases conduction velocity but not repolarization rate. Class II drugs decrease the heart rate, myocardial contractility, blood pressure, and AV node conduction. Class IV drugs decrease myocardial contractility and oxygen demand by inhibiting calcium ion influx; they also dilate coronary arteries and arterioles.

ADVERSE REACTIONS
Most antiarrhythmics can aggravate existing arrhythmias or cause new ones. They also may produce CNS disturbances, such as dizziness or fatigue; GI problems, such as nausea, vomiting, or altered bowel elimination; hypersensitivity reactions; and hypotension. Some antiarrhythmics may worsen heart failure. Class II drugs may cause bronchoconstriction.

CONTRAINDICATIONS AND CAUTIONS
• Contraindicated in patients hypersensitive to these drugs.
• Many antiarrhythmics are contraindicated or require cautious use in patients with cardiogenic shock, digitalis toxicity, and second- or third-degree heart block (unless patient has a pacemaker or implantable cardioverter defibrillator).
• In pregnant women, use only if potential benefits to the mother outweigh risks to the fetus. In breast-feeding women, use cautiously; many antiarrhythmics appear in breast milk. In children, monitor closely because they have an increased risk of adverse reactions. In elderly patients, use these drugs cautiously because these patients may exhibit physiologic alterations in CV system.

amiodarone hydrochloride
am-ee-OH-dah-rohn

Cordarone, Nexterone, Pacerone

Pharmacologic class: Benzofuran derivative

INDICATIONS
➤ Life-threatening recurrent ventricular fibrillation or recurrent hemodynamically unstable ventricular tachycardia unresponsive to adequate doses of other antiarrhythmics or when alternative drugs can't be tolerated

ACTION
Effects result from blockade of potassium chloride leading to a prolongation of action potential duration.

ADVERSE REACTIONS
CNS: fatigue, malaise, tremor
CV: hypotension, bradycardia, arrhythmias, heart failure, heart block, sinus arrest
EENT: asymptomatic corneal microdeposits, visual disturbances
GI: nausea, vomiting
Hematologic: coagulation abnormalities
Hepatic: hepatic failure, hepatic dysfunction
Metabolic: hypothyroidism, hyperthyroidism
Respiratory: acute respiratory distress syndrome, severe pulmonary toxicity
Skin: photosensitivity, blue-gray skin

NURSING CONSIDERATIONS
• Give drug I.V. only if continuous ECG and electrophysiologic monitoring are available.
• Be aware of the high risk of adverse reactions
• Obtain baseline pulmonary, liver, and thyroid function test results and baseline chest X-ray.
• Watch carefully for pulmonary toxicity.
• Monitor liver and thyroid function test results and electrolyte levels, particularly potassium and magnesium.
• Don't confuse amiodarone with amiloride.

PATIENT TEACHING
• Advise patient to wear sunscreen or protective clothing to prevent sensitivity reaction to the sun.
• Tell patient to take oral drug with food if GI reactions occur.

flecainide acetate
FLEH-kay-nighd

Tambocor

Pharmacologic class: Benzamide derivative

INDICATIONS
➤ Prevention of paroxysmal supraventricular tachycardia in patients without structural heart disease
➤ Life-threatening ventricular arrhythmias

ACTION
A class IC antiarrhythmic that decreases excitability, conduction velocity, and automaticity by slowing atrial, AV node, His-Purkinje system, and intraventricular conduction; prolongs refractory periods in these tissues.

ADVERSE REACTIONS
CNS: dizziness, headache, light-headedness
CV: new or worsened arrhythmias
EENT: blurred vision and other visual disturbances
GI: nausea, constipation, abdominal pain, vomiting, diarrhea
Respiratory: dyspnea

NURSING CONSIDERATIONS
• Check that pacing threshold was determined 1 week before and after starting therapy in a patient with a pacemaker; flecainide can alter endocardial pacing thresholds.
• Correct hypokalemia or hyperkalemia before giving flecainide because these electrolyte disturbances may alter drug's effect.
• Monitor ECG rhythm for proarrhythmic effects.
• Monitor flecainide level, especially if patient has renal or heart failure. Therapeutic flecainide levels range from 0.2 to 1 mcg/ml. Risk of adverse effects increases when trough blood level exceeds 1 mcg/ml.

PATIENT TEACHING
• Stress importance of taking drug exactly as prescribed.
• Instruct patient to report adverse reactions promptly and to limit fluid and sodium intake to minimize fluid retention.

lidocaine hydrochloride

LYE-doe-kane

LidoPen Auto-Injector, Xylocaine

Pharmacologic class: Amide derivative

INDICATIONS
➤Ventricular arrhythmias caused by MI, cardiac manipulation, or cardiac glycosides

ACTION
A class IB antiarrhythmic that decreases the depolarization, automaticity, and excitability in the ventricles during the diastolic phase by direct action on the tissues, especially the Purkinje network.

ADVERSE REACTIONS
CNS: confusion, tremor, stupor, restlessness, light-headedness, seizures, muscle twitching
CV: hypotension, bradycardia, new or worsened arrhythmias, cardiac arrest
EENT: tinnitus, blurred or double vision
Respiratory: respiratory depression and arrest
Other: anaphylaxis

NURSING CONSIDERATIONS
• Patients receiving infusions must be on a cardiac monitor. Use an infusion control device for giving infusion precisely.
• Monitor drug level. Therapeutic levels are 2 to 5 mcg/ml.
• Monitor patient for toxicity. In many severely ill patients, seizures may be the first sign of toxicity. If signs of toxicity occur, stop drug at once and notify prescriber. Keep oxygen and cardiopulmonary resuscitation equipment available.
• Monitor patient's response, especially blood pressure and electrolytes, BUN, and creatinine levels.
• If arrhythmias worsen or ECG changes (e.g., QRS complex widens or PR interval substantially prolongs), stop infusion and notify prescriber.

PATIENT TEACHING
• Tell patient to report adverse reactions promptly because toxicity can occur.

procainamide hydrochloride
proe-KANE-a-myed

Pharmacologic class: Procaine derivative

INDICATIONS
➤ Symptomatic PVCs, life-threatening ventricular tachycardia
➤ To convert atrial fibrillation or paroxysmal atrial tachycardia

ACTION
Decreases excitability, conduction velocity, automaticity, and membrane responsiveness with prolonged refractory period. Larger than usual doses may induce AV block.

ADVERSE REACTIONS
CNS: fever, seizures, hallucinations, psychosis, confusion, dizziness
CV: hypotension, bradycardia, AV block, ventricular fibrillation, ventricular asystole
GI: abdominal pain, nausea, vomiting, anorexia, diarrhea
Skin: maculopapular rash, urticaria, pruritus, flushing
Other: lupuslike syndrome, angioneurotic edema

NURSING CONSIDERATIONS
• May increase ALT, AST, alkaline phosphatase, LDH, and bilirubin levels.
• Patients receiving infusions must be on a cardiac monitor. Use an infusion control device for giving infusion precisely.
• Monitor ECG closely. If QRS widens more than 25% or marked prolongation of the QTc interval occurs, check for overdosage.

PATIENT TEACHING
• Tell patient not to crush or break extended-release tablets.
• Reassure patient who is taking extended-release form that a wax-matrix "ghost" from the tablet may be passed in stools. Drug is completely absorbed before this occurs.

propafenone hydrochloride
proe-PAF-a-non

Rythmol, Rythmol SR

Pharmacologic class: Sodium channel antagonist

INDICATIONS
➤ To suppress life-threatening ventricular arrhythmias; to prevent paroxysmal supraventricular tachycardia and paroxysmal atrial fibrillation or flutter
➤ To prolong time until recurrence of symptomatic atrial fibrillation

ACTION
Reduces inward sodium current in cardiac cells, prolongs refractory period in AV node, and decreases excitability, conduction velocity, and automaticity in cardiac tissue.

ADVERSE REACTIONS
CNS: dizziness, anxiety, ataxia, drowsiness, fatigue, headache
CV: heart failure, bradycardia, arrhythmias, ventricular tachycardia, premature ventricular contractions, ventricular fibrillation
GI: nausea, vomiting

NURSING CONSIDERATIONS
• Perform continuous cardiac monitoring at start of therapy and during dosage adjustments.
• Grapefruit juice may increase drug level. Discourage use together.

PATIENT TEACHING
• Instruct patient to notify prescriber if prolonged diarrhea, sweating, vomiting, or loss of appetite or thirst occurs; these may cause an electrolyte imbalance.
• Tell patient not to crush, chew, or open the extended-release capsules.

quinidine gluconate/quinidine sulfate
KWIN-i-deen

Pharmacologic class: Cinchona alkaloid

INDICATIONS
➤ Atrial flutter or fibrillation
➤ Paroxysmal supraventricular tachycardia
➤ Premature atrial and ventricular contractions, paroxysmal AV junctional rhythm, paroxysmal atrial tachycardia, paroxysmal ventricular tachycardia, maintenance after cardioversion of atrial fibrillation or flutter
➤ Severe *Plasmodium falciparum* malaria

ACTION
A class IA antiarrhythmic with direct and indirect (anticholinergic) effects on cardiac tissue. Decreases automaticity, conduction velocity, and membrane responsiveness; prolongs effective refractory period; and reduces vagal tone.

ADVERSE REACTIONS
CNS: vertigo, fever, headache, light-headedness
CV: ECG changes, tachycardia, PVCs, ventricular tachycardia, atypical ventricular tachycardia, complete AV block, aggravated heart failure
EENT: tinnitus, blurred vision, diplopia, photophobia
GI: diarrhea, nausea, vomiting
Hematologic: thrombocytopenia, agranulocytosis, hemolytic anemia.
Hepatic: hepatotoxicity
Respiratory: acute asthmatic attack, respiratory arrest
Other: cinchonism, angioedema, lupus erythematosus

NURSING CONSIDERATIONS
• May increase digoxin level.
• Monitor patient for atypical ventricular tachycardia, such as torsades de pointes and ECG changes, particularly widening of QRS complex, widened QT and PR intervals. Monitor liver function test results during first 4 to 8 weeks of therapy.
• Watch for signs and symptoms of quinidine toxicity (ringing in the ears, visual disturbances, dizziness, headache, nausea).
• Don't confuse quinidine with quinine or clonidine.

PATIENT TEACHING
• Instruct patient not to crush or chew extended-release tablets.
• Tell patient to avoid grapefruit juice because it may delay drug absorption and inhibit drug metabolism.

Antiasthmatics

fluticasone propionate and salmeterol inhalation powder
mometasone furoate
montelukast sodium

INDICATIONS
➤ Maintenance therapy for asthma

ACTION
The antiasthmatic drugs are beta$_2$-adrenergic agonists, corticosteroids, glucocorticoids, and leukotriene-receptor antagonists. Beta$_2$-adrenergic agonists increase levels of cyclic adenosine monophosphate through the stimulation of beta$_2$-adrenergic receptors in the smooth muscle, resulting in bronchodilation. Corticosteroids inhibit the production of cytokines, leukotrienes, and prostaglandins, the recruitment of eosinophils, and the release of other inflammatory mediators. Glucocorticoids suppress hypersensitivity and immune responses. Leukotriene-receptor antagonists inhibit leukotriene from interacting with its receptor and blocking its action.

ADVERSE REACTIONS
Headache, pharyngitis, upper respiratory tract infection, cough, rash, dry throat, and abdominal pain.

CONTRAINDICATIONS AND CAUTIONS
• Contraindicated in patients hypersensitive to these drugs or their components.
• Contraindicated as primary treatment of status asthmaticus or other acute asthmatic episodes (fluticasone propionate and salmeterol inhalation powder).
• Use cautiously in patients at high risk for decreased bone mineral content (those with a family history of osteoporosis, prolonged immobilization, long-term use of drugs that reduce bone mass), patients switching from a systemic to an inhaled corticosteroid, and patients with active or dormant tuberculosis, untreated systemic infections, ocular herpes simplex, or immunosuppression (mometasone furoate).

fluticasone propionate and salmeterol inhalation powder

FLOO-tih-ka-sone and sal-MEE-ter-ol

Advair Diskus 100/50, Advair Diskus 250/50, Advair Diskus 500/50, Advair HFA 45/21, Advair HFA 115/21, Advair HFA 230/21

Pharmacologic class: Corticosteroid, long-acting beta$_2$-adrenergic agonist

INDICATIONS

➤ Long-term maintenance of asthma

➤ Maintenance therapy for airflow obstruction in patients with COPD from chronic bronchitis; to reduce exacerbations of COPD in patients with a history of exacerbations

ACTION

Fluticasone is a synthetic corticosteroid with potent anti-inflammatory activity. Salmeterol xinafoate, a long-acting beta agonist, relaxes bronchial smooth muscle and inhibits release of mediators.

ADVERSE REACTIONS

CNS: headache
EENT: pharyngitis, hoarseness or dysphonia
GI: diarrhea, nausea, oral discomfort and pain, oral candidiasis, unusual taste, vomiting
Musculoskeletal: arthralgia, muscle pain
Respiratory: upper respiratory tract infection
Other: allergic reactions, viral or bacterial infections

NURSING CONSIDERATIONS

• Closely monitor children for growth suppression.

PATIENT TEACHING

• Instruct patient to keep the dry-powder multidose inhaler in a dry place, away from direct heat or sunlight, and to avoid washing the mouthpiece or other parts of the device.

• Instruct patient to rinse mouth after inhalation to prevent oral candidiasis.

• Inform patient that improvement may occur within 30 minutes after dose, but the full benefit may not occur for 1 week or more.

• Advise patient not to exceed recommended prescribing dose.

• Instruct patient not to relieve acute symptoms with Advair. Treat acute symptoms with an inhaled short-acting beta$_2$ agonist.

mometasone furoate/mometasone furoate monohydrate

moe-MEH-tah-zone

Asmanex Twisthaler/Nasonex

Pharmacologic class: Glucocorticoid

INDICATIONS

➤ Asthma
➤ Allergic rhinitis
➤ Nasal polyps

ACTION

Unknown, although corticosteroids inhibit many cells and mediators involved in inflammation and the asthmatic response.

ADVERSE REACTIONS

CNS: headache, depression, fatigue, insomnia, pain
EENT: allergic rhinitis, pharyngitis
GI: dyspepsia, flatulence, nausea, oral candidiasis, vomiting
Respiratory: upper respiratory tract infection, respiratory disorder
Other: accidental injury, flulike symptoms, infection

NURSING CONSIDERATIONS

• Use cautiously in patients at high risk for decreased bone mineral content (those with a family history of osteoporosis, prolonged immobilization, long-term use of drugs that reduce bone mass).
• Monitor lung function tests.
• Watch for evidence of localized mouth infections, glaucoma, and immunosuppression.

PATIENT TEACHING

• Instruct patient on proper use and routine care of the inhaler or nasal spray pump.
• Tell patient to use drug regularly and at the same time each day. If he uses it only once daily, tell him to do so in the evening.
• Caution patient not to use drug for immediate relief of an asthma attack or bronchospasm.
• Warn patient to avoid exposure to chickenpox or measles and to notify prescriber if such contact occurs.
• Long-term use of an inhaled corticosteroid may increase the risk of cataracts or glaucoma; tell patient to report vision changes.

montelukast sodium

mon-tell-OO-kast

Singulair

Pharmacologic class: Leukotriene-receptor antagonist

INDICATIONS
➤ Asthma, seasonal allergic rhinitis, perennial allergic rhinitis
➤ Prevention of exercise-induced bronchospasm

ACTION
Reduces early and late-phase bronchoconstriction from antigen challenge.

ADVERSE REACTIONS
CNS: headache, asthenia, dizziness, fatigue, fever
EENT: dental pain, nasal congestion
GI: abdominal pain, dyspepsia, infectious gastroenteritis
GU: pyuria
Hematologic: systemic eosinophilia
Respiratory: cough
Skin: rash
Other: influenza, trauma

NURSING CONSIDERATIONS
• Give oral granules directly in the mouth mixed with a spoonful of cold or room-temperature soft foods.
• Give oral granules without regard for food.

PATIENT TEACHING
• Inform caregiver that the oral granules may be given directly into the child's mouth, dissolved in 1 teaspoon of cold or room-temperature baby formula or breast milk, or mixed in a spoonful of applesauce, carrots, rice, or ice cream.
• Tell caregiver not to open packet until ready to use and, after opening, to give the full dose within 15 minutes. Tell her that if she's mixing the drug with food, not to store excess for future use and to discard the unused portion.
• Advise patient to take drug daily, even if asymptomatic, and to contact his prescriber if asthma isn't well controlled.
• Advise patient with known aspirin sensitivity to continue to avoid using aspirin and NSAIDs during drug therapy.

Anticholinergics

atropine sulfate
benztropine mesylate
dicyclomine hydrochloride

INDICATIONS
➤ Prevention of motion sickness, preoperative reduction of secretions and blockage of cardiac reflexes, adjunct treatment of peptic ulcers and other GI disorders, blockage of cholinomimetic effects of cholinesterase inhibitors or other drugs, and (for benztropine) various spastic conditions, including acute dystonic reactions, muscle rigidity, parkinsonism, and extrapyramidal disorders

ACTION
Anticholinergics competitively antagonize the actions of acetylcholine and other cholinergic agonists at muscarinic receptors.

ADVERSE REACTIONS
Therapeutic doses commonly cause blurred vision, constipation, cycloplegia, decreased sweating or anhidrosis, dry mouth, headache, mydriasis, palpitations, tachycardia, and urinary hesitancy and retention. These reactions usually disappear when therapy stops. Toxicity can cause signs and symptoms resembling psychosis (disorientation, confusion, hallucinations, delusions, anxiety, agitation, and restlessness); dilated, nonreactive pupils; blurred vision; hot, dry, flushed skin; dry mucous membranes; dysphagia; decreased or absent bowel sounds; urine retention; hyperthermia; tachycardia; hypertension; and increased respirations.

CONTRAINDICATIONS AND CAUTIONS
• Contraindicated in patients hypersensitive to these drugs and in those with angle-closure glaucoma, renal or GI obstructive disease, reflux esophagitis, or myasthenia gravis.
• Use cautiously in patients with heart disease, GI infection, open-angle glaucoma, prostatic hypertrophy, hypertension, hyperthyroidism, ulcerative colitis, autonomic neuropathy, or hiatal hernia with reflux esophagitis.
• In pregnant women, safe use hasn't been established. In breast-feeding women, avoid anticholinergics because they may decrease milk production; some may appear in breast milk and cause infant toxicity. In children, safety and effectiveness haven't been established. Patients older than age 40 may be more sensitive to these drugs. In elderly patients, use cautiously and give a reduced dosage, as indicated.

atropine sulfate

AT-troe-peen

AtroPen, Sal-Tropine

Pharmacologic class: Anticholinergic, belladonna alkaloid

INDICATIONS

➤ Symptomatic bradycardia, bradyarrhythmia (junctional or escape rhythm)

➤ Antidote for anticholinesterase-insecticide poisoning

➤ Preoperatively to diminish secretions and block cardiac vagal reflexes

➤ Adjunct treatment of peptic ulcer disease; functional GI disorders such as irritable bowel syndrome; salivation and bronchial secretion reduction; CNS conditions such as parkinsonism; ureteral and biliary colic

ACTION

Inhibits acetylcholine at parasympathetic neuroeffector junction, blocking vagal effects on SA and AV nodes, enhancing conduction through AV node and increasing heart rate.

ADVERSE REACTIONS

CNS: headache, restlessness, insomnia, dizziness

CV: bradycardia, palpitations, tachycardia

EENT: blurred vision, mydriasis, photophobia, cycloplegia, increased intraocular pressure

GI: dry mouth, constipation, thirst, nausea, vomiting

GU: urine retention

Other: anaphylaxis

NURSING CONSIDERATIONS

• In adults, avoid doses less than 0.5 mg because of risk of paradoxical bradycardia.

• Monitor fluid intake and urine output.

PATIENT TEACHING

• Teach patient receiving oral form of drug how to handle distressing anticholinergic effects such as dry mouth.

• Instruct patient to report serious or persistent adverse reactions promptly.

• Tell patient about potential for sensitivity of the eyes to the sun and suggest use of sunglasses.

benztropine mesylate

BENZ-troe-peen

Cogentin

Pharmacologic class: Anticholinergic

INDICATIONS
➤ Drug-induced extrapyramidal disorders (except tardive dyskinesia)
➤ Transient extrapyramidal disorders
➤ Acute dystonic reaction
➤ Parkinsonism; postencephalitic parkinsonism

ACTION
Unknown. May block central cholinergic receptors, helping to balance cholinergic activity in the basal ganglia.

ADVERSE REACTIONS
CNS: confusion, memory impairment, nervousness, depression
CV: tachycardia
EENT: dilated pupils, blurred vision
GI: dry mouth, constipation, nausea, vomiting, paralytic ileus
GU: urine retention, dysuria
Musculoskeletal: muscle weakness
Skin: decreased sweating

NURSING CONSIDERATIONS
• Drug may be given before or after meals depending on patient reaction. If patient is prone to excessive salivation, give drug after meal. If his mouth dries excessively, give drug before meals unless it causes nausea.
• Monitor vital signs carefully. Watch closely for adverse reactions, especially in elderly or debilitated patients.
• Don't confuse benztropine with bromocriptine.

PATIENT TEACHING
• Warn patient to avoid activities that require alertness until CNS effects of drug are known.
• If patient takes a single daily dose, tell him to do so at bedtime.
• Advise patient to report signs and symptoms of urinary hesitancy or urine retention.
• Tell patient to relieve dry mouth with cool drinks, ice chips, sugarless gum, or hard candy.
• Advise patient to limit hot weather activities because drug-induced lack of sweating may cause overheating.

dicyclomine hydrochloride

dye-SYE-kloe-meen

Bentyl, Di-Spaz

Pharmacologic class: Anticholinergic, antimuscarinic

INDICATIONS

➤ Irritable bowel syndrome, other functional GI disorders

ACTION

Inhibits action of acetylcholine on postganglionic, parasympathetic muscarinic receptors, decreasing GI motility. Drug possesses local anesthetic properties that may be partly responsible for spasmolysis.

ADVERSE REACTIONS

CNS: headache, dizziness
CV: palpitations, tachycardia
EENT: blurred vision, increased intraocular pressure, mydriasis
GI: constipation, dry mouth, thirst, vomiting, nausea
GU: urinary hesitancy or retention, impotence
Skin: urticaria, decreased sweating or inability to sweat, local irritation
Other: allergic reactions, heat prostration

NURSING CONSIDERATIONS

• Antacids may interfere with dicyclomine absorption. Give dicyclomine at least 1 hour before antacid.
• Give drug 30 to 60 minutes before meals and at bedtime. Bedtime dose can be larger; give at least 2 hours after last meal of day.
• Monitor patient's vital signs and urine output carefully.
• Don't confuse dicyclomine with dyclonine or doxycycline; don't confuse Bentyl with Aventyl or Benadryl.

PATIENT TEACHING

• Advise patient to avoid driving and other hazardous activities if drowsiness, dizziness, or blurred vision occurs; to drink plenty of fluids to help prevent constipation; and to report rash or other skin eruption.

Anticoagulants

dalteparin sodium
enoxaparin sodium
fondaparinux sodium
heparin sodium
warfarin sodium

INDICATIONS
➤ Pulmonary emboli, deep vein thrombosis, thrombus, blood clotting, DIC, unstable angina, MI, atrial fibrillation

ACTION
Heparin derivatives accelerate formation of an antithrombin III–thrombin complex. It inactivates thrombin and prevents conversion of fibrinogen to fibrin. The coumarin derivative warfarin inhibits vitamin K–dependent activation of clotting factors II, VII, IX, and X, which are formed in the liver. Thrombin inhibitors directly bind to thrombin and inhibit its action. Selective factor Xa inhibitors bind to antithrombin III, which in turn initiates the neutralization of factor Xa.

ADVERSE REACTIONS
Anticoagulants commonly cause bleeding and may cause hypersensitivity reactions. Warfarin may cause agranulocytosis, alopecia (long-term use), anorexia, dermatitis, fever, nausea, tissue necrosis or gangrene, urticaria, and vomiting. Heparin derivatives may cause thrombocytopenia and may increase liver enzyme levels.

Nonhemorrhagic adverse reactions associated with thrombin inhibitors may include back pain, bradycardia, and hypotension.

CONTRAINDICATIONS AND CAUTIONS
• Contraindicated in patients hypersensitive to these drugs or any of their components; in patients with aneurysm, active bleeding, CV hemorrhage, hemorrhagic blood dyscrasias, hemophilia, severe hypertension, pericardial effusions, or pericarditis; and in patients undergoing major surgery, neurosurgery, or ophthalmic surgery.
• Use cautiously in patients with severe diabetes, renal impairment, severe trauma, ulcerations, or vasculitis.
• Most anticoagulants (except warfarin) may be used in pregnancy only if clearly necessary. In pregnant women and those who have just had a threatened or complete spontaneous abortion, warfarin is contraindicated. Women should avoid breastfeeding during therapy. Infants, especially neonates, may be more susceptible to anticoagulants because of vitamin K deficiency. Elderly patients are at greater risk for hemorrhage because of altered hemostatic mechanisms or deterioration of hepatic and renal functions.

dalteparin sodium

DAHL-tep-ah-rin

Fragmin

Pharmacologic class: Low–molecular-weight heparin

INDICATIONS

➤ DVT prevention in patients undergoing abdominal or hip replacement surgery
➤ Unstable angina; non–Q-wave MI
➤ DVT prevention in patients at risk for thromboembolic complications because of severely restricted mobility during acute illness
➤ Symptomatic venous thromboembolism in cancer patients

ACTION

Enhances inhibition of factor Xa and thrombin by antithrombin.

ADVERSE REACTIONS

CNS: fever
GU: hematuria
Hematologic: thrombocytopenia, hemorrhage, ecchymoses, bleeding complications
Skin: pruritus, rash, hematoma at injection site, injection site pain
Other: anaphylaxis

NURSING CONSIDERATIONS

• Before giving injection, obtain complete list of all prescribed and OTC medications, and supplements, including herbs.
• Have patient sit or lie supine when giving drug.
• Injection sites include a U-shaped area around the navel, upper outer side of thigh, and upper outer quadrangle of buttock. Rotate sites daily.
• Periodic, routine CBC and fecal occult blood tests are recommended during therapy. Monitor patient closely for thrombocytopenia.

PATIENT TEACHING

• Instruct patient and family to watch for and report signs of bleeding (bruising and blood in stools).
• Tell patient to avoid OTC drugs containing aspirin or other salicylates unless ordered by prescriber.
• Tell patient to use a soft toothbrush and electric razor during treatment.

enoxaparin sodium
en-OCKS-a-par-in

Lovenox

Pharmacologic class: Low–molecular-weight heparin

INDICATIONS
➤ PE and DVT prevention after hip or knee replacement surgery or abdominal surgery and in patients with acute illness who have decreased mobility
➤ To prevent ischemic complications of unstable angina and non–Q-wave MI with oral aspirin therapy
➤ Acute ST-segment elevation MI
➤ Treatment of acute DVT when given with warfarin sodium

ACTION
Accelerates formation of antithrombin III–thrombin complex and deactivates thrombin, preventing conversion of fibrinogen to fibrin. Drug has a higher antifactor-Xa-to-antifactor-IIa activity ratio than heparin.

ADVERSE REACTIONS
Hematologic: thrombocytopenia, hemorrhage, ecchymoses, bleeding complications, hypochromic anemia
Skin: rash, urticaria
Other: angioedema, anaphylaxis

NURSING CONSIDERATIONS
• Never give drug I.M. Avoid I.M. injections of other drugs to prevent or minimize hematoma.
• Monitor platelet counts regularly.
• Regularly inspect patient for bleeding gums, bruises on arms or legs, petechiae, nosebleeds, melena, tarry stools, hematuria, hematemesis.
• To treat severe overdose, give protamine sulfate.

PATIENT TEACHING
• Instruct patient and family to watch for signs of bleeding or abnormal bruising.
• Tell patient to avoid OTC drugs containing aspirin or other salicylates unless ordered by prescriber.
• Advise patient to consult with prescriber before initiating any herbal therapy.

fondaparinux sodium

fon-dah-PEAR-ah-nucks

Arixtra

Pharmacologic class: Activated factor X inhibitor

INDICATIONS
➤ DVT prevention in patients undergoing surgery for hip fracture, hip replacement, knee replacement, or abdominal surgery
➤ Acute DVT (with warfarin); acute pulmonary embolism (with warfarin) when treatment is started in the hospital

ACTION
Binds to antithrombin III (AT-III) and potentiates the neutralization of factor Xa by AT-III, which interrupts coagulation and inhibits formation of thrombin and blood clots.

ADVERSE REACTIONS
CNS: fever, insomnia, dizziness, confusion, headache, pain
CV: hypotension, edemas
GI: nausea, constipation, vomiting, diarrhea, dyspepsia
Hematologic: hemorrhage, anemia, hematoma, postoperative hemorrhage, thrombocytopenia
Metabolic: hypokalemia

NURSING CONSIDERATIONS
• Routinely assess patient for signs and symptoms of bleeding, and regularly monitor CBC, platelet count, creatinine level, and stool occult blood test results.
• Anticoagulant effects may last for 2 to 4 days after stopping drug in patients with normal renal function.
• Give subcutaneously only, never I.M, rotating injection sites.

PATIENT TEACHING
• Tell patient to report signs and symptoms of bleeding.
• Instruct patient to avoid OTC products that contain aspirin or other salicylates.
• Advise patient to consult with prescriber before starting herbal therapy.
• Teach patient the correct technique for subcutaneous use, if needed.

heparin sodium
HEP-ah-rin

Heparin Lock Flush Solution, Heparin Sodium Injection, Hep-Lock, Hep-Pak

Pharmacologic class: Anticoagulant

INDICATIONS
➤ DVT, MI, PE
➤ Prevention of venous thrombosis, PE, embolism associated with atrial fibrillation, and postoperative DVT
➤ Consumptive coagulopathy (such as DIC)
➤ Patency maintenance of I.V. indwelling catheters

ACTION
Accelerates formation of antithrombin III—thrombin complex and deactivates thrombin, preventing conversion of fibrinogen to fibrin.

ADVERSE REACTIONS
CNS: fever
Hematologic: hemorrhage, overly prolonged clotting time, thrombocytopenia, white clot syndrome
Metabolic: hyperkalemia, hypoaldosteronism
Skin: irritation, mild pain, hematoma

NURSING CONSIDERATIONS
• Measure PTT regularly. Anticoagulation is present when PTT values are 1½ to 2 times the control values.
• Regularly inspect patient for bleeding gums, bruises on arms or legs, petechiae, nosebleeds, melena, tarry stools, hematuria, and hematemesis.
• To treat overdose, use protamine sulfate
• Don't confuse heparin with Hespan.

PATIENT TEACHING
• Instruct patient and family to watch for signs of bleeding or bruising and to notify prescriber immediately if any occur.
• Tell patient to avoid OTC drugs containing aspirin, other salicylates, or drugs that may interact with heparin, unless ordered by prescriber.
• Advise patient to consult with prescriber before starting herbal therapy.

warfarin sodium
WAR-far-in

Coumadin, Jantoven

Pharmacologic class: Coumarin derivative

INDICATIONS
➤ Pulmonary embolism, deep vein thrombosis, MI, rheumatic heart disease with heart valve damage, prosthetic heart valves, chronic atrial fibrillation

ACTION
Inhibits vitamin K–dependent activation of clotting factors II, VII, IX, and X, formed in the liver.

ADVERSE REACTIONS
CNS: fever, headache, dizziness, fatigue, syncope
CV: angina syndrome, hypotension
Hematologic: hemorrhage
Hepatic: hepatitis, jaundice, cholestatic hepatic injury
Skin: dermatitis, urticaria, necrosis, alopecia, rash
Other: hypersensitivity, allergic reactions, anaphylactic reactions

NURSING CONSIDERATIONS
• Regularly monitor INR in all patients. INR should be 2.0 to 3.0.
• Check patient for bleeding gums, bruises, nosebleeds, melena, tarry stools, hematuria, and hematemesis.
• Effect can be neutralized by oral or parenteral vitamin K.
• Elderly patients and patients with renal or hepatic failure are especially sensitive to drug's effect.
• Don't confuse Coumadin with Avandia, Cardura, or Kemadrin.

PATIENT TEACHING
• Tell patient to carry a card that identifies his increased risk of bleeding.
• Tell patient and family to watch for signs of bleeding or abnormal bruising and to call prescriber at once if they occur.
• Warn patient to avoid OTC products containing aspirin, other salicylates, or drugs that may interact with warfarin.
• Advise patient to consult with prescriber before initiating any herbal therapy.
• Tell patient to read labels. Food, nutritional supplements, and multivitamins that contain vitamin K may impair anticoagulation.

Anticonvulsants

carbamazepine
clonazepam
gabapentin
lamotrigine
oxcarbazepine
phenobarbital/phenobarbital sodium
phenytoin/phenytoin sodium/phenytoin sodium (extended)
pregabalin
topiramate
valproate sodium/valproic acid/divalproex sodium

INDICATIONS

➤ Seizure disorders; acute, isolated seizures not caused by seizure disorders; status epilepticus; prevention of seizures after trauma or craniotomy; neuropathic pain

ACTION

Anticonvulsants include six classes of drugs: selected hydantoin derivatives, barbiturates, benzodiazepines, succinimides, iminostilbene derivatives (carbamazepine), and carboxylic acid derivatives. Some hydantoin derivatives and carbamazepine inhibit the spread of seizure activity in the motor cortex. Some barbiturates and succinimides limit seizure activity by increasing the threshold for motor cortex stimuli. Selected benzodiazepines and carboxylic acid derivatives may increase inhibition of GABA in brain neurons.

ADVERSE REACTIONS

Anticonvulsants can cause adverse CNS effects, such as ataxia, confusion, somnolence, and tremor. Many anticonvulsants also cause CV disorders, such as arrhythmias and hypotension; GI effects, such as vomiting; and hematologic disorders, such as agranulocytosis, bone marrow depression, leukopenia, and thrombocytopenia.

CONTRAINDICATIONS AND CAUTIONS

• Contraindicated in patients hypersensitive to these drugs.
• In pregnant women, therapy usually continues despite the fetal risks caused by some anticonvulsants (barbiturates, phenytoin). In breast-feeding women, the safety of many anticonvulsants hasn't been established. Children are sensitive to the CNS depression of some anticonvulsants; use cautiously. Elderly patients are sensitive to CNS effects and may require lower doses.

carbamazepine

kar-ba-MAZ-e-peen

Carbatrol, Epitol, Equetro, Tegretol, Tegretol-XR, Teril

Pharmacologic class: Iminostilbene derivative

INDICATIONS

➤ Generalized tonic-clonic and complex partial seizures, mixed seizure patterns

➤ Trigeminal neuralgia

ACTION

Thought to stabilize neuronal membranes and limit seizure activity by either increasing efflux or decreasing influx of sodium ions across cell membranes in the motor cortex during generation of nerve impulses.

ADVERSE REACTIONS

CNS: ataxia, dizziness, drowsiness, somnolence, vertigo, worsening of seizures, pain, depression including suicidal ideation
CV: arrhythmias, AV block, heart failure
EENT: blurred vision, conjunctivitis, diplopia, dry pharynx, nystagmus
GI: nausea, vomiting, abdominal pain, diarrhea, dry mouth, dyspepsia
Hematologic: agranulocytosis, aplastic anemia, thrombocytopenia
Hepatic: hepatitis
Skin: erythema multiforme, Stevens-Johnson syndrome

NURSING CONSIDERATIONS

• Obtain baseline determinations of urinalysis, BUN and iron levels, liver function, CBC, and platelet and reticulocyte counts. Monitor these values periodically thereafter.
• Never stop drug suddenly; gradually decrease dosage.
• Don't confuse Tegretol or Tegretol-XR with Topamax, Toprol-XL, or Toradol. Don't confuse Carbatrol with carvedilol.

PATIENT TEACHING

• Instruct patient to take drug with food to minimize GI distress.
• Tell patient not to crush or chew extended-release form and not to take broken or chipped tablets.
• Tell patient that drug may cause mild to moderate dizziness and drowsiness when first taken. Advise him to avoid hazardous activities until effects disappear, usually within 3 to 4 days.
• Advise patient that periodic eye examinations are recommended.

clonazepam
kloe-NAZ-e-pam

Klonopin

Pharmacologic class: Benzodiazepine

INDICATIONS
➤ Lennox-Gastaut syndrome, atypical absence seizures, akinetic and myoclonic seizures
➤ Panic disorder

ACTION
Unknown. Probably acts by facilitating the effects of the inhibitory neurotransmitter GABA.

ADVERSE REACTIONS
CNS: drowsiness, agitation, ataxia, behavioral disturbances, confusion, depression, slurred speech, tremor
GI: anorexia, constipation, diarrhea, gastritis, nausea, sore gums
Hematologic: leukopenia, thrombocytopenia, eosinophilia
Respiratory: respiratory depression, shortness of breath

NURSING CONSIDERATIONS
• Closely monitor all patients for changes in behavior that may indicate worsening of suicidal thoughts or behavior or depression.
• Don't stop drug abruptly because this may worsen seizures.
• Assess elderly patient's response closely. Elderly patients are more sensitive to drug's CNS effects.
• Monitor patient for oversedation.
• Monitor CBC and liver function tests.

PATIENT TEACHING
• Advise patient to avoid driving and other hazardous activities that require mental alertness until drug's CNS effects are known.
• Instruct parent to monitor child's school performance because drug may interfere with attentiveness.
• Warn patient and parents not to stop drug abruptly because seizures may occur.
• Tell patient that ODTs can be taken with or without water.

gabapentin

gab-ah-PEN-tin

Neurontin

Pharmacologic class: Gamma-aminobutyric acid (GABA) structural analogue

INDICATIONS
➤ Seizures
➤ Postherpetic neuralgia

ACTION
Unknown. Structurally related to GABA but doesn't interact with GABA receptors, isn't converted into GABA or GABA agonist, doesn't inhibit GABA reuptake, and doesn't prevent degradation.

ADVERSE REACTIONS
CNS: ataxia, dizziness, fatigue, somnolence, depression, dysarthria, incoordination, nervousness, tremor
EENT: amblyopia, diplopia, dry throat, pharyngitis, rhinitis
GI: constipation, dry mouth, dyspepsia, , nausea, vomiting
Hematologic: leukopenia
Musculoskeletal: back pain, fractures, myalgia

NURSING CONSIDERATIONS
• Antacids may decrease absorption of gabapentin. Separate dosage times by at least 2 hours.
• If drug is to be stopped or an alternative drug substituted, do so gradually over at least 1 week to minimize risk of precipitating seizures.
• Don't confuse Neurontin with Noroxin.

PATIENT TEACHING
• Instruct patient to take first dose at bedtime to minimize adverse reactions.
• Warn patient to avoid driving and operating heavy machinery until drug's CNS effects are known.
• Advise patient not to stop drug abruptly.

lamotrigine
la-MO-tri-geen

Lamictal, Lamictal CD, Lamictal ODT, Lamictal XR

Pharmacologic class: Phenyltriazine

INDICATIONS
➤ Seizures
➤ Bipolar disorder

ACTION
Unknown. May inhibit release of glutamate and aspartate (excitatory neurotransmitters) in the brain via an action at voltage-sensitive sodium channels.

ADVERSE REACTIONS
CNS: ataxia, dizziness, headache, somnolence, seizures
EENT: blurred vision, diplopia, rhinitis
GI: nausea, vomiting, abdominal pain, anorexia
Skin: rash, Stevens-Johnson syndrome, toxic epidermal necrolysis, acne, alopecia, hot flashes, pruritus

NURSING CONSIDERATIONS
• Orally disintegrating tablets may be swallowed with or without water and without regard to food.
• Give extended-release tablets once daily with or without food. Patient must swallow tablets whole and must not chew, crush, or divide them.
• Don't stop drug abruptly because this may increase seizure frequency. Instead, taper drug over at least 2 weeks.
• Stop drug at first sign of rash, unless rash is clearly not drug-related.
• Don't confuse lamotrigine with lamivudine or Lamictal with Lamisil, Ludiomil, labetalol, or Lomotil.

PATIENT TEACHING
• Inform patient that drug may cause rash. Combination therapy of valproic acid and lamotrigine may cause a serious rash. Tell patient to report rash or signs or symptoms of hypersensitivity promptly.
• Warn patient not to engage in hazardous activity until drug's CNS effects are known.
• Warn patient that the drug may trigger sensitivity to the sun and to take precautions until tolerance is determined.

oxcarbazepine

oks-car-BAZ-e-peen

Trileptal

Pharmacologic class: Carboxamide derivative

INDICATIONS
➤ Seizures

ACTION
Thought to prevent seizure spread in the brain by blocking voltage-sensitive sodium channels, and to produce anticonvulsant effects by increasing potassium conduction and modulating high-voltage activated calcium channels.

ADVERSE REACTIONS
CNS: abnormal gait, ataxia, dizziness, fatigue, headache, somnolence, tremor, vertigo, aggravated seizures, abnormal coordination
EENT: abnormal vision, diplopia, nystagmus
GI: abdominal pain, nausea, vomiting, rectal hemorrhage
Metabolic: hypernatremia
Respiratory: upper respiratory tract infection, bronchitis, coughing

NURSING CONSIDERATIONS
• Withdraw drug gradually to minimize potential for increased seizure frequency.
• Monitor sodium level.

PATIENT TEACHING
• Advise patient not to stop drug abruptly.
• Advise patient to report signs and symptoms of low sodium in the blood, such as nausea, malaise, headache, lethargy, and confusion.
• Multiorgan hypersensitivity reactions may occur. Tell patient to report fever and swollen lymph nodes to his prescriber.
• Serious skin reactions, including Stevens-Johnson syndrome and toxic epidermal necrosis, can occur. Advise patient to immediately report skin rashes to his prescriber.
• Warn patient not to engage in hazardous activity until drug's CNS effects are known.
• Tell patient to avoid alcohol while taking drug.

phenobarbital/phenobarbital sodium
fee-noe-BAR-bi-tal

Solfoton/Luminal Sodium

Pharmacologic class: Barbiturate

INDICATIONS
➤ Seizures
➤ Status epilepticus
➤ Sedation
➤ Short-term treatment of insomnia

ACTION
As a barbiturate, may depress CNS and increase seizure threshold. As a sedative, may interfere with transmission of impulses from thalamus to cortex of brain.

ADVERSE REACTIONS
CNS: drowsiness, lethargy, hangover, paradoxical excitement in elderly patients, somnolence, changes in EEG patterns
CV: bradycardia, hypotension, syncope
GI: nausea, vomiting
Respiratory: respiratory depression, apnea
Other: injection-site reactions, angioedema

NURSING CONSIDERATIONS
• Don't stop drug abruptly because this may worsen seizures.
• Give I.V. dose slowly (no more than 60 mg/minute) under close supervision. Have resuscitation equipment available. Monitor respirations closely.
• Give I.M. injection deeply into large muscle. Superficial injection may cause pain, sterile abscess, and tissue sloughing.
• Don't confuse phenobarbital with pentobarbital.

PATIENT TEACHING
• Advise patient to avoid driving and other potentially hazardous activities that require mental alertness until drug's CNS effects are known.
• Warn patient and parents not to stop drug abruptly.

phenytoin/phenytoin sodium/phenytoin sodium (extended)

FEN-i-toe-in

Dilantin 125, Dilantin Infatabs/Dilantin/Phenytek

Pharmacologic class: Hydantoin derivative

INDICATIONS
➤ Seizures
➤ Status epilepticus

ADVERSE REACTIONS
CNS: ataxia, decreased coordination, mental confusion, slurred speech, dizziness, headache, insomnia, nervousness, twitching
EENT: diplopia, nystagmus, blurred vision
GI: gingival hyperplasia, nausea, vomiting, constipation
Hematologic: agranulocytosis, leukopenia, pancytopenia, thrombocytopenia, macrocythemia, megaloblastic anemia
Hepatic: toxic hepatitis
Skin: Stevens-Johnson syndrome, toxic epidermal necrolysis

NURSING CONSIDERATIONS
• Give P.O. divided doses with or after meals to decrease adverse GI reactions.
• Mix with normal saline solution and give as slow infusion over 30 minutes to 1 hour, when possible. In adults, don't exceed 50 mg/minute I.V. In neonates, administer drug at a rate not exceeding 1 to 3 mg/kg/minute.
• Monitor vital signs and ECG closely during I.V. administration.
• Don't stop drug suddenly because this may worsen seizures.
• Watch for gingival hyperplasia, especially in children.
• Don't confuse phenytoin with mephenytoin or fosphenytoin or Dilantin with Dilaudid.

PATIENT TEACHING
• Tell patient to notify prescriber if skin rash develops.
• Advise patient to avoid driving and other potentially hazardous activities that require mental alertness until drug's CNS effects are known.
• Serious skin reactions, including Stevens-Johnson syndrome and toxic epidermal necrosis, can occur. Advise patient to immediately report skin rashes to his prescriber.
• Advise patient to avoid alcohol.
• Warn patient and parents not to stop drug abruptly.
• Caution patient that drug may color urine pink, red, or reddish brown.

pregabalin
pray-GAB-ah-lin

Lyrica

Pharmacologic class: CNS drug

INDICATIONS
➤ Fibromyalgia
➤ Diabetic peripheral neuropathy
➤ Postherpetic neuralgia
➤ Partial onset seizures

ACTION
May contribute to analgesic and anticonvulsant effects by binding to sites in CNS.

ADVERSE REACTIONS
CNS: ataxia, dizziness, somnolence, tremor
CV: edema, PR interval prolongation
GI: dry mouth, abdominal pain, constipation
GU: anorgasmia, impotence, urinary incontinence, urinary frequency
Metabolic: hypoglycemia, weight gain

NURSING CONSIDERATIONS
• Monitor patient for signs and symptoms of angioedema (including swelling of face, mouth, and neck), which may compromise breathing. Discontinue drug immediately if angioedema occurs.
• Monitor patient's weight and fluid status, especially if he has heart failure.
• Watch for signs of rhabdomyolysis, such as dark, red, or cola-colored urine; muscle tenderness; generalized weakness; or muscle stiffness or aching.

PATIENT TEACHING
• Explain that drug may be taken without regard to food.
• Warn patient not to stop drug abruptly.
• Caution patient to avoid hazardous activities until drug's effects are known.
• Instruct patient to watch for weight changes and water retention.
• Advise patient to report vision changes and malaise or fever accompanied by muscle pain, tenderness, or weakness.
• Tell patient to avoid alcohol while taking drug.

topiramate
toe-PIE-rah-mate

Topamax

Pharmacologic class: Sulfamate-substituted monosaccharide

INDICATIONS
➤ Seizures
➤ Lennox-Gastaut syndrome
➤ To prevent migraine headache

ACTION
Unknown. May block a sodium channel, potentiate the activity of GABA, and inhibit kainate's ability to activate an amino acid receptor.

ADVERSE REACTIONS
CNS: anxiety, asthenia, ataxia, confusion, difficulty with memory, dizziness, fatigue, nervousness, paresthesia, psychomotor slowing, somnolence, speech disorders, tremor, generalized tonic-clonic seizures, suicide attempts.
EENT: abnormal vision, diplopia, nystagmus
GI: anorexia, nausea
Hematologic: leukopenia, anemia
Respiratory: upper respiratory tract infection, bronchitis, coughing

NURSING CONSIDERATIONS
• Don't stop drug suddenly because this may worsen seizures.
• Stop drug if patient experiences acute myopia and secondary angle-closure glaucoma.
• Don't confuse Topamax with Toprol-XL, Tegretol, or Tegretol-XR.

PATIENT TEACHING
• Tell patient to drink plenty of fluids during therapy to minimize risk of forming kidney stones.
• Caution patient to avoid hazardous activities until drug's effects are known.
• Tell patient that capsules may either be swallowed whole or carefully opened and contents sprinkled on a teaspoonful of soft food.
• Tell patient to swallow immediately without chewing.
• Tell patient to notify prescriber immediately if he experiences changes in vision.

valproate sodium/valproic acid/divalproex sodium
val-PROH-ayt

Depacon/Depakene, Stavzor/Depakote, Depakote ER, Depakote Sprinkle

Pharmacologic class: Carboxylic acid derivative

INDICATIONS
➤ Seizures
➤ Mania
➤ To prevent migraine headache

ADVERSE REACTIONS
CNS: asthenia, dizziness, headache, insomnia, nervousness, somnolence, tremor, abnormal thinking, amnesia, ataxia, depression
EENT: blurred vision, diplopia, nystagmus, pharyngitis, rhinitis, tinnitus
GI: diarrhea, dyspepsia, nausea, vomiting, pancreatitis
Hematologic: bone marrow suppression, hemorrhage, thrombocytopenia, bruising, petechiae
Hepatic: hepatotoxicity
Skin: alopecia, erythema multiforme, hypersensitivity reactions, Stevens-Johnson syndrome, rash, photosensitivity reactions, pruritus

NURSING CONSIDERATIONS
• Obtain liver function test results, platelet count, and PT and INR before starting therapy, and monitor these values periodically.
• Don't stop drug suddenly because this may worsen seizures.
• Perform liver function tests prior to therapy and at frequent intervals, especially during the first 6 months.
• Don't confuse Depakote with Depakote ER.

PATIENT TEACHING
• Tell patient to take drug with food or milk.
• Advise patient not to chew capsules; irritation may result.
• Tell patient that capsules may be either swallowed whole or carefully opened and contents sprinkled on a teaspoonful of soft food.
• Warn patients and guardians that abdominal pain, nausea, vomiting, and anorexia can be symptoms of pancreatitis that require prompt medical evaluation.

Antidepressants

buPROPion hydrochloride/buPROPion hydrobromide
duloxetine hydrochloride
mirtazapine
trazodone hydrochloride
venlafaxine hydrochloride

INDICATIONS
▶ Major depressive disorder (bupropion, duloxetine), depression; generalized anxiety disorder (duloxetine, venlafaxine); fibromyalgia, neuropathic pain related to diabetic peripheral neuropathy, chronic musculoskeletal pain (duloxetine); insomnia, prevention of migraine (trazodone); panic disorder, social anxiety disorder, hot flashes (venlafaxine)

ACTION
Other antidepressant drugs include aminoketones, serotonin-norepinephrine reuptake inhibitors, tetracyclic antidepressants, and triazolopyridine derivatives. Much about how these drugs work has yet to be fully understood.

ADVERSE REACTIONS
Headache, dizziness, insomnia, suicidal thoughts or behavior, dry mouth, constipation, abnormal dreams (bupropion), seizures (bupropion), arrhythmias (bupropion), hypoglycemia (duloxetine).

CONTRAINDICATIONS AND CAUTIONS
• Contraindicated in patients hypersensitive to drug or within 14 days of MAO inhibitor therapy.
• Use cautiously in patients at risk for suicide.
• Use cautiously in patients with recent history of MI, unstable heart disease, renal or hepatic impairment, a history of seizures, head trauma, or other predisposition to seizures, and in those being treated with drugs that lower seizure threshold (bupropion).
• Use cautiously in patients with a history of mania or seizures, patients who drink substantial amounts of alcohol, patients with hypertension, patients with controlled angle-closure glaucoma, and those with conditions that slow gastric emptying (duloxetine).
• Use cautiously in patients with conditions that predispose them to hypotension, such as dehydration (mirtazapine).
• Use cautiously in patients with cardiac disease or in the initial recovery phase of MI (trazodone).
• Use cautiously in patients with renal impairment, diseases or conditions that could affect hemodynamic responses or metabolism, and in those with history of mania or seizures (venlafaxine).

buPROPion hydrochloride/buPROPion hydrobromide

byoo-PROE-pee-on

Aplenzin/Wellbutrin, Wellbutrin SR, Wellbutrin XL, Zyban

Pharmacologic class: Aminoketone

INDICATIONS
➤ Major depressive disorder (Aplenzin only)
➤ Seasonal affective disorder (Wellbutrin XL only)
➤ Depression
➤ Aid to smoking-cessation treatment

ACTION
Unknown. Drug doesn't inhibit MAO, but it weakly inhibits norepinephrine, dopamine, and serotonin reuptake. Noradrenergic or dopaminergic mechanisms, or both, may cause drug's effect.

ADVERSE REACTIONS
CNS: abnormal dreams, insomnia, headache, sedation, tremor, agitation, dizziness, seizures, suicidal behavior, anxiety
CV: tachycardia, arrhythmias, palpitations, chest pain
EENT: blurred vision, rhinitis
GI: constipation, nausea, vomiting, anorexia, dry mouth
Skin: excessive sweating, pruritus, rash

NURSING CONSIDERATIONS
• Don't crush, split, or allow patients to chew tablets.
• Begin smoking-cessation treatment while patient is still smoking; about 1 week is needed to achieve steady-state drug levels.
• Don't confuse bupropion with buspirone or Wellbutrin with Wellcovorin.

PATIENT TEACHING
• Advise families and caregivers to closely observe patient for increased suicidal thinking and behavior and hostility, agitation, and depressed mood.
• Advise patient to report mood swings or suicidal thoughts immediately.
• Explain that excessive use of alcohol, abrupt withdrawal from alcohol or other sedatives, and addiction to cocaine, opiates, or stimulants during therapy may increase risk of seizures. Tell patient that it may take 4 weeks to reach full antidepressant effect.

duloxetine hydrochloride
do-LOCKS-ah-teen

Cymbalta

Pharmacologic class: SSNRI

INDICATIONS
➤ Major depressive disorder
➤ Generalized anxiety disorder
➤ Fibromyalgia
➤ Neuropathic pain related to diabetic peripheral neuropathy
➤ Chronic musculoskeletal pain

ACTION
May inhibit serotonin and norepinephrine reuptake in the CNS.

ADVERSE REACTIONS
CNS: dizziness, fatigue, headache, insomnia, somnolence, suicidal thoughts, fever, lethargy, nervousness, nightmares
EENT: blurred vision, nasopharyngitis, pharyngolaryngeal pain
GI: constipation, diarrhea, dry mouth, nausea, vomiting
Metabolic: decreased appetite, hypoglycemia

NURSING CONSIDERATIONS
• Monitor patient for worsening of depression or suicidal behavior, especially when therapy starts or dosage changes.
• Decrease dosage gradually, and watch for symptoms that may arise when drug is stopped, such as dizziness, nausea, headache, paresthesia, vomiting, irritability, and nightmares.
• Combining triptans with an SSRI or an SSNRI may cause serotonin syndrome or neuroleptic malignant syndrome–like reactions.

PATIENT TEACHING
• Advise families and caregivers to closely observe patient for increased suicidal thinking and behavior and hostility, agitation, and depressed mood.
• Instruct patient to swallow capsules whole and not to chew, crush, or open them because they have an enteric coating.
• Urge patient to avoid activities that are hazardous or require mental alertness until he knows how the drug affects him.
• Warn against drinking alcohol during therapy.
• If patient takes drug for depression, explain that it may take 1 to 4 weeks to notice an effect.

mirtazapine
mer-TAH-zah-peen

Remeron, Remeron Soltab

Pharmacologic class: Tetracyclic antidepressant

INDICATIONS
➤ Depression

ACTION
Thought to enhance central noradrenergic and serotonergic activity.

ADVERSE REACTIONS
CNS: somnolence, suicidal behavior, dizziness, asthenia, abnormal dreams, abnormal thinking, tremors, confusion
GI: increased appetite, dry mouth, constipation, nausea
Metabolic: weight gain
Musculoskeletal: back pain, myalgia

NURSING CONSIDERATIONS
• ODT may be given with or without water.
• Don't split or crush ODT.
• Don't use within 14 days of MAO inhibitor therapy.
• Record mood changes. Watch for suicidal tendencies.

PATIENT TEACHING
• Advise families and caregivers to closely observe patient for increasing suicidal thinking and behavior.
• Caution patient not to perform hazardous activities if he gets too sleepy.
• Instruct patient not to use alcohol or other CNS depressants while taking drug.
• Instruct patient to remove ODTs from blister pack and place immediately on tongue. Tell the patient to be sure his hands are clean and dry if he touches the tablet.
• Advise patient not to break or split tablet.

trazodone hydrochloride
TRAYZ-oh-dohn

Oleptro

Pharmacologic class: Triazolopyridine derivative

INDICATIONS
➤ Depression
➤ Insomnia
➤ Prevention of migraine

ACTION
Unknown. Inhibits CNS neuronal uptake of serotonin; not a tricyclic derivative.

ADVERSE REACTIONS
CNS: drowsiness, dizziness, nervousness, fatigue, confusion, tremor, hostility, nightmares, vivid dreams, headache, insomnia, syncope
CV: orthostatic hypotension, tachycardia, hypertension, ECG changes
EENT: blurred vision, tinnitus, nasal congestion
GI: dry mouth, dysgeusia, constipation, nausea, vomiting, anorexia
Skin: rash, urticaria, diaphoresis

NURSING CONSIDERATIONS
• Give drug after meals or a light snack for optimal absorption and to decrease risk of dizziness.
• Give extended-release tablets at the same time each day, preferably at bedtime, on an empty stomach.
• Don't crush or allow patient to chew extended-release tablets.
• Monitor patient for signs and symptoms of serotonin syndrome (mental status changes, tachycardia, labile blood pressure, hyperreflexia, incoordination, nausea, vomiting, diarrhea) or neuroleptic malignant syndrome (hyperthermia, muscle rigidity, rapidly fluctuating vital signs, mental status change).
• Monitor patient for suicidal tendencies.
• Don't confuse trazodone hydrochloride with tramadol hydrochloride.

PATIENT TEACHING
• Caution patient not to perform hazardous activities if he gets too sleepy.
• Teach caregivers how to recognize signs and symptoms of suicidal tendency or suicidal thoughts.

venlafaxine hydrochloride

vin-lah-FACKS-in

Effexor, Effexor XR

Pharmacologic class: SSNRI

INDICATIONS
➤ Depression
➤ Generalized anxiety disorder
➤ Panic disorder
➤ Social anxiety disorder

ACTION
May increase the amount of norepinephrine, serotonin, or both in the CNS by blocking their reuptake by the presynaptic neurons.

ADVERSE REACTIONS
CNS: asthenia, headache, somnolence, dizziness, nervousness, insomnia, suicidal behavior, anxiety, tremor, abnormal dreams
GI: nausea, constipation, dry mouth, anorexia, vomiting, diarrhea
GU: abnormal ejaculation, impotence, impaired urination
Skin: diaphoresis, rash

NURSING CONSIDERATIONS
• Give drug with food and a full glass of water.
• Give capsule whole. If patient can't swallow whole, open and sprinkle contents on spoonful of applesauce; mix and give immediately. Follow with a full glass of water.
• Carefully monitor blood pressure. Drug therapy may cause sustained, dose-dependent increases in blood pressure. Monitor patient's weight, particularly underweight, depressed patients.

PATIENT TEACHING
• If medication is to be stopped, inform patient who has received drug for 6 weeks or longer that drug will be stopped gradually by tapering dosage over a 2-week period, as instructed by prescriber. Patient shouldn't abruptly stop taking the drug.
• Warn patient to avoid hazardous activities that require alertness and good coordination until effects of drug are known.
• Tell patient to avoid alcohol and to consult prescriber before taking other prescription or OTC drugs.

Antidepressants, selective serotonin reuptake inhibitors

citalopram hydrobromide
escitalopram oxalate
fluoxetine hydrochloride
paroxetine hydrochloride/paroxetine mesylate
sertraline hydrochloride

INDICATIONS

➤ Major depression, obsessive-compulsive disorder, bulimia nervosa, premenstrual dysphoric disorders, panic disorders, posttraumatic stress disorder (sertraline)

ACTION

SSRIs selectively inhibit the reuptake of serotonin with little or no effects on other neurotransmitters, such as norepinephrine or dopamine, in the CNS.

ADVERSE REACTIONS

Common adverse effects include headache, tremor, dizziness, sleep disturbances, GI disturbances, and sexual dysfunction. Less common adverse effects include bleeding (ecchymoses, epistaxis), akathisia, breast tenderness or enlargement, extrapyramidal effects, dystonia, fever, hyponatremia, mania or hypomania, palpitations, serotonin syndrome, weight gain or loss, rash, urticaria, or pruritus.

CONTRAINDICATIONS AND CAUTIONS

• Contraindicated in patients hypersensitive to these drugs or their components.
• Use cautiously in patients with hepatic, renal, or cardiac insufficiency.
• In pregnant women, use drug only if benefits outweigh risks; use of certain SSRIs in the first trimester may cause birth defects. Neonates born to women who took an SSRI during the third trimester may develop complications that warrant prolonged hospitalization, respiratory support, and tube feeding. In breast-feeding women, use isn't recommended. SSRIs appear in breast milk and may cause diarrhea and sleep disturbance in neonates. However, risks and benefits to both the woman and infant must be considered. Children and adolescents may be more susceptible to increased suicidal tendencies when taking SSRIs or other antidepressants. Elderly patients may be more sensitive to the insomniac effects of SSRIs.

citalopram hydrobromide

si-TAL-oh-pram

Celexa

Pharmacologic class: SSRI

INDICATIONS
➤ Depression

ACTION
Probably linked to potentiation of serotonergic activity in the CNS resulting from inhibition of neuronal reuptake of serotonin.

ADVERSE REACTIONS
CNS: somnolence, insomnia, suicide attempt, anxiety, agitation
CV: tachycardia, orthostatic hypotension, hypotension
GI: dry mouth, nausea, diarrhea, anorexia, dyspepsia, vomiting
Respiratory: upper respiratory tract infection, coughing
Other: increased sweating, yawning, decreased libido

NURSING CONSIDERATIONS
• At least 14 days should elapse between MAO inhibitor therapy and citalopram therapy.
• Combining triptans with an SSRI or an SSNRI may cause serotonin syndrome or neuroleptic malignant syndrome–like reactions.
• Aspirin, NSAIDs, and other drugs known to affect coagulation may increase the risk of bleeding. Use together cautiously.
• Don't confuse Celexa with Celebrex or Cerebyx.

PATIENT TEACHING
• Advise families and caregivers to closely observe patient for increased suicidal thinking and behavior.
• Inform patient that, although improvement may take 1 to 4 weeks, he should continue therapy as prescribed.
• Advise patient not to stop drug abruptly.
• Tell patient that drug may be taken in the morning or evening without regard to meals. If drowsiness occurs, he should take drug in evening.
• Tell patient to allow orally disintegrating tablet to dissolve on his tongue and then to swallow, with or without water. Tell him not to cut, crush, or chew the tablet.
• Warn patient to avoid alcohol during drug therapy.

escitalopram oxalate
ess-si-TAL-oh-pram

Lexapro

Pharmacologic class: SSRI

INDICATIONS
➤ Major depressive disorder
➤ Generalized anxiety disorder

ACTION
Action may be linked to increase of serotonergic activity in the CNS from inhibition of neuronal reuptake of serotonin. Drug is closely related to citalopram, which may be the active component.

ADVERSE REACTIONS
CNS: suicidal behavior, fever, insomnia, dizziness, lethargy
CV: palpitations, hypertension, flushing, chest pain
GI: nausea, diarrhea, constipation, indigestion, vomiting
Respiratory: bronchitis, cough

NURSING CONSIDERATIONS
• Closely monitor patients at high risk of suicide.
• Aspirin, NSAIDs, and other drugs known to affect coagulation may increase the risk of bleeding. Use together cautiously.
• Evaluate patient for history of drug abuse and observe for signs of misuse or abuse.
• Combining triptans with an SSRI or an SSNRI may cause serotonin syndrome or neuroleptic malignant syndrome–like reactions.
• Don't confuse escitalopram with estazolam.

PATIENT TEACHING
• Inform patient that symptoms should improve gradually over several weeks, rather than immediately.
• Tell patient that although improvement may occur within 1 to 4 weeks, he should continue drug as prescribed.
• Caution patient and patient's family to report signs of worsening depression and signs of suicidal behavior.
• Tell patient that drug may be taken in the morning or evening without regard to meals.
• Encourage patient to avoid alcohol while taking drug.

fluoxetine hydrochloride

floo-OX-e-teen

Prozac, Prozac Weekly, Sarafem

Pharmacologic class: SSRI

INDICATIONS
➤ Depression, obsessive–compulsive disorder (excluding Sarafem)
➤ Bulimia nervosa (excluding Sarafem)
➤ Premenstrual dysphoric disorder

ACTION
Thought to be linked to drug's inhibition of CNS neuronal uptake of serotonin.

ADVERSE REACTIONS
CNS: nervousness, somnolence, anxiety, insomnia, headache, drowsiness, tremor, dizziness, asthenia, suicidal behavior
CV: palpitations
GI: nausea, diarrhea, dry mouth, anorexia, constipation, vomiting
Respiratory: cough, respiratory distress
Skin: rash, pruritus, diaphoresis

NURSING CONSIDERATIONS
• Closely monitor patients at high risk of suicide.
• Avoid giving drug in the afternoon, whenever possible; doing so commonly causes nervousness and insomnia.
• Delayed-release capsules must be swallowed whole; don't crush or open.
• Drug has a long half-life; monitor patient for adverse effects for up to 2 weeks after drug is stopped.
• Combining triptans with an SSRI or an SSNRI may cause serotonin syndrome or neuroleptic malignant syndrome–like reactions.
• When discontinuing drug, taper dosage over 2 weeks to 1 month to avoid withdrawal syndrome.
• Don't confuse fluoxetine with fluvoxamine or fluvastatin. Don't confuse Prozac with Proscar, Prilosec, or ProSom.

PATIENT TEACHING
• Advise patient that full therapeutic effect may not be seen for 4 weeks or longer.
• Advise families and caregivers to carefully observe patient for worsening suicidal thinking or behavior.

paroxetine hydrochloride/paroxetine mesylate
pah-ROX-a-teen

Paxil, Paxil CR/Pexeva

Pharmacologic class: SSRI

INDICATIONS
➤ Depression, obsessive–compulsive disorder
➤ Panic disorder
➤ Anxiety (excluding Pexeva)
➤ Premenstrual dysphoric disorder (PMDD)

ACTION
Linked to drug's inhibition of CNS neuronal uptake of serotonin.

ADVERSE REACTIONS
CNS: asthenia, dizziness, headache, insomnia, somnolence, tremor, nervousness, suicidal behavior, anxiety, confusion, agitation
CV: palpitations, vasodilation, orthostatic hypotension
GI: dry mouth, nausea, constipation, diarrhea, flatulence, vomiting
GU: ejaculatory disturbances, sexual dysfunction, urinary frequency
Skin: diaphoresis, rash, pruritus
Other: decreased libido, yawning

NURSING CONSIDERATIONS
• May decrease digoxin level. Use together cautiously.
• Record mood changes. Monitor patient for suicidal tendencies, and allow only a minimum supply of drug.
• Monitor patient for complaints of sexual dysfunction. In men, they include anorgasmia, erectile difficulties, delayed ejaculation or orgasm, or impotence; in women, they include anorgasmia or difficulty with orgasm.
• Don't stop drug abruptly; taper drug slowly over 1 to 2 weeks.
• Combining triptans with an SSRI or an SSNRI may cause serotonin syndrome or neuroleptic malignant syndrome–like reactions.
• Don't confuse paroxetine with paclitaxel, or Paxil with Doxil, paclitaxel, Plavix, or Taxol.

PATIENT TEACHING
• Caution patient and patient's family to report signs of worsening depression and signs of suicidal behavior.
• Warn patient to avoid activities that require alertness and good coordination until effects of drug are known.
• Tell patient to avoid alcohol and to consult prescriber before taking other prescription or OTC drugs or herbal medicines.

sertraline hydrochloride
SIR-trah-leen

Zoloft

Pharmacologic class: SSRI

INDICATIONS
➤ Depression, obsessive–compulsive disorder
➤ Panic disorder
➤ Posttraumatic stress disorder
➤ Premenstrual dysphoric disorder
➤ Social anxiety disorder

ACTION
Linked to drug's inhibition of CNS neuronal uptake of serotonin.

ADVERSE REACTIONS
CNS: fatigue, headache, tremor, dizziness, insomnia, somnolence, suicidal behavior, paresthesia, hypesthesia, nervousness, anxiety
GI: dry mouth, nausea, diarrhea, dyspepsia, vomiting, constipation
GU: male sexual dysfunction

NURSING CONSIDERATIONS
• Record mood changes. Monitor patient for suicidal tendencies and allow only a minimum supply of drug.
• Don't use the oral concentrate dropper, which is made of rubber, for a patient with latex allergy.
• Combining triptans with an SSRI or an SSNRI may cause serotonin syndrome or neuroleptic malignant syndrome-like reactions.

PATIENT TEACHING
• Caution patient and patient's family to report signs of worsening depression and signs of suicidal behavior.
• Advise patient to use caution when performing hazardous tasks that require alertness.
• Tell patient to avoid alcohol and to consult prescriber before taking OTC drugs.
• Advise patient to mix the oral concentrate with 4 oz (½ cup) of water, ginger ale, lemon-lime soda, lemonade, or orange juice only, and to take the dose right away.

Antidepressants, tricyclic

amitriptyline hydrochloride
doxepin hydrochloride
imipramine hydrochloride/imipramine pamoate
nortriptyline hydrochloride

INDICATIONS
➤ Depression, anxiety (doxepin hydrochloride), enuresis in children older than age 6 (imipramine), neuropathic pain

ACTION
Tricyclic antidepressants may inhibit reuptake of norepinephrine and serotonin in CNS nerve terminals (presynaptic neurons), thus enhancing the concentration and activity of neurotransmitters in the synaptic cleft. Tricyclic antidepressants also exert antihistaminic, sedative, anticholinergic, vasodilatory, and quinidine-like effects.

ADVERSE REACTIONS
Adverse reactions include anticholinergic effects, orthostatic hypotension, and sedation. The tertiary amines (amitriptyline, doxepin, and imipramine) exert the strongest sedative effects; tolerance usually develops in a few weeks. Tricyclic antidepressants may cause CV effects, such as T-wave abnormalities, conduction disturbances, and arrhythmias.

CONTRAINDICATIONS AND CAUTIONS
• Contraindicated in patients hypersensitive to these drugs and in patients with urine retention or angle-closure glaucoma.
• Tricyclic antidepressants are contraindicated within 2 weeks of MAO inhibitor therapy.
• Use cautiously in patients with suicidal tendencies, schizophrenia, paranoia, seizure disorders, CV disease, or impaired hepatic function.
• In pregnant and breast-feeding women, safety hasn't been established; use cautiously. In children younger than age 12, tricyclic antidepressants aren't recommended. Elderly patients are more sensitive to therapeutic and adverse effects; they need lower dosages.

amitriptyline hydrochloride

a-mee-TRIP-ti-leen

Pharmacologic class: Tricyclic antidepressant

INDICATIONS

➤ Depression

ACTION

Unknown. A tricyclic antidepressant that increases the amount of norepinephrine, serotonin, or both in the CNS by blocking their reuptake by the presynaptic neurons.

ADVERSE REACTIONS

CNS: stroke, seizures, coma, ataxia, tremor

CV: orthostatic hypotension, tachycardia, heart block, arrhythmias, MI, ECG changes, hypertension, edema

GI: dry mouth, nausea, vomiting, anorexia, diarrhea, constipation

GU: urine retention, altered libido, impotence

Hematologic: agranulocytosis, thrombocytopenia, leukopenia

Metabolic: hypoglycemia, hyperglycemia

NURSING CONSIDERATIONS

• Amitriptyline has strong anticholinergic effects and is one of the most sedating tricyclic antidepressants. Anticholinergic effects have rapid onset even though therapeutic effect is delayed for weeks.

• Record mood changes. Monitor patient for suicidal tendencies and allow only minimum supply of drug.

• Because patients using tricyclic antidepressants may suffer hypertensive episodes during surgery, stop drug gradually several days before surgery.

• Monitor glucose level.

• Don't withdraw drug abruptly.

• Don't confuse amitriptyline with nortriptyline or aminophylline.

PATIENT TEACHING

• Whenever possible, advise patient to take full dose at bedtime, but warn him of possible morning orthostatic hypotension.

• Tell patient to avoid alcohol during drug therapy.

• To prevent photosensitivity reactions, advise patient to use a sunblock, wear protective clothing, and avoid prolonged exposure to strong sunlight.

• Advise patient that it may take as long as 30 days to achieve full therapeutic effect.

doxepin hydrochloride

DOKS-eh-pin

Silenor

Pharmacologic class: Tricyclic antidepressant

INDICATIONS

➤ Depression; anxiety
➤ Insomnia

ACTION

Unknown. Increases amount of norepinephrine, serotonin, or both in the CNS by blocking their reuptake by the presynaptic neurons.

ADVERSE REACTIONS

CNS: drowsiness, dizziness, seizures, confusion, numbness
CV: orthostatic hypotension, tachycardia, ECG changes
EENT: blurred vision, tinnitus
GI: dry mouth, constipation, nausea, vomiting, anorexia
Metabolic: hypoglycemia, hyperglycemia
Skin: diaphoresis, rash, urticaria, photosensitivity reactions

NURSING CONSIDERATIONS

• Don't withdraw drug abruptly.
• Record mood changes. Monitor patient for suicidal tendencies and allow only a minimum supply of drug.
• Don't confuse doxepin with doxazosin, digoxin, doxapram, or Doxidan.

PATIENT TEACHING

• Tell patient to dilute oral concentrate with 4 oz (120 ml) of water, milk, or juice (orange, grapefruit, tomato, prune, or pineapple, but not grape); preparation shouldn't be mixed with carbonated beverages.
• Tell patient to take full dose at bedtime whenever he can, but warn him of possible morning dizziness on standing up quickly.
• Tell patient that, to minimize the potential for next-day effect, not to take Silenor within 3 hours of a meal.
• Tell patient to avoid alcohol during drug therapy.
• Tell patient that maximal effect may not be evident for 2 to 3 weeks.
• To prevent sensitivity to the sun, advise patient to use sunblock, wear protective clothing, and avoid prolonged exposure to strong sunlight.

imipramine hydrochloride/imipramine pamoate

im-IP-ra-meen

Tofranil/Tofranil-PM

Pharmacologic class: Tricyclic antidepressant (TCA)

INDICATIONS
➤ Depression
➤ Childhood enuresis

ACTION
Unknown. Increases norepinephrine, serotonin, or both in the CNS by blocking their reuptake by the presynaptic neurons.

ADVERSE REACTIONS
CNS: drowsiness, dizziness, seizures, stroke, excitation, tremor
CV: orthostatic hypotension, tachycardia, ECG changes, MI, arrhythmias, heart block, hypertension, precipitation of heart failure
EENT: blurred vision, tinnitus, mydriasis
GI: dry mouth, constipation, nausea, vomiting, anorexia
GU: urine retention
Hematologic: bone marrow depression
Metabolic: hypoglycemia, hyperglycemia

NURSING CONSIDERATIONS
• Monitor WBCs during therapy and monitor patient for fever and sore throat. Discontinue drug if pathological neutrophil depression occurs.
• Don't withdraw drug abruptly.
• Record mood changes. Monitor patient for suicidal tendencies and allow only a minimum supply of drug.
• To prevent relapse in children receiving drug for enuresis, withdraw drug gradually.
• Don't confuse imipramine with desipramine.

PATIENT TEACHING
• Tell patient to take full dose at bedtime whenever possible, but warn him of possible morning dizziness upon standing up quickly.
• If child is an early-night bed-wetter, tell parents it may be more effective to divide dose and give the first dose earlier in day.
• Tell patient to avoid alcohol while taking this drug.
• To prevent oversensitivity to the sun, advise patient to use sunblock, wear protective clothing, and avoid prolonged exposure to strong sunlight.

nortriptyline hydrochloride
nor-TRIP-ti-leen

Aventyl, Pamelor

Pharmacologic class: Tricyclic antidepressant

INDICATIONS
➤ Depression

ACTION
Unknown. Increases the amount of norepinephrine, serotonin, or both in the CNS by blocking reuptake by the presynaptic neurons.

ADVERSE REACTIONS
CNS: drowsiness, dizziness, seizures, stroke, tremor, weakness
CV: tachycardia, heart block, MI, ECG changes
EENT: blurred vision, tinnitus, mydriasis
GI: constipation, dry mouth, nausea, vomiting, anorexia
GU: urine retention
Hematologic: agranulocytosis, thrombocytopenia
Metabolic: hypoglycemia, hyperglycemia

NURSING CONSIDERATIONS
• Record mood changes. Monitor patient for suicidal tendencies and allow only a minimum supply of drug.
• Don't stop drug suddenly.
• Don't confuse nortriptyline with amitriptyline.

PATIENT TEACHING
• Advise patient to take full dose at bedtime whenever possible to reduce risk of dizziness upon standing quickly.
• Warn patient to avoid activities that require alertness and good coordination until effects of drug are known. Drowsiness and dizziness usually subside after a few weeks.
• To prevent oversensitivity to the sun, advise patient to use sunblock, wear protective clothing, and avoid prolonged exposure to strong sunlight.

Antidiabetics

acarbose
glimepiride
glipizide
glyburide
insulin aspart (rDNA origin)
insulin aspart (rDNA origin) protamine suspension and insulin
aspart (rDNA origin)
insulin detemir (rDNA origin)
insulin glargine (rDNA origin)
insulin glulisine (rDNA origin)
insulin (lispro)/insulin lispro protamine and insulin lispro
insulin, regular
isophane insulin suspension
metformin hydrochloride
pioglitazone hydrochloride
repaglinide
rosiglitazone maleate
sitagliptin phosphate

INDICATIONS
➤ Type 1 and type 2 diabetes mellitus

ACTION
Oral antidiabetics come in several types and lower glucose levels by
stimulating insulin release from the pancreas; decreasing hepatic
glucose production, reducing intestinal glucose absorption, and
improving insulin sensitivity; delaying digestion of carbohydrates; slowing the rate at which food leaves the stomach, decreasing postprandial
increase in glucose level, and reducing appetite or improving insulin
sensitivity. Insulin increases glucose transport across muscle and fat
cell membranes.

ADVERSE REACTIONS
Oral antidiabetics: anorexia, headache, heartburn, nausea, vomiting,
and weakness. Hypoglycemia may follow excessive dosage, increased
exercise, decreased food intake, or alcohol use.
Insulin: hypoglycemia, dry mouth, hypokalemia, increased cough,
lipoatrophy, or anaphylaxis.

CONTRAINDICATIONS AND CAUTIONS
• Contraindicated in patients hypersensitive to these drugs and in
patients with diabetic ketoacidosis with or without coma.
• Use of oral hypoglycemics may carry a higher risk of CV mortality
than use of diet alone or of diet and insulin therapy.

acarbose

a-KAR-boz

Precose

Pharmacologic class: Alpha-glucosidase inhibitor

INDICATIONS
➤ Type 2 diabetes

ACTION
Delays digestion of carbohydrates, resulting in a smaller increase in glucose level after meals.

ADVERSE REACTIONS
GI: abdominal pain, diarrhea, flatulence

NURSING CONSIDERATIONS
• Closely monitor patients receiving a sulfonylurea or insulin; drug may increase risk of hypoglycemia. If hypoglycemia occurs, give oral glucose (dextrose). Severe hypoglycemia may require I.V. glucose infusion or glucagon administration.
• Insulin therapy may be needed during increased stress (infection, fever, surgery, or trauma). Monitor patient closely for hyperglycemia.
• Monitor patient's 1-hour postprandial glucose level to determine therapeutic effectiveness of drug and to identify appropriate dose. Report hyperglycemia to prescriber. Thereafter, measure glycosylated hemoglobin level every 3 months.
• Monitor transaminase level every 3 months in first year of therapy and periodically thereafter in patients receiving more than 50 mg t.i.d. Report abnormalities; dosage adjustment or drug withdrawal may be needed.

PATIENT TEACHING
• Tell patient to take drug daily with first bite of each of three main meals.
• Stress importance of adhering to therapeutic regimen, specific diet, weight reduction, exercise, and hygiene programs. Show patient how to monitor glucose level and how to recognize and treat hyperglycemia.
• Teach patient taking a sulfonylurea how to recognize hypoglycemia. Advise treating symptoms with a form of dextrose rather than with a product containing table sugar.
• Urge patient to wear or carry medical identification at all times.

glimepiride
glye-MEH-per-ide

Amaryl

Pharmacologic class: Sulfonylurea

INDICATIONS
➤ Type 2 diabetes
➤ Adjunct to diet and exercise in conjunction with insulin or metformin therapy in patients with type 2 diabetes

ACTION
Lowers glucose level, possibly by stimulating release of insulin from functioning pancreatic beta cells, and may lead to increased sensitivity of peripheral tissues to insulin.

ADVERSE REACTIONS
CNS: dizziness, asthenia, headache
EENT: changes in accommodation
GI: nausea
Hematologic: leukopenia, hemolytic anemia, agranulocytosis, thrombocytopenia, aplastic anemia, pancytopenia
Metabolic: hypoglycemia, dilutional hyponatremia

NURSING CONSIDERATIONS
• Monitor fasting glucose level periodically to determine therapeutic response. Also monitor glycosylated hemoglobin level, usually every 3 to 6 months, to precisely assess long-term glycemic control.
• Don't confuse glimepiride with glyburide or glipizide. Don't confuse Amaryl with Altace.

PATIENT TEACHING
• Tell patient to take drug with first meal of the day.
• Stress importance of adhering to diet, weight reduction, exercise, and personal hygiene programs. Explain to patient and family how and when to monitor glucose level, and teach recognition of and intervention for signs and symptoms of high- and low-glucose levels.
• Advise patient to wear or carry medical identification at all times.
• Teach patient to carry candy or other simple sugars to treat mild episodes of low-glucose level. Patient experiencing severe episode may need hospital treatment.
• Advise patient to avoid alcohol, which lowers glucose level.

glipiZIDE
GLIP-i-zide

Glucotrol, Glucotrol XL

Pharmacologic class: Sulfonylurea

INDICATIONS
➤ Type 2 diabetes

ACTION
Unknown. Probably stimulates insulin release from pancreatic beta cells, reduces glucose output by the liver, and increases peripheral sensitivity to insulin.

ADVERSE REACTIONS
CNS: dizziness, drowsiness, headache, syncope, asthenia, nervousness
GI: nausea, dyspepsia, flatulence, constipation, diarrhea
Hematologic: leukopenia, hemolytic anemia, agranulocytosis, thrombocytopenia, aplastic anemia
Metabolic: hypoglycemia

NURSING CONSIDERATIONS
• Give immediate-release tablet about 30 minutes before meals. Give extended-release tablet with breakfast.
• During periods of increased stress, patient may need insulin therapy. Monitor patient closely for hyperglycemia in these situations.
• Don't confuse glipizide with glyburide or glimepiride.

PATIENT TEACHING
• Tell patient to carry candy or other simple sugars to treat mild low-glucose episodes. Patient experiencing severe episode may need hospital treatment.
• Instruct patient not to change drug dosage without prescriber's consent and to report abnormal blood or urine glucose test results.
• Advise patient to wear or carry medical identification at all times.
• Advise patient to avoid alcohol, which lowers glucose level.
• Tell patient that he may occasionally notice something in his stool that looks like a tablet and that it's the nonabsorbable shell of the extended-release tablet.

glyBURIDE (glibenclamide)

GLYE-byoor-ide

DiaBeta, Glynase PresTab

Pharmacologic class: Sulfonylurea

INDICATIONS
➤ Type 2 diabetes

ACTION
Unknown. Probably stimulates insulin release from pancreatic beta cells, reduces glucose output by the liver, and increases peripheral sensitivity to insulin.

ADVERSE REACTIONS
Hematologic: leukopenia, hemolytic anemia, agranulocytosis, thrombocytopenia, aplastic anemia
Hepatic: cholestatic jaundice, hepatitis
Metabolic: hypoglycemia, hyponatremia
Other: angioedema

NURSING CONSIDERATIONS
• Give with breakfast or first main meal.
• During periods of increased stress, such as infection, fever, surgery, or trauma, patient may need insulin therapy. Monitor patient closely for hyperglycemia in these situations.
• Don't confuse glyburide with glimepiride or glipizide.

PATIENT TEACHING
• Teach patient to carry candy or other simple sugars for mild low-glucose level. Patient experiencing severe episode may need hospital treatment.
• Advise patient to wear or carry medical identification at all times.
• Instruct patient to report episodes of low glucose to prescriber immediately; a severely low-glucose level is sometimes fatal in patients receiving as little as 2.5 to 5 mg daily.
• Advise patient to avoid alcohol, which may lower glucose level.

insulin aspart (rDNA origin) injection
IN-su-lin AS-part

NovoLog

Pharmacologic class: Human insulin analogue

INDICATIONS
➤ Control of hyperglycemia in patients with diabetes

ACTION
Regulates glucose metabolism with the same glucose-lowering effect as regular human insulin, but its effect is more rapid and of shorter duration.

ADVERSE REACTIONS
Metabolic: hypoglycemia, hypokalemia
Skin: injection site reactions, lipodystrophy, pruritus, rash
Other: allergic reactions

NURSING CONSIDERATIONS
• Adjustments in the dose of NovoLog or of any insulin may be needed with changes in physical activity or meal routine. Insulin requirements also may be altered during emotional disturbances, illness, or other stresses.
• Adjust dose regularly, according to patient's glucose measurements. Monitor glucose level regularly.
• Be aware that when administered subcutaneously, onset of action is 15 minutes, peak is 1 to 3 hours, and duration is 3 to 5 hours.
• Periodically monitor glycosylated hemoglobin level.
• Monitor patient with an external insulin pump for erythematous, pruritic, or thickened skin at injection site.

PATIENT TEACHING
• Tell patient not to stop insulin therapy without medical approval.
• Advise patient of the warning signs of low-glucose level (shaking, sweating, moodiness, irritability, confusion, or agitation). Tell patient to carry sugar (candy, sugar packets) to counteract low-glucose level.
• Tell patient not to dilute or mix insulin aspart with any other insulin when using an external insulin pump.
• Instruct patient to monitor glucose level regularly.
• Urge patient to carry medical identification at all times.

insulin aspart (rDNA origin) protamine suspension and insulin aspart (rDNA origin) injection

IN-su-lin AS-part

NovoLog Mix 70/30

Pharmacologic class: Human insulin analogue

INDICATIONS

➤ Control of hyperglycemia in patients with diabetes

ACTION

Regulates glucose metabolism with the same glucose-lowering effect as regular human insulin, but its effect is more rapid and of shorter duration.

ADVERSE REACTIONS

Metabolic: hypoglycemia, hypokalemia
Skin: injection site reactions, lipodystrophy, pruritus, rash
Other: allergic reactions

NURSING CONSIDERATIONS

• Adjustments in the dose of NovoLog or of any insulin may be needed with changes in physical activity or meal routine. Insulin requirements also may be altered during emotional disturbances, illness, or other stresses.
• Adjust dose regularly, according to patient's glucose measurements. Monitor glucose level regularly.
• When administered subcutaneously, onset of action is rapid, peak is 1 to 4 hours, and duration is less than or equal to 24 hours.
• Periodically monitor glycosylated hemoglobin level.
• Monitor patient with an external insulin pump for erythematous, pruritic, or thickened skin at injection site.
• Don't confuse NovoLog Mix 70/30 with Novolin 70/30.

PATIENT TEACHING

• Tell patient not to stop insulin therapy without medical approval.
• Advise patient of the warning signs of low-glucose level (shaking, sweating, moodiness, irritability, confusion, or agitation). Tell patient to carry sugar (candy, sugar packets) to counteract low-glucose level.
• Tell patient not to dilute or mix insulin aspart with any other insulin when using an external insulin pump.
• Instruct patient to monitor glucose level regularly.
• Urge patient to carry medical identification at all times.

insulin detemir (rDNA origin) injection

IN-su-lin DEH-teh-meer

Levemir

Pharmacologic class: Insulin analogue

INDICATIONS

➤ Hyperglycemia in patients with diabetes mellitus who need basal (long-acting) insulin

ACTION

Regulates glucose metabolism by binding to insulin receptors, facilitating cellular uptake of glucose into muscle and fat, and inhibiting release of glucose from liver.

ADVERSE REACTIONS

CV: edema
Metabolic: hypoglycemia, sodium retention, weight gain
Skin: injection site reactions, lipodystrophy, pruritus, rash
Other: allergic reactions

NURSING CONSIDERATIONS

• Don't give I.V. or I.M. Don't mix or dilute with other insulins.
• Give by subcutaneous injection in the thigh, abdominal wall, or upper arm. Rotate injection sites within the same region.
• Monitor glucose level routinely in all patients receiving insulin.
• Measure patient's glycosylated hemoglobin level periodically.
• Watch for hyperglycemia, especially if patient's diet or exercise pattern changes.
• Assess patient for signs and symptoms of hypoglycemia. Insulin doses may need adjustment.
• When administered subcutaneously, onset of action is unknown, peak is 6 to 8 hours, and duration is 6 to 23 hours.

PATIENT TEACHING

• Instruct patient to use only solution that's clear and colorless, with no visible particles.
• Tell patient to recognize and report signs and symptoms of hyperglycemia, such as nausea, vomiting, drowsiness, flushed dry skin, dry mouth, increased urination, thirst, and loss of appetite.
• Teach patient to recognize and report signs and symptoms of hypoglycemia, such as sweating, dizziness, light-headedness, headache, drowsiness, and irritability.
• Advise patient to carry a quick source of simple sugar, such as hard candy or glucose tablets, in case of hypoglycemia.

insulin glargine (rDNA origin) injection

IN-su-lin GLAR-gene

Lantus

Pharmacologic class: Pancreatic hormone

INDICATIONS
➤ To manage type 1 (insulin-dependent) diabetes in patients who need basal (long-acting) insulin to control hyperglycemia
➤ To manage type 2 (non–insulin-dependent) diabetes in patients who need basal (long-acting) insulin to control hyperglycemia

ACTION
Reduces glucose level by stimulating peripheral glucose uptake, especially by skeletal muscle and fat, and by inhibiting hepatic glucose production.

ADVERSE REACTIONS
Metabolic: hypoglycemia
Skin: lipodystrophy, pruritus, rash

NURSING CONSIDERATIONS
• Don't give I.V. or with an insulin pump.
• Don't mix or dilute with other insulins or solutions.
• Rotate injection sites with each dose.
• Because of prolonged duration, this isn't the insulin of choice for diabetic ketoacidosis.
• When administered subcutaneously, onset of action is 1 hour, with no peak, and duration is 24 hours.
• Don't confuse Lantus with Lente.

PATIENT TEACHING
• Tell patient to take dose once daily at the same time each day.
• Urge patient to wear or carry medical identification at all times.
• Advise patient to treat mild hypoglycemia with oral glucose tablets. Encourage patient to always carry glucose tablets in case of a low-glucose episode.
• Advise patient not to dilute or mix any other insulin or solution with insulin glargine. If the solution is cloudy, urge patient to discard the vial.
• Inform patient to avoid alcohol, which lowers glucose level.

insulin glulisine (rDNA origin) injection
IN-su-lin GLUE-lih-seen

Apidra, Apidra SoloStar

Pharmacologic class: Human insulin analogue

INDICATIONS
➤ Diabetes mellitus

ACTION
Lowers glucose level by increasing peripheral glucose uptake and decreasing hepatic glucose production.

ADVERSE REACTIONS
CNS: headache, seizures
CV: hypertension, peripheral edema
EENT: nasopharyngitis
Metabolic: hypoglycemia
Respiratory: upper respiratory tract infection
Skin: injection site reactions, lipodystrophy, pruritus, rash
Other: allergic reactions, anaphylaxis, insulin antibody production, influenza

NURSING CONSIDERATIONS
• Give within 15 minutes before or within 20 minutes after the start of a meal.
• Don't mix drug in a syringe with any other insulin except NPH.
• When used in an external subcutaneous infusion pump, don't mix drug with any other insulin or diluent.
• Use with a longer-acting or basal insulin analogue.
• Early warning signs of hypoglycemia may be different or less pronounced in patients who take beta blockers, who have had an oral antidiabetic added to the regimen, or who have long-term diabetes or diabetic nerve disease.
• When administered subcutaneously, onset of action is 15 minutes, peak is 55 minutes, and duration is unknown.

PATIENT TEACHING
• Tell patient not to mix insulin glulisine in a syringe with any insulin other than NPH.
• If patient is mixing insulin glulisine with NPH, tell patient to use U-100 syringes, to draw insulin glulisine into the syringe first, followed by NPH insulin, and to inject the mixture immediately.

insulin (lispro)/insulin lispro protamine and insulin lispro

IN-su-lin

Humalog/Humalog Mix 75/25, Humalog Mix 50/50

Pharmacologic class: Pancreatic hormone

INDICATIONS
➤ Type 1 diabetes
➤ Type 2 diabetes in combination with a sulfonylurea

ACTION
Increases glucose transport across muscle and fat cell membranes to reduce glucose level. Helps convert glucose to glycogen.

ADVERSE REACTIONS
GI: dry mouth
Metabolic: hypoglycemia, hyperglycemia, hypomagnesemia, hypokalemia
Skin: rash, swelling, redness, stinging, warmth at injection site
Respiratory: increased cough, respiratory tract infection, dyspnea
Other: lipoatrophy, lipohypertrophy, anaphylaxis

NURSING CONSIDERATIONS
• Lispro insulin may be mixed with Humulin N; give within 15 minutes before a meal to prevent a hypoglycemic reaction.
• Injection dosage is expressed in USP units. Use only the syringes calibrated for that concentration of insulin.
• Don't use insulin that changes color or becomes clumped or granular in appearance.
• Check expiration date on vial before using contents.
• Drug is usually given subcutaneously. To give, pinch a fold of skin with fingers at least 3 inches (7.5 cm) apart and insert needle at a 45- to 90-degree angle.
• Press, don't rub, site after injection. Rotate injection sites to avoid overuse of one area.
• Store injectable insulin in cool area. Refrigeration is desirable. Don't freeze.
• Monitor patient's blood sugar.

PATIENT TEACHING
• Stress that accuracy of measurement is important. A magnifying sleeve or dose magnifier may improve accuracy. Show patient and caregivers how to measure and give insulin.
• Teach patient to avoid alcohol because it lowers glucose level.
• Advise patient to wear or carry medical identification.

insulin, regular

IN-su-lin

Humulin R, Humulin R Regular U-500 (concentrated), Novolin R, Novolin R PenFill, Novolin R Prefilled

Pharmacologic class: Pancreatic hormone

INDICATIONS
➤ Management of diabetes

ACTION
Increases glucose transport across muscle and fat cell membranes to reduce glucose level. Helps convert glucose to glycogen.

ADVERSE REACTIONS
GI: dry mouth
Metabolic: hypoglycemia, hyperglycemia, hypomagnesemia, hypokalemia
Skin: rash, swelling, redness, stinging, warmth at injection site
Respiratory: increased cough, respiratory tract infection, dyspnea
Other: lipoatrophy, lipohypertrophy, anaphylaxis

NURSING CONSIDERATIONS
• For continuous infusion, dilute drug in normal saline solution and give at prescribed rate.
• When mixing regular insulin with NPH, always draw up regular insulin into syringe first.
• Don't use insulin that changes color or becomes clumped or granular in appearance.
• Check expiration date on vial before using contents.
• Drug is usually given subcutaneously. To give, pinch a fold of skin with fingers at least 3 inches (7.5 cm) apart and insert needle at a 45- to 90-degree angle.
• Press, don't rub, site after injection. Rotate injection sites to avoid overuse of one area.
• Store injectable insulin in cool area. Refrigeration is desirable. Don't freeze.
• Monitor patient's blood sugar.

PATIENT TEACHING
• Stress that accuracy of measurement is important. A magnifying sleeve or dose magnifier may improve accuracy. Show patient and caregivers how to measure and give insulin.
• Teach patient to avoid alcohol because it lowers glucose level.
• Advise patient to wear or carry medical identification.

isophane insulin suspension

IN-su-lin

(NPH)Humulin N, Novolin N, Novolin N PenFill, Novolin N Prefilled

Pharmacologic class: Pancreatic hormone

INDICATIONS

➤ Management of diabetes

ACTION

Increases glucose transport across muscle and fat cell membranes to reduce glucose level. Helps convert glucose to glycogen.

ADVERSE REACTIONS

GI: dry mouth

Metabolic: hypoglycemia, hyperglycemia, hypomagnesemia, hypokalemia

Skin: rash, swelling, redness, stinging, warmth at injection site

Respiratory: increased cough, respiratory tract infection, dyspnea

Other: lipoatrophy, lipohypertrophy, anaphylaxis

NURSING CONSIDERATIONS

• Switching from separate injections to a prepared mixture may alter patient response. When NPH is mixed with regular insulin in the same syringe, give immediately to avoid loss of potency.

• Don't use insulin that changes color or becomes clumped or granular in appearance.

• Check expiration date on vial before using contents.

• Drug is usually given subcutaneously. To give, pinch a fold of skin with fingers at least 3 inches (7.5 cm) apart and insert needle at a 45- to 90-degree angle.

• Press, don't rub, site after injection. Rotate injection sites to avoid overuse of one area.

• Store injectable insulin in cool area. Refrigeration is desirable. Don't freeze.

• Monitor patient's blood sugar.

PATIENT TEACHING

• Stress that accuracy of measurement is important. A magnifying sleeve or dose magnifier may improve accuracy. Show patient and caregivers how to measure and give insulin.

• Teach patient to avoid alcohol because it lowers glucose level.

• Advise patient to wear or carry medical identification.

metformin hydrochloride
met-FORE-min

Fortamet, Glucophage, Glucophage XR, Glumetza, Riomet

Pharmacologic class: Biguanide

INDICATIONS
➤ Type 2 diabetes

ACTION
Decreases hepatic glucose production and intestinal absorption of glucose and improves insulin sensitivity (increases peripheral glucose uptake and use).

ADVERSE REACTIONS
CNS: asthenia, headache, dizziness, chills, light-headedness
GI: diarrhea, nausea, vomiting
Metabolic: lactic acidosis, hypoglycemia
Other: accidental injury, infection

NURSING CONSIDERATIONS
• Monitor patient's glucose level regularly to evaluate effectiveness of therapy.
• If patient hasn't responded to 4 weeks of therapy with maximum dosage, an oral sulfonylurea can be added while keeping metformin at maximum dosage. If patient still doesn't respond after several months of therapy with both drugs at maximum dosage, prescriber may stop both and start insulin therapy.
• Monitor patient closely during times of increased stress, such as infection, fever, surgery, or trauma. Insulin therapy may be needed in these situations.
• Monitor for signs of lactic acidosis.
• Don't confuse Glucophage with Glucovance or Glucotrol.

PATIENT TEACHING
• Warn patient not to consume excessive alcohol while taking drug.
• Advise patient not to cut, crush, or chew extended-release tablets; instead, he should swallow them whole.
• Tell patient that inactive ingredients may be eliminated in the stool as a soft mass resembling the original tablet.
• Instruct patient to carry medical identification at all times.

pioglitazone hydrochloride
pie-oh-GLIT-ah-zohn

Actos

Pharmacologic class: Thiazolidinedione

INDICATIONS
➤ Type 2 diabetes

ACTION
Lowers glucose level by decreasing insulin resistance and hepatic glucose production. Improves sensitivity of insulin in muscle and adipose tissue.

ADVERSE REACTIONS
CNS: headache
CV: edema, heart failure
EENT: sinusitis, pharyngitis, macular edema
Metabolic: hypoglycemia with combination therapy, aggravated diabetes, weight gain
Respiratory: upper respiratory tract infection

NURSING CONSIDERATIONS
• Measure liver enzyme levels at start of therapy, every 2 months for first year of therapy, and periodically thereafter. Obtain liver function test results in patients who develop signs and symptoms of liver dysfunction.
• Observe patients carefully for signs and symptoms of heart failure.
• Hemoglobin level and hematocrit may drop.
• Monitor glucose level regularly.
• Risk of fractures in female patients receiving long-term treatment is increased. Give only if risk outweighs benefits.
• Don't confuse pioglitazone with rosiglitazone.

PATIENT TEACHING
• Instruct patient to adhere to dietary instructions and to have glucose and glycosylated hemoglobin levels tested regularly.
• Tell patient to report unexplained nausea, vomiting, abdominal pain, fatigue, anorexia, and dark urine immediately because these symptoms may indicate liver problems.
• Warn patient to contact his health care provider if he has signs or symptoms of heart failure (unusually rapid increase in weight or swelling, shortness of breath).
• Tell patient to have regular eye exams and to report any visual changes immediately.

repaglinide
re-PAG-lah-nyde

Prandin

Pharmacologic class: Meglitinide

INDICATIONS
➤ Type 2 diabetes

ACTION
Stimulates insulin release from beta cells in the pancreas by closing ATP-dependent potassium channels in beta cell membranes, which causes calcium channels to open. Increased calcium influx induces insulin secretion; the overall effect is to lower glucose level.

ADVERSE REACTIONS
CNS: headache, paresthesia
Metabolic: hypoglycemia, hyperglycemia
Respiratory: bronchitis, upper respiratory tract infection

NURSING CONSIDERATIONS
• Give drug before meals, usually 15 minutes before start of meal; however, time can vary from immediately preceding meal to up to 30 minutes before meal.
• Increase dosage carefully in patients with impaired renal function or renal failure requiring dialysis.
• Don't confuse Prandin with Avandia.

PATIENT TEACHING
• Encourage patient to keep regular appointments and have his HbA_{1c} level checked every 3 months to determine long-term glucose control.
• Tell patient that, if a meal is skipped or added, he should skip dose or add an extra dose of drug for that meal, respectively.
• Instruct patient to monitor glucose level carefully.
• Teach patient to carry candy or other simple sugars to treat mild hypoglycemia episodes. Patient experiencing severe episode may need emergency treatment.
• Advise patient to avoid alcohol, which lowers glucose level.

rosiglitazone maleate
roh-zee-GLIT-ah-zohn

Avandia

Pharmacologic class: Thiazolidinedione

INDICATIONS
➤ Type 2 diabetes

ACTION
Lowers glucose level by improving insulin sensitivity.

ADVERSE REACTIONS
CV: edema, worsening heart failure
Metabolic: hyperglycemia, weight gain

NURSING CONSIDERATIONS
• Monitor liver enzyme levels every 2 months for first 12 months and periodically thereafter. If ALT level becomes elevated, recheck as soon as possible.
• Observe patients carefully for signs and symptoms of heart failure.
• Check glucose and glycosylated hemoglobin levels periodically to monitor therapeutic response to drug.
• Hemoglobin level and hematocrit may drop during therapy.
• For patients inadequately controlled with a maximum dose of a sulfonylurea or metformin, add rosiglitazone to, rather than substitute it for, a sulfonylurea or metformin.
• Drug may increase the incidence of bone fractures (most common in the arm, hand, and foot) in women.
• Don't confuse rosiglitazone with pioglitazone, or Avandia with Prandin.

PATIENT TEACHING
• Advise patient that drug can be taken with or without food.
• Tell patient to immediately notify prescriber about unexplained signs and symptoms, such as nausea, vomiting, abdominal pain, fatigue, anorexia, or dark urine; these may indicate liver problems.
• Tell patient to immediately notify prescriber of changes in vision as this may indicate macular edema.
• Warn patient to contact his health care provider about signs or symptoms of heart failure.
• Instruct patient to monitor glucose level carefully.

sitagliptin phosphate
sit-ah-GLIP-ten

Januvia

Pharmacologic class: Dipeptidyl peptidase-4 (DPP-4) enzyme inhibitor

INDICATIONS
➤ Type 2 diabetes

ACTION
Inhibits DPP-4, an enzyme that rapidly inactivates incretin hormones, which play a part in the body's regulation of glucose. By increasing and prolonging active incretin levels, the drug helps to increase insulin release and decrease circulating glucose.

ADVERSE REACTIONS
CNS: headache
GI: abdominal pain, nausea, diarrhea
Metabolic: hypoglycemia

NURSING CONSIDERATIONS
• In elderly patients and those at risk for renal insufficiency, periodically assess renal function.
• Monitor glycosylated hemoglobin level periodically to assess long-term glycemic control.
• Watch for hypoglycemia, especially in patients receiving combination therapy.
• Don't confuse sitagliptin with saxagliptin.

PATIENT TEACHING
• Inform patient and family members of the signs and symptoms of hyperglycemia and hypoglycemia.
• Tell patient drug may be taken without regard for food.

Antidiarrheals

bismuth subsalicylate
loperamide

INDICATIONS
➤ Mild, acute, or chronic diarrhea

ACTION
Bismuth preparations may have a mild water-binding capacity, may absorb toxins, and provide a protective coating for the intestinal mucosa. Piperidine derivatives inhibit peristalsis.

ADVERSE REACTIONS
Bismuth preparations may cause salicylism (with high doses) or temporary darkening of tongue and stools.

CONTRAINDICATIONS AND CAUTIONS
• Contraindicated in patients hypersensitive to these drugs.
• Some antidiarrheals may appear in breast milk; check individual drugs for specific recommendations. For children or teenagers recovering from flu or chickenpox, consult prescriber before giving bismuth subsalicylate.
• For elderly patients, use caution when giving antidiarrheal drugs.

bismuth subsalicylate
BIS-mith

Bismatrol, Kaopectate, Kao-Tin, Maalox Total Stomach Relief Liquid, Peptic Relief, Pepto-Bismol, Pink Bismuth

Pharmacologic class: Adsorbent

INDICATIONS
➤ Mild, nonspecific diarrhea

ACTION
May have antisecretory, antimicrobial, and anti-inflammatory effects against bacterial and viral enteropathogens.

ADVERSE REACTIONS
GI: temporary darkening of tongue and stools
Other: salicylism with high doses

NURSING CONSIDERATIONS
• Avoid use before GI radiologic procedures because drug is radiopaque and may interfere with X-rays.
• Liquid form is preferred for children, to give more accurate dosing.

PATIENT TEACHING
• Advise patient that drug contains salicylate.
• Instruct patient to shake liquid before measuring dose and to chew tablets well before swallowing.
• Tell patient to call prescriber if diarrhea lasts longer than 2 days or is accompanied by high fever.
• Advise patient to drink plenty of clear fluids to help prevent dehydration, which may accompany diarrhea.
• Tell patient that tongue and stools may temporarily turn gray-black.
• Urge patient to consult with prescriber before giving drug to children or teenagers during or after recovery from the flu or chickenpox.

loperamide
loe-PER-a-mide

Diar-aid Caplets, Imodium A-D, Imodium A-D EZ chews, K-pec II, Neo-Diaral

Pharmacologic class: Piperidine derivative

INDICATIONS
➤ Acute, nonspecific diarrhea
➤ Chronic diarrhea associated with chronic bowel disease

ACTION
Inhibits peristalsis

ADVERSE REACTIONS
CNS: dizziness, drowsiness, fatigue
GI: constipation, abdominal pain, distention or discomfort, dry mouth, nausea, vomiting
Skin: hypersensitivity reactions, rash

NURSING CONSIDERATIONS
• Monitor children closely for CNS effects; children may be more sensitive to these effects than adults.
• Don't confuse Imodium with Ionamin.

PATIENT TEACHING
• Advise patient not to exceed recommended dosage.
• Tell patient with acute diarrhea to stop drug and seek medical attention if no improvement occurs within 48 hours. In chronic diarrhea, tell patient to notify prescriber and to stop drug if no improvement occurs after taking 16 mg daily for at least 10 days.
• Advise patient with acute colitis to stop drug immediately and notify prescriber about abdominal distention.
• Warn patient to avoid activities that require mental alertness until CNS effects of drug are known.

Antiemetics

meclizine hydrochloride
metoclopramide hydrochloride
ondansetron/ondansetron hydrochloride
prochlorperazine/prochlorperazine maleate

INDICATIONS
➤ Nausea, vomiting, motion sickness, and vertigo

ACTION
For antihistamines (meclizine hydrochloride) the mechanism of action is unclear. Phenothiazines (prochlorperazine) work by blocking the dopaminergic receptors in the chemoreceptor trigger zone of the brain. Serotonin-receptor antagonists (ondansetron) block serotonin stimulation centrally in the chemoreceptor trigger zone and peripherally in vagal nerve terminals.

ADVERSE REACTIONS
Antiemetics may cause asthenia, fatigue, dizziness, headache, insomnia, abdominal pain, anorexia, constipation, diarrhea, epigastric discomfort, gastritis, heartburn, nausea, vomiting, neutropenia, hiccups, tinnitus, dehydration, and fever.

CONTRAINDICATIONS AND CAUTIONS
• Contraindicated in patients hypersensitive to any of the drug components.
• Contraindicated in severe vomiting until etiology of vomiting is established.
• Use cautiously in patients with tartrazine and sulfite sensitivities. Antiemetics may cause allergic-type reactions, including hives, itching, wheezing, asthma, and anaphylaxis.

meclizine hydrochloride (meclozine hydrochloride)

MEK-li-zeen

Antivert, Antivert/25, Bonine, Dramamine Less Drowsy Formula, Meni-D

Pharmacologic class: Anticholinergic

INDICATIONS

➤ Vertigo
➤ Motion sickness

ACTION

Unknown. May affect neural pathways originating in the labyrinth to inhibit nausea and vomiting.

ADVERSE REACTIONS

CNS: drowsiness, auditory and visual hallucinations, excitation, nervousness, restlessness
CV: hypotension, palpitations, tachycardia
EENT: blurred vision, diplopia, dry nose and throat, tinnitus
GI: anorexia, constipation, diarrhea, dry mouth, nausea, vomiting
GU: urinary frequency, urine retention
Skin: rash, urticaria

NURSING CONSIDERATIONS

• Stop drug 4 days before diagnostic skin tests to avoid interference with test response.
• Drug may mask signs and symptoms of ototoxicity, brain tumor, or intestinal obstruction.
• Don't confuse Antivert with Axert. Don't confuse Dramamine Less Drowsy with other Dramamine formulations.

PATIENT TEACHING

• Advise patient to avoid hazardous activities that require alertness until CNS effects of drug are known.
• Urge patient to report persistent or serious adverse reactions promptly.

metoclopramide hydrochloride
met-oh-KLOE-pra-mide

Octamide PFS, Reglan

Pharmacologic class: Dopamine antagonist

INDICATIONS
➤ To prevent or reduce nausea and vomiting from emetogenic cancer chemotherapy
➤ To prevent or reduce postoperative nausea and vomiting
➤ To facilitate small-bowel intubation, to aid in radiologic examinations
➤ Delayed gastric emptying secondary to diabetic gastroparesis
➤ Gastroesophageal reflux disease

ACTION
Stimulates motility of upper GI tract, increases lower esophageal sphincter tone, and blocks dopamine receptors at the chemoreceptor trigger zone.

ADVERSE REACTIONS
CNS: anxiety, drowsiness, dystonic reactions, fatigue, lassitude, restlessness, neuroleptic malignant syndrome, seizures, suicide ideation, akathisia, confusion, depression, dizziness
CV: bradycardia, supraventricular tachycardia
GI: bowel disorders, diarrhea, nausea
Hematologic: agranulocytosis, neutropenia

NURSING CONSIDERATIONS
• Give drug before each meal and at bedtime.
• Give doses of 10 mg or less by direct injection over 1 to 2 minutes.
• Monitor bowel sounds.
• Monitor patient for involuntary movements of face, tongue, and extremities, which may indicate tardive dyskinesia.
• Use 25 mg diphenhydramine I.V. to counteract extrapyramidal adverse effects from high doses.

PATIENT TEACHING
• Tell patient to avoid activities that require alertness for 2 hours after doses.
• Advise patient not to drink alcohol during therapy.

ondansetron/ondansetron hydrochloride
on-DAN-sah-tron

Zuplenz/Zofran, Zofran ODT

Pharmacologic class: Selective serotonin (5-HT$_3$) receptor antagonist

INDICATIONS
➤ To prevent nausea and vomiting from emetogenic chemotherapy
➤ To prevent postoperative nausea and vomiting
➤ To prevent nausea and vomiting from radiation therapy

ACTION
May block 5-HT$_3$ in the CNS in the chemoreceptor trigger zone and in the peripheral nervous system on nerve terminals of the vagus nerve.

ADVERSE REACTIONS
CNS: dizziness, fatigue, headache, malaise, sedation, extrapyramidal syndrome, fever, pain
CV: arrhythmias, chest pain
GI: constipation, diarrhea, abdominal pain, decreased appetite
GU: gynecologic disorders, urine retention
Respiratory: hypoxia
Skin: pruritus, rash

NURSING CONSIDERATIONS
• Monitor liver function test results. Don't exceed 8 mg in patients with hepatic impairment.
• Don't confuse Zofran with Zosyn, Zantac, or Zoloft.

PATIENT TEACHING
• Instruct patient to immediately report difficulty breathing after drug administration.
• Tell patient receiving drug I.V. to report discomfort at insertion site.
• For patient taking ODTs, tell him to open blister just before use by peeling backing off and not by pushing through foil blister, and tell him that taking it with liquid isn't required.
• Teach patient to place ODTs on tongue, allow to dissolve, then swallow with saliva.

prochlorperazine/prochlorperazine maleate

proe-klor-PER-a-zeen

Compro/Procomp

Pharmacologic class: Dopamine antagonist

INDICATIONS
➤ To control preoperative nausea
➤ Severe nausea and vomiting

ACTION
Acts on the chemoreceptor trigger zone to inhibit nausea and vomiting; in larger doses, it partially depresses vomiting center.

ADVERSE REACTIONS
CNS: extrapyramidal reactions
CV: orthostatic hypotension, ECG changes, tachycardia
EENT: blurred vision, ocular changes
GI: constipation, dry mouth, increased appetite
GU: urine retention, dark urine
Hematologic: agranulocytosis, transient leukopenia
Skin: mild photosensitivity reactions

NURSING CONSIDERATIONS
• Dilute oral solution with tomato juice, fruit juice, milk, coffee, carbonated beverage, tea, water, or soup. Or, mix with pudding.
• Protect from light.
• Monitor CBC and liver function studies during long-term therapy.
• Use drug only when vomiting can't be controlled by other measures or when only a few doses are needed. If more than four doses are needed in 24 hours, notify prescriber.

PATIENT TEACHING
• Teach patient what to use to dilute oral solution.
• Advise patient to wear protective clothing when exposed to sunlight.
• Tell patient to call prescriber if more than four doses are needed within 24 hours.

Antifungals

amphotericin B lipid complex
amphotericin B liposomal
fluconazole
ketoconazole
nystatin
terconazole

INDICATIONS
➤ Various fungal infections

ACTION
The amphotericin products bind to sterols in the fungal cell membrane, altering permeability and allowing intracellular components to leak out. These drugs usually inhibit fungal growth and multiplication, but if the level is high enough, the drugs can destroy fungi. The azole class of drugs includes fluconazole, ketoconazole, and terconazole. Fluconazole inhibits fungal cytochrome P450, which weakens fungal cell walls. Ketoconazole interferes with sterol synthesis in fungal cells, damaging cell membranes and increasing permeability. Terconazole may increase *Candida* cell membrane permeability. Nystatin binds to sterols in fungal cell membranes and alters membrane permeability.

ADVERSE REACTIONS
Antifungals cause dizziness, nausea, vomiting, abdominal pain, diarrhea, rash, headache, hypokalemia, and elevated BUN and creatinine levels.

CONTRAINDICATIONS AND CAUTIONS
• Contraindicated in patients hypersensitive to any of the drug components.
• The amphotericin drugs aren't interchangeable and are each prescribed differently.

amphotericin B lipid complex

am-foe-TER-i-sin

Abelcet

Pharmacologic class: Polyene antibiotic

INDICATIONS

➤ Invasive fungal infections, including *Aspergillus* and *Candida* species

ACTION

Binds to sterols of fungal cell membranes, altering cell permeability and causing cell death.

ADVERSE REACTIONS

CNS: fever, headache, pain

CV: cardiac arrest, chest pain, hypertension, hypotension

GI: GI hemorrhage, abdominal pain, diarrhea, nausea, vomiting

GU: renal failure

Hematologic: leukopenia, thrombocytopenia, anemia

Respiratory: respiratory failure, dyspnea, respiratory disorder

Other: multiple organ failure, chills, sepsis, infection

NURSING CONSIDERATIONS

• May increase alkaline phosphatase, ALT, AST, bilirubin, BUN, creatinine, GGT, and LDH levels. May decrease hemoglobin and potassium levels.

• Use an infusion pump, and give by continuous infusion at 2.5 mg/kg/hour.

• Monitor vital signs closely. Fever, shaking chills, and hypotension may appear within 2 hours of starting infusion.

• If severe respiratory distress occurs, stop infusion, provide supportive therapy for anaphylaxis, and notify prescriber. Don't restart drug.

• Hydrate before infusion to reduce risk of nephrotoxicity.

• Monitor creatinine and electrolyte levels (especially magnesium and potassium), liver function, and CBC during therapy.

PATIENT TEACHING

• Warn patient that therapy may take several months.

• Tell patient to expect frequent laboratory testing to monitor kidney and liver function.

amphotericin B liposomal
am-foe-TER-i-sin

AmBisome

Pharmacologic class: Polyene antibiotic

INDICATIONS
➤ Presumed fungal infection in febrile, neutropenic patients
➤ Systemic fungal infections caused by *Aspergillus* species, *Candida* species, or *Cryptococcus* species
➤ Visceral leishmaniasis in immunocompetent patients
➤ Cryptococcal meningitis in patients with HIV infection

ACTION
Binds to sterols of fungal cell membranes, altering cell permeability and causing cell death.

ADVERSE REACTIONS
CNS: fever, anxiety, confusion, headache, insomnia, asthenia, pain
CV: chest pain, hypotension, tachycardia, hypertension, edema
GI: nausea, vomiting, abdominal pain, diarrhea, GI hemorrhage
GU: hematuria, renal failure
Hepatic: bilirubinemia, hepatotoxicity
Metabolic: hypocalcemia, hypokalemia, hypomagnesemia
Respiratory: increased cough, dyspnea, hypoxia, pleural effusion
Other: chills, infection, anaphylaxis, sepsis

NURSING CONSIDERATIONS
• Don't reconstitute with bacteriostatic water for injection, and don't allow bacteriostatic product in solution.
• After reconstitution, shake vial vigorously for 30 seconds or until particulate matter disperses.
• Flush existing I.V. line with D_5W before infusing drug. If this isn't possible, give drug through a separate line.
• Use a controlled infusion device and an in-line filter with a mean pore diameter of 1 micron or larger.
• Initially, infuse drug over at least 2 hours. If drug is tolerated well, reduce infusion time to 1 hour.
• Hydrate before infusion to reduce the risk of nephrotoxicity.
• Observe patient closely. If anaphylaxis occurs, stop infusion, provide supportive therapy, and notify prescriber.

PATIENT TEACHING
• Advise patient that frequent laboratory testing will be needed.

fluconazole
floo-KON-a-zole

Diflucan

Pharmacologic class: Bis-triazole derivative

INDICATIONS
➤ Oropharyngeal, esophageal, systemic, or vulvovaginal candidiasis
➤ Cryptococcal meningitis
➤ To prevent candidiasis in bone marrow transplant and cancer patients

ACTION
Inhibits fungal cytochrome P-450 (responsible for fungal sterol synthesis); weakens fungal cell walls

ADVERSE REACTIONS
CNS: headache, dizziness
GI: nausea, vomiting, abdominal pain, diarrhea, dyspepsia, taste perversion
Hematologic: leukopenia, thrombocytopenia
Skin: rash
Other: anaphylaxis

NURSING CONSIDERATIONS
• Give drug without regard for food.
• Add 24 ml of distilled or purified water to the bottle and shake oral suspension well before giving.
• For IV administration, use an infusion pump and give by continuous infusion at no more than 200 mg/hour.
• Serious hepatotoxicity has occurred in patients with underlying medical conditions.
• If patient develops mild rash, monitor him closely. Stop drug if lesions progress.
• Likelihood of adverse reactions may be greater in HIV-infected patients.

PATIENT TEACHING
• Tell patient to take drug as directed, even after he feels better.

ketoconazole (oral)

kee-toe-KOE-na-zole

Nizoral

Pharmacologic class: Imidazole derivative

INDICATIONS

➤ Systemic candidiasis, chronic mucocutaneous candidiasis, oral candidiasis, candiduria, coccidioidomycosis, blastomycosis, histoplasmosis, chromomycosis, and paracoccidioidomycosis; severe cutaneous dermatophyte infections that are resistant to topical therapy

ACTION

Interferes with fungal cell-wall synthesis by inhibiting formation of ergosterol and increasing cell-wall permeability that makes the fungus susceptible to osmotic instability.

ADVERSE REACTIONS

CNS: suicidal tendencies, severe depression
GI: nausea, vomiting, abdominal pain, diarrhea
Hematologic: leukopenia, thrombocytopenia
Hepatic: fatal hepatotoxicity

NURSING CONSIDERATIONS

• Due to increased risk of hepatotoxicity, monitor patient for signs and symptoms of hepatotoxicity.
• Drug is a potent inhibitor of the cytochrome P-450 enzyme system. Giving this drug with drugs metabolized by the cytochrome P-450 3A4 enzyme system may lead to increased drug levels.

PATIENT TEACHING

• Instruct patient with achlorhydria to dissolve each tablet in 4 ml aqueous solution of 0.2N hydrochloric acid, sip mixture through a glass or plastic straw, and then drink a glass of water because drug needs gastric acidity for dissolution and absorption.
• Instruct patient to wait at least 2 hours after dose before taking antacids, anticholinergics, or H_2 blockers.
• Make sure patient understands that treatment should continue until all tests indicate that active fungal infection has subsided. If drug is stopped too soon, infection will recur.
• Reassure patient that nausea is common early in therapy but will subside. To minimize nausea, instruct patient to divide daily amount into two doses or take drug with meals.

nystatin
nye-STAT-in

Mycostatin, Nilstat

Pharmacologic class: Polyene macrolide

INDICATIONS
➤ Intestinal, oral, or vaginal candidiasis

ACTION
Probably binds to sterols in fungal cell membrane, altering cell permeability and allowing leakage of intracellular components.

ADVERSE REACTIONS
GI: transient nausea, vomiting, diarrhea
GU: irritation, sensitization, vulvovaginal burning (vaginal form)
Skin: rash

NURSING CONSIDERATIONS
• Drug isn't effective against systemic infections.

PATIENT TEACHING
• Advise patient to continue taking drug for at least 2 days after signs and symptoms disappear. Consult prescriber for exact length of therapy.
• Instruct patient to continue therapy during menstruation.
• Explain that factors predisposing women to vaginal infection include use of antibiotics, hormonal contraceptives, and corticosteroids; diabetes; reinfection by sexual partner; and tight-fitting pantyhose. Encourage woman to wear cotton underwear.
• Instruct woman in careful hygiene for affected areas, including cleaning perineal area from front to back.
• Advise patient to report redness, swelling, or irritation.
• Tell patient, especially an older patient, that overusing mouthwash or wearing poorly fitting dentures may promote infection.

terconazole
ter-CONE-uh-zole

Terazol 3, Terazol 7

Pharmacologic class: Triazole derivative

INDICATIONS
➤ Vulvovaginal candidiasis

ACTION
May increase *Candida* cell membrane permeability.

ADVERSE REACTIONS
CNS: headache, fever
GI: abdominal pain
GU: dysmenorrhea, genital pain, vulvovaginal burning
Skin: pruritus, irritation, photosensitivity
Other: body aches

NURSING CONSIDERATIONS
• Therapeutic effect of drug is unaffected by menstruation or hormonal contraceptive use.
• Don't confuse terconazole with tioconazole.

PATIENT TEACHING
• Advise patient to continue treatment during menstrual period. However, tell her not to use tampons.
• Instruct patient to insert drug high in vagina (except during pregnancy).
• Tell patient to use drug for full treatment period prescribed. Explain how to prevent reinfection.
• Instruct patient to notify prescriber and stop drug if fever, chills, other flulike signs and symptoms, or sensitivity develops.
• Caution patient to refrain from sexual intercourse during treatment.
• Tell patient that drug base may react with latex, causing decreased effectiveness of condoms and diaphragms (for up to 72 hours after treatment is completed).
• Instruct patient to store drug at room temperature.

Antiglaucomas

brimonidine tartrate
dorzolamide hydrochloride
latanoprost
levobunolol hydrochloride
timolol maleate
travoprost

INDICATIONS
➤ To reduce intraocular pressure (IOP) in open-angle glaucoma or ocular hypertension

ACTION
The antiglaucoma drugs are selective alpha$_2$ agonists, carbonic anhydrase inhibitors, prostaglandin analogues, and nonselective beta blockers. Selective alpha$_2$ agonists reduce aqueous humor production and increase uveoscleral outflow. Carbonic anhydrase inhibitors decrease aqueous humor secretion, presumably by slowing the formation of bicarbonate ions. This reduces sodium and fluid transport, reducing IOP. Prostaglandin analogues are thought to increase outflow of aqueous humor, thereby lowering IOP. Nonselective beta blockers are thought to reduce formation, and possibly increase outflow, of aqueous humor.

ADVERSE REACTIONS
Burning; stinging; blurred vision; syncope, hypotension, arrhythmias (levobunolol, timolol); ocular allergic reaction (brimonidine, dorzolamide).

CONTRAINDICATIONS AND CAUTIONS
• Contraindicated in patients hypersensitive to drug or its components.
• Contraindicated in patients taking MAO inhibitors. Use cautiously in patients with CV disease, cerebral or coronary insufficiency, hepatic or renal impairment, depression, Raynaud phenomenon, orthostatic hypotension, or thromboangiitis obliterans (selective alpha$_2$ agonist).
• Use cautiously in patients with impaired renal or hepatic function (prostaglandin analogue).
• Contraindicated in patients with bronchial asthma, sinus bradycardia, second- or third-degree AV block, cardiac failure, cardiogenic shock, or history of bronchial asthma or severe COPD (nonselective beta blocker).

brimonidine tartrate

bri-MOE-ni-deen

Alphagan P

Pharmacologic class: Selective alpha$_2$ agonist

INDICATIONS

➤ To reduce IOP in open-angle glaucoma or ocular hypertension

ACTION

Reduces aqueous humor production and increases uveoscleral outflow.

ADVERSE REACTIONS

CNS: asthenia, dizziness, headache
CV: hypertension, hypotension
EENT: allergic conjunctivitis, ocular hyperemia, pruritus
GI: dyspepsia, oral dryness
Respiratory: bronchitis, cough, dyspnea
Skin: rash
Other: flulike syndrome

NURSING CONSIDERATIONS

• Monitor IOP because drug effect may reverse after first month of therapy.

PATIENT TEACHING

• Tell patient to wait at least 15 minutes after instilling drug before wearing soft contact lenses.
• Caution patient to avoid hazardous activities because of risk of decreased mental alertness, fatigue, or drowsiness.
• Advise patient to avoid alcohol.
• If patient is using more than one ophthalmic drug, tell him to apply them at least 5 minutes apart.

dorzolamide hydrochloride
dor-ZOLE-ah-mide

Trusopt

Pharmacologic class: Carbonic anhydrase inhibitor, sulfonamide

INDICATIONS
➤ Increased IOP in patients with ocular hypertension or open-angle glaucoma

ACTION
Decreases aqueous humor secretion, presumably by slowing the formation of bicarbonate ions. This reduces sodium and fluid transport, reducing IOP.

ADVERSE REACTIONS
CNS: asthenia, fatigue, headache
EENT: blurred vision; dryness; lacrimation; ocular allergic reaction; ocular burning, stinging, and discomfort; photophobia; superficial punctate keratitis; iridocyclitis
GI: bitter taste, nausea
GU: urolithiasis
Skin: rash

NURSING CONSIDERATIONS
• Normal IOP is 10 to 21 mm Hg.
• Monitor patient who is hypersensitive to sulfonamides carefully. Drug may cause reactions similar to oral sulfonamides.

PATIENT TEACHING
• Tell patient that drug is a sulfonamide and, although it's given topically, it can be absorbed systemically. Advise patient to apply light finger pressure on lacrimal sac for 1 minute after drug instillation to minimize systemic absorption.
• Tell patient to stop drug and notify prescriber immediately if signs or symptoms of serious adverse reactions or hypersensitivity occur, including eye inflammation and eyelid reactions.
• Tell patient not to wear soft contact lenses during therapy.
• Stress importance of compliance with recommended therapy.

latanoprost
lah-TAN-oh-prost

Xalatan

Pharmacologic class: Prostaglandin analogue

INDICATIONS
➤ Increased IOP in patients with ocular hypertension or open-angle glaucoma

ACTION
Thought to increase outflow of aqueous humor, thereby lowering IOP.

ADVERSE REACTIONS
EENT: blurred vision, burning, foreign body sensation, increased brown pigmentation of the iris, itching, stinging, conjunctival hyperemia, dry eye, excessive tearing, eye pain, eyelash changes, lid crusting or edema, lid discomfort, photophobia
Musculoskeletal: muscle, joint, or back pain
Respiratory: upper respiratory tract infection
Skin: allergic skin reaction, rash
Other: cold, flulike syndrome

NURSING CONSIDERATIONS
• Don't give drug while patient is wearing contact lenses.
• Giving drug more frequently than recommended may decrease its IOP-lowering effects; don't exceed once-daily dosing.
• Drug may gradually change eye color, increasing amount of brown pigment in iris. Increased pigmentation may be permanent.

PATIENT TEACHING
• Instruct patient to report reactions in the eye, especially eye inflammation and lid reactions.
• Tell patient who wears contact lenses to remove them before instilling solution and not to reinsert the lenses until 15 minutes have elapsed.
• If patient is using more than one topical ophthalmic drug, tell him to apply them at least 5 minutes apart.
• Stress importance of compliance with recommended therapy.

levobunolol hydrochloride

LEE-voe-BYOO-no-lahl

AKBeta, Betagan

Pharmacologic class: Nonselective beta blocker

INDICATIONS

➤ Chronic open-angle glaucoma, ocular hypertension

ACTION

Thought to reduce formation, and possibly increase outflow, of aqueous humor.

ADVERSE REACTIONS

CNS: syncope, depression, headache, insomnia
CV: hypotension, bradycardia, heart failure, slight reduction in resting heart rate
EENT: transient eye stinging and burning, blepharoconjunctivitis, corneal punctate staining, decreased corneal sensitivity, erythema, itching, keratitis, photophobia, tearing
GI: nausea
Respiratory: bronchospasm
Skin: urticaria

NURSING CONSIDERATIONS

• Use cautiously in patients with chronic bronchitis, emphysema, diabetes mellitus, hyperthyroidism, or myasthenia gravis.

PATIENT TEACHING

• Advise elderly patient to report shortness of breath, chest pain, or heart irregularities to prescriber. Drug may be absorbed systemically and produce signs and symptoms of beta blockade.
• Advise patient to carry medical identification at all times during therapy.
• *Sun exposure:* May cause photophobia. Advise patient to wear sunglasses.

timolol maleate

tye-MOE-lol

Betimol, Istalol, Timoptic, Timoptic-XE

Pharmacologic class: Nonselective beta blocker

INDICATIONS

➤ To reduce IOP in ocular hypertension or open-angle glaucoma

ACTION

Thought to reduce formation, and possibly increase outflow, of aqueous humor.

ADVERSE REACTIONS

CNS: syncope, stroke, confusion, depression, dizziness, fatigue
CV: hypotension, arrhythmia, bradycardia, cardiac arrest, heart block, heart failure, palpitations, hypertension
EENT: burning and stinging, blepharitis, conjunctivitis, decreased corneal sensitivity with long-term use, diplopia, visual disturbances, discharge, tearing, ocular pain, itching
Respiratory: bronchospasm in patients with history of asthma

NURSING CONSIDERATIONS

• Monitor diabetic patients carefully. Systemic beta-blocking effects can mask some signs and symptoms of hypoglycemia.
• Some patients may need a few weeks of treatment to stabilize pressure-lowering response. Determine IOP after 4 weeks of treatment.
• Drug can be used safely in patients with glaucoma who wear hard contact lenses.
• Don't confuse timolol with atenolol, or Timoptic with Viroptic.

PATIENT TEACHING

• Instruct patient using gel to invert container and shake once before each use. Also tell him to use other ophthalmic drugs at least 10 minutes before applying gel.
• Tell patient to instill drug without contact lenses in place. Lenses may be reinserted about 15 minutes after drug use.
• Drug may be absorbed systemically and produce signs and symptoms of beta blockade. Advise patient to monitor pulse rate and report slow rate to prescriber.

travoprost
TRA-voe-prost

Travatan, Travatan Z

Pharmacologic class: Prostaglandin analogue

INDICATIONS
➤ To reduce IOP in patients with open-angle glaucoma or ocular hypertension

ACTION
Thought to reduce IOP by increasing uveoscleral outflow.

ADVERSE REACTIONS
CNS: anxiety, depression, headache, pain
CV: bradycardia, angina pectoris, chest pain
EENT: eye discomfort, eye pain, eye pruritus, decreased visual acuity, foreign body sensation, ocular hyperemia, abnormal vision
GU: prostate disorder, urinary incontinence, UTI
Respiratory: bronchitis

NURSING CONSIDERATIONS
• Temporary or permanent increased pigmentation of the iris and eyelid may occur as well as increased pigmentation and growth of eyelashes.
• Patient should remove contact lenses before instilling drug and reinsert them 15 minutes after administration.

PATIENT TEACHING
• Tell patient to remove contact lenses before administration, and explain that he can reinsert them 15 minutes afterward.
• Tell patient receiving treatment in only one eye about potential for increased iris pigmentation, eyelid darkening, and increased length, thickness, pigmentation, or number of lashes in the treated eye.
• Advise patient to immediately report eye inflammation or lid reactions.
• Stress importance of compliance with recommended therapy.
• If a pregnant woman or a woman attempting to become pregnant accidentally comes in contact with drug, tell her to thoroughly clean the exposed area with soap and water immediately.

Antigouts

allopurinol/allopurinol sodium
colchicine
probenecid

INDICATIONS
➤ Gout or hyperuricemia; to prevent acute gout attacks (allopurinol and colchicine); gouty arthritis (probenecid)

ACTION
Antigout drugs include xanthine oxidase inhibitors, colchicum autumnale alkaloids, and sulfonamide derivatives.

Xanthine oxidase inhibitors reduce uric acid production by inhibiting xanthine oxidase, the enzyme responsible for the production of uric acid. Colchicum autumnale alkaloids' exact mechanism of action is not fully known; thought to involve a reduction in lactic acid produced by leukocytes, reducing uric acid deposits and phagocytosis, thereby decreasing the inflammatory process. Sulfonamide derivatives block renal tubular reabsorption of uric acid, increasing excretion.

ADVERSE REACTIONS
Rash, nausea, vomiting, diarrhea, aplastic anemia (probenecid).

CONTRAINDICATIONS AND CAUTIONS
• Contraindicated in patients hypersensitive to drug.
• Contraindicated in patients with idiopathic hemochromatosis (allopurinol).
• Contraindicated in patients with renal or hepatic impairment who are taking P-gp or strong CYP3A4 inhibitors (colchicine).
• Use cautiously in patients with peptic ulcer or renal impairment (probenecid).

allopurinol/allopurinol sodium
al-oh-PURE-i-nole

Lopurin, Zyloprim/Aloprim

Pharmacologic class: Xanthine oxidase inhibitor

INDICATIONS
➤ Gout or hyperuricemia
➤ To prevent acute gout attacks
➤ To prevent uric acid nephropathy during cancer chemotherapy
➤ Recurrent calcium oxalate calculi

ACTION
Reduces uric acid production by inhibiting xanthine oxidase.

ADVERSE REACTIONS
GI: nausea, diarrhea
Musculoskeletal: acute gout attack
Skin: rash, maculopapular rash

NURSING CONSIDERATIONS
• Monitor uric acid level to evaluate drug's effectiveness.
• Monitor fluid intake and output; daily urine output of at least 2 L and maintenance of neutral or slightly alkaline urine are desirable.
• Optimal benefits may need 2 to 6 weeks of therapy. Because acute gout attacks may occur during this time, concurrent use of colchicine may be prescribed prophylactically.
• Don't confuse Zyloprim with ZORprin.

PATIENT TEACHING
• To minimize GI adverse reactions, tell patient to take drug with or immediately after meals.
• Encourage patient to drink plenty of fluids while taking drug unless otherwise contraindicated.
• If patient is taking drug for recurrent calcium oxalate stones, advise him also to reduce his dietary intake of animal protein, sodium, refined sugars, oxalate-rich foods, and calcium.
• Tell patient to stop drug at first sign of rash, which may precede severe hypersensitivity or other adverse reactions.
• Advise patient to avoid alcohol during therapy.
• Teach patient importance of continuing drug even if asymptomatic.

colchicine
KOL-chih-seen

Colcrys

Pharmacologic class: Colchicum autumnale alkaloid

INDICATIONS
➤ Prevention of gout flares
➤ Gout flares
➤ Familial Mediterranean fever (FMF)

ACTION
Exact mechanism of action is not fully known; thought to involve a reduction in lactic acid produced by leukocytes, reducing uric acid deposits and phagocytosis, thereby decreasing the inflammatory process.

ADVERSE REACTIONS
CNS: fatigue, headache
GI: diarrhea, nausea, vomiting

NURSING CONSIDERATIONS
• Obtain baseline laboratory studies, including CBC, before starting therapy and periodically thereafter; watch for myelosuppression, leukopenia, granulocytopenia, thrombocytopenia, pancytopenia, and aplastic anemia.
• Monitor patient who has used drug for a prolonged period for neuromuscular toxicity and rhabdomyolysis.
• When used for gout prophylaxis, colchicine must be given with allopurinol or a uricosuric drug (such as probenecid) to decrease serum uric acid level. However, colchicine should be started before the other agent because a sudden change in uric acid level may cause a gout attack.

PATIENT TEACHING
• Grapefruit juice may increase drug level. Discourage use together.
• Advise female patient not to breast-feed and to use an alternative method for feeding the baby.

probenecid
proe-BEN-e-sid

Pharmacologic class: Sulfonamide derivative

INDICATIONS
➤ Hyperuricemia of gout, gouty arthritis
➤ Adjunct to penicillin therapy
➤ Alternate therapy for uncomplicated gonorrhea

ACTION
Blocks renal tubular reabsorption of uric acid, increasing excretion, and inhibits active renal tubular secretion of many weak organic acids, such as penicillins and cephalosporins.

ADVERSE REACTIONS
CNS: fever, headache, dizziness
Hematologic: aplastic anemia, hemolytic anemia, anemia
Hepatic: hepatic necrosis
Other: worsening of gout, hypersensitivity reactions, anaphylaxis

NURSING CONSIDERATIONS
• Force fluids to maintain minimum daily output of 2 to 3 L. Alkalinize urine with sodium bicarbonate or potassium citrate. These measures prevent hematuria, renal colic, urate stone development, and costovertebral pain.
• Don't use to treat gout until acute attack subsides. Drug has no analgesic or anti-inflammatory effects and is of no value during acute gout attacks.
• Don't confuse probenecid with Procanbid.

PATIENT TEACHING
• Instruct patient with gout to take drug regularly to prevent recurrence.
• Advise patient with gout to avoid all drugs that contain aspirin, which may precipitate gout.
• Instruct patient to drink at least 6 to 8 glasses of water per day.
• Urge patient with gout to avoid alcohol; it increases urate level.
• Tell patient with gout to limit intake of foods high in purine, such as anchovies, liver, sardines, kidneys, sweetbreads, peas, and lentils. Also tell him to identify and avoid other foods that may trigger gout attacks.

Antihistamines

cetirizine hydrochloride
fexofenadine hydrochloride
loratadine
promethazine hydrochloride

INDICATIONS
➤ Allergic rhinitis, urticaria, pruritus, vertigo, motion sickness, nausea and vomiting, sedation, dyskinesia, parkinsonism

ACTION
Antihistamines are structurally related chemicals that compete with histamine for histamine-1 (H_1) receptor sites on smooth muscle of bronchi, GI tract, and large blood vessels, binding to cellular receptors and preventing access to and subsequent activity of histamine. They don't directly alter histamine or prevent its release.

ADVERSE REACTIONS
Most antihistamines cause drowsiness and impaired motor function early in therapy. They also can cause blurred vision, constipation, and dry mouth and throat. Promethazine may also cause extrapyramidal reactions with high doses.

CONTRAINDICATIONS AND CAUTIONS
• Contraindicated in patients hypersensitive to these drugs and in those with angle closure glaucoma, stenosing peptic ulcer, pyloroduodenal obstruction, or bladder neck obstruction. Also contraindicated in those taking MAO inhibitors.
• In pregnant women, safe use hasn't been established. During breastfeeding, antihistamines shouldn't be used because many of these drugs appear in breast milk and may cause unusual excitability in the infant. Neonates, especially premature infants, may experience seizures. Children, especially those younger than age 6, may experience paradoxical hyperexcitability with restlessness, insomnia, nervousness, euphoria, tremors, and seizures; give cautiously. Elderly patients usually are more sensitive to the adverse effects of antihistamines, especially dizziness, sedation, hypotension, and urine retention; use cautiously and monitor these patients closely.

cetirizine hydrochloride
se-TEER-i-zeen

Zyrtec

Pharmacologic class: Piperazine derivative

INDICATIONS
➤ Seasonal allergic rhinitis
➤ Perennial allergic rhinitis, chronic urticaria

ACTION
A long-acting, nonsedating antihistamine that selectively inhibits peripheral H_1 receptors.

ADVERSE REACTIONS
CNS: somnolence, fatigue, dizziness, headache
EENT: pharyngitis
GI: dry mouth, nausea, vomiting, abdominal distress

NURSING CONSIDERATIONS
• Stop drug 4 days before diagnostic skin testing because antihistamines can prevent, reduce, or mask positive skin test response.
• Don't confuse Zyrtec with Zyprexa or Zantac.

PATIENT TEACHING
• Warn patient not to perform hazardous activities until CNS effects of drug are known. Somnolence is a common adverse reaction.
• Advise patient not to use alcohol or other CNS depressants while taking drug.
• Inform patient that sugarless gum, hard candy, or ice chips may relieve dry mouth.

fexofenadine hydrochloride
fecks-oh-FEN-a-deen

Allegra, Allegra ODT

Pharmacologic class: Piperidine

INDICATIONS
➤ Seasonal allergic rhinitis
➤ Chronic idiopathic urticaria

ACTION
A long-acting nonsedating antihistamine that selectively inhibits peripheral H_1 receptors.

ADVERSE REACTIONS
CNS: fatigue, drowsiness, fever, headache
GI: nausea, dyspepsia, vomiting
Musculoskeletal: back pain
Respiratory: cough, rhinorrhea, upper respiratory tract infection

NURSING CONSIDERATIONS
• Don't give antacid within 2 hours of this drug.
• Give orally disintegrating tablets (ODTs) to patient with an empty stomach. Allow ODT to disintegrate on the patient's tongue; and it may be swallowed with or without water.
• Stop drug 4 days before patient undergoes diagnostic skin tests because drug can prevent, reduce, or mask positive skin test response.

PATIENT TEACHING
• Instruct patient or parent not to exceed prescribed dosage and to use drug only when needed.
• Warn patient to avoid alcohol and hazardous activities that require alertness until CNS effects of drug are known. Explain that drug may cause drowsiness.
• Advise patient with dry mouth to try sugarless gum, hard candy, or ice chips.
• Tell parents to keep the oral suspension in a cool, dry place, tightly closed, and to shake well before using.
• Tell patient to keep ODT in original blister package until time of use.

loratadine
lor-AT-a-deen

Alavert, Alavert Children's, Children's Claritin Allergy, Claritin, Claritin Hives Relief, Claritin 24-Hour Allergy, Claritin Liqui-Gels, Claritin RediTabs, Clear-Atadine, Dimetapp Children's Non-Drowsy Allergy, Triaminic Allerchews

Pharmacologic class: Piperidine

INDICATIONS
➤ Allergic rhinitis

ACTION
Blocks effects of histamine at H_1-receptor sites. Drug is a nonsedating antihistamine; its chemical structure prevents entry into the CNS.

ADVERSE REACTIONS
CNS: headache, drowsiness, fatigue, insomnia, nervousness
GI: dry mouth

NURSING CONSIDERATIONS
• Stop drug 4 days before patient undergoes diagnostic skin tests because drug can prevent, reduce, or mask positive skin test response.

PATIENT TEACHING
• Make sure patient understands to take drug once daily. If symptoms persist or worsen, tell him to contact prescriber.
• Tell patient taking Claritin RediTabs to use tablet immediately after opening individual blister.
• Advise patient taking Claritin RediTabs to place tablet on the tongue, where it disintegrates within a few seconds. It can be swallowed with or without water.
• Warn patient to avoid alcohol and hazardous activities that require alertness until CNS effects of drug are known.
• Tell patient that dry mouth can be relieved with sugarless gum, hard candy, or ice chips.

promethazine hydrochloride
proe-METH-a-zeen

Phenadoz, Promethegan

Pharmacologic class: Phenothiazine

INDICATIONS
➤ Motion sickness
➤ Nausea and vomiting
➤ Rhinitis, allergy symptoms
➤ Nighttime sedation
➤ Adjunct to analgesics for routine preoperative or postoperative sedation

ACTION
Phenothiazine derivative that competes with histamine for H_1-receptor sites on effector cells. Prevents, but doesn't reverse, histamine-mediated responses.

ADVERSE REACTIONS
CNS: drowsiness, sedation, confusion, sleepiness, dizziness, disorientation, extrapyramidal symptoms
EENT: dry mouth, blurred vision
GI: nausea, vomiting
GU: urine retention
Hematologic: leukopenia, agranulocytosis, thrombocytopenia
Respiratory: respiratory depression, apnea

NURSING CONSIDERATIONS
• Stop drug 4 days before diagnostic skin testing because antihistamines can prevent, reduce, or mask positive skin test response.
• In patients scheduled for a myelogram, stop drug 48 hours before procedure. Don't resume drug until 24 hours after procedure because of the risk of seizures.

PATIENT TEACHING
• Tell patient to take oral form with food or milk.
• When treating motion sickness, tell patient to take first dose 30 to 60 minutes before travel; dose may be repeated in 8 to 12 hours, if necessary. On succeeding days of travel, patient should take dose upon arising and with evening meal.
• Warn patient about possible photosensitivity reactions. Advise use of a sunblock.

Antihypoglycemic

Glucagon

INDICATIONS
➤ Hypoglycemia; diagnostic aid for radiologic examination of the GI tract

ACTION
Glucagon regulates the rate of glucose production through glycogenolysis (conversion of glycogen back into glucose by the liver), glucogenesis (formation of glucose from free fatty acids and proteins), and lipolysis (release of fatty acids from adipose tissue for conversion to glucose).

ADVERSE REACTIONS
Nausea, vomiting, hypersensitivity reactions

CONTRAINDICATIONS AND CAUTIONS
• Contraindicated in patients hypersensitive to drug and in those with pheochromocytoma.
• Use cautiously in patients with history of insulinoma or pheochromocytoma.

glucagon
GLOO-ka-gon

GlucaGen Diagnostic Kit, GlucaGen HypoKit, Glucagon
Emergency Kit

Pharmacologic class: Antihypoglycemic

INDICATIONS
➤ Hypoglycemia
➤ Diagnostic aid for radiologic examination of the GI tract

ACTION
Raises glucose level by promoting catalytic depolymerization of hepatic glycogen to glucose. Relaxes the smooth muscle of the stomach, duodenum, small bowel, and colon.

ADVERSE REACTIONS
CV: hypotension
GI: nausea, vomiting
Other: hypersensitivity reactions

NURSING CONSIDERATIONS
• For hypoglycemia, use drug only in emergency situations.
• Store at room temperature before reconstituting. Avoid freezing and protect from light. After reconstitution, use immediately.
• Monitor glucose level before, during, and after administration.
• As soon as patient regains consciousness and is able to swallow, give additional carbohydrates orally to prevent secondary hypoglycemic reactions.

PATIENT TEACHING
• Instruct patient and caregivers how to give glucagon and recognize a low glucose episode.
• Explain importance of calling prescriber immediately in emergencies.
• Teach patient and caregivers how to prevent hypoglycemia.

Antilipemics

atorvastatin calcium
cholestyramine
ezetimibe
fenofibrate
gemfibrozil
lovastatin
pravastatin sodium
rosuvastatin calcium
simvastatin

INDICATIONS
➤ Hyperlipidemia, hypercholesterolemia

ACTION
Antilipemics lower elevated lipid levels. Bile-sequestering drugs (cholestyramine) lower LDL level by forming insoluble complexes with bile salts, thus triggering cholesterol to leave the bloodstream and other storage areas to make new bile acids. Fibric acid derivatives (gemfibrozil) reduce cholesterol formation, increase sterol excretion, and decrease lipoprotein and triglyceride synthesis. HMG-CoA reductase inhibitors (atorvastatin, lovastatin, pravastatin, rosuvastatin, simvastatin) interfere with the activity of enzymes that generate cholesterol in the liver. Selective cholesterol absorption inhibitors (ezetimibe) inhibit cholesterol absorption by the small intestine, reducing hepatic cholesterol stores and increasing cholesterol clearance from the blood.

ADVERSE REACTIONS
Antilipemics commonly cause GI upset. Bile-sequestering drugs may cause bloating, cholelithiasis, constipation, and steatorrhea. Fibric acid derivatives may cause cholelithiasis and have other GI or CNS effects. HMG-CoA reductase inhibitors may affect liver function or cause rash, pruritus, increased CK levels, rhabdomyolysis, and myopathy.

CONTRAINDICATIONS AND CAUTIONS
• Contraindicated in patients hypersensitive to these drugs.
• In pregnant women, use bile-sequestering drugs and fibric acid derivatives cautiously and avoid using HMG-CoA inhibitors. In breast-feeding women, avoid using fibric acid derivatives and HMG-CoA inhibitors; give bile-sequestering drugs cautiously. In children ages 10 to 17, certain antilipemics have been approved to treat heterozygous familial hypercholesterolemia. Elderly patients have an increased risk of severe constipation; use bile-sequestering drugs cautiously and monitor patients closely.

atorvastatin calcium

ah-TOR-va-stah-tin

Lipitor

Pharmacologic class: HMG-CoA reductase inhibitor

INDICATIONS
➤ To reduce the risk of MI or stroke in patients with type 2 diabetes
➤ Adjunct to diet to reduce LDL, total cholesterol, apolipoprotein B, and triglyceride levels and to increase HDL levels
➤ Heterozygous familial hypercholesterolemia

ACTION
Inhibits HMG-CoA reductase, an early (and rate-limiting) step in cholesterol biosynthesis.

ADVERSE REACTIONS
CNS: headache, asthenia, insomnia
GI: constipation, diarrhea, dyspepsia, flatulence, nausea
Musculoskeletal: rhabdomyolysis, arthritis, arthralgia, myalgia
Skin: rash

NURSING CONSIDERATIONS
• Grapefruit juice may increase drug levels, increasing risk of adverse reactions. Discourage use together.
• Patient should follow a standard cholesterol-lowering diet before and during therapy.
• Before treatment, assess patient for underlying causes for hypercholesterolemia and obtain a baseline lipid profile. Obtain periodic liver function test results and lipid levels.
• Watch for signs of myositis.
• Don't confuse Lipitor with Levatol.

PATIENT TEACHING
• Teach patient about proper dietary management, weight control, and exercise. Explain their importance in controlling high fat levels.
• Warn patient to avoid alcohol.
• Tell patient to inform prescriber of adverse reactions, such as muscle pain, malaise, and fever.
• Advise patient that drug can be taken at any time of day, without regard for meals.

cholestyramine

koe-LESS-tir-a-meen

Locholest, Locholest Light, Prevalite, Questran, Questran Light

Pharmacologic class: Bile acid sequestrant

INDICATIONS

➤ Primary hyperlipidemia or pruritus caused by partial bile obstruction, adjunct for reduction of increased cholesterol level in patients with primary hypercholesterolemia

ACTION

Binds bile acids in the intestinal tract, impeding their absorption and causing their elimination in feces. In response to this bile acid depletion, LDL cholesterol levels decrease as the liver uses LDL cholesterol to replenish reduced bile acid stores.

ADVERSE REACTIONS

CNS: dizziness, headache, vertigo, anxiety, fatigue, syncope, tinnitus
GI: abdominal discomfort, constipation, fecal impaction, nausea, anorexia, diarrhea, flatulence, GI bleeding, vomiting
Musculoskeletal: backache, muscle and joint pains, osteoporosis
Other: vitamin A, D, E, and K deficiencies from decreased absorption

NURSING CONSIDERATIONS

• Give other drugs 1 hour before or at least 4 hours after cholestyramine to avoid impeding absorption.
• Monitor cholesterol and triglyceride levels regularly.
• Monitor levels of cardiac glycosides in patients receiving cardiac glycosides and cholestyramine together.
• Long-term use may lead to deficiencies of vitamins A, D, E, and K, and folic acid.
• Don't confuse Questran with Quarzan.

PATIENT TEACHING

• Tell patient never to take drug in its dry form because it may irritate the esophagus or cause severe constipation.
• Tell patient to prepare drug in a large glass containing water, milk, or juice (especially pulpy fruit juice). Tell him to sprinkle powder on the surface of the beverage, let the mixture stand for a few minutes, and then stir thoroughly.
• Tell patient to avoid sipping or holding the suspension in the mouth because drug may damage tooth surfaces. Advise patient to maintain good oral hygiene.
• Advise patient to take at mealtime, if possible.

ezetimibe

ee-ZET-ah-mibe

Zetia

Pharmacologic class: Selective cholesterol absorption inhibitor

INDICATIONS

➤ Adjunct to diet and exercise to reduce total-cholesterol (C), LDL-C, and apolipoprotein B (Apo B) levels in patients with primary hypercholesterolemia

ACTION

Inhibits absorption of cholesterol by the small intestine, unlike other drugs used for cholesterol reduction; causes reduced hepatic cholesterol stores and increased cholesterol clearance from the blood.

ADVERSE REACTIONS

CNS: dizziness, fatigue, headache
GI: abdominal pain, diarrhea
Musculoskeletal: arthralgia, back pain, myalgia
Respiratory: upper respiratory tract infection, cough

NURSING CONSIDERATIONS

• Check liver function test values when therapy starts and thereafter according to the HMG-CoA reductase inhibitor manufacturer's recommendations.
• Patient should maintain a cholesterol-lowering diet during treatment.

PATIENT TEACHING

• Emphasize importance of following a cholesterol-lowering diet during drug therapy.
• Tell patient he may take drug without regard for meals.
• Advise patient to notify prescriber of unexplained muscle pain, weakness, or tenderness.
• Urge patient to tell his prescriber about any herbal or dietary supplements he's taking.
• Advise patient to visit his prescriber for routine follow-ups and blood tests.
• Tell woman to notify prescriber if she becomes pregnant.

fenofibrate
fee-no-FYE-brate

Antara, Fenoglide, Lipofen, TriCor, Triglide

Pharmacologic class: Fibric acid derivative

INDICATIONS
➤ Hypertriglyceridemia
➤ Primary hypercholesterolemia or mixed dyslipidemia

ACTION
May lower triglyceride levels by inhibiting triglyceride synthesis with less very–low-density lipoproteins released into circulation. Drug may also stimulate breakdown of triglyceride-rich protein.

ADVERSE REACTIONS
CNS: dizziness, headache, asthenia, fatigue, insomnia, paresthesia
CV: arrhythmias
EENT: blurred vision, conjunctivitis, earache, eye discomfort, eye floaters, rhinitis, sinusitis
GI: constipation, diarrhea, dyspepsia, nausea, vomiting
Musculoskeletal: arthralgia
Respiratory: cough

NURSING CONSIDERATIONS
• Monitor liver function periodically during therapy. Stop drug if enzyme levels persist above three times normal.
• Watch for signs and symptoms of pancreatitis, myositis, rhabdomyolysis, cholelithiasis, and renal failure. Monitor patient for muscle pain, tenderness, or weakness, especially with malaise or fever.
• Beta blockers, estrogens, and thiazide diuretics may increase triglyceride levels; evaluate need for continued use of these drugs.

PATIENT TEACHING
• Inform patient that drug therapy doesn't reduce need for following a triglyceride-lowering diet.
• Advise patient to promptly report unexplained muscle weakness, pain, or tenderness, especially with malaise or fever.
• Tell patient to take capsules with meals for best drug absorption.
• Instruct patient who is also taking a bile-acid resin to take fenofibrate 1 hour before or 4 to 6 hours after resin.

gemfibrozil
jem-FI-broe-zil

Lopid

Pharmacologic class: Fibric acid derivative

INDICATIONS
➤ Types IV and V hyperlipidemia unresponsive to diet and other drugs

ACTION
Inhibits peripheral lipolysis and reduces triglyceride synthesis in the liver; lowers triglyceride levels and increases HDL cholesterol levels.

ADVERSE REACTIONS
GI: abdominal and epigastric pain, dyspepsia, acute appendicitis, constipation, diarrhea, nausea, vomiting
Hematologic: leukopenia, thrombocytopenia, anemia, eosinophilia
Metabolic: hypokalemia
Skin: dermatitis, eczema, pruritus, rash

NURSING CONSIDERATIONS
• Check CBC and test liver function periodically during the first 12 months of therapy.
• Patient shouldn't take drug together with repaglinide or itraconazole.

PATIENT TEACHING
• Instruct patient to take drug 30 minutes before breakfast and dinner.
• Teach patient about proper dietary management of cholesterol and triglycerides. When appropriate, recommend weight control, exercise, and smoking cessation programs.
• Tell patient to observe bowel movements and to report evidence of excess fat in feces or other signs of bile duct obstruction.
• Advise patient to report muscle pain to prescriber if occurs during therapy.

lovastatin (mevinolin)
loe-va-STA-tin

Altoprev, Mevacor

Pharmacologic class: HMG-CoA reductase inhibitor

INDICATIONS
➤ To prevent and treat coronary heart disease; hyperlipidemia
➤ Heterozygous familial hypercholesterolemia in adolescents

ACTION
Inhibits HMG-CoA reductase, an early (and rate-limiting) step in cholesterol biosynthesis.

ADVERSE REACTIONS
CNS: headache, dizziness, insomnia, peripheral neuropathy
EENT: blurred vision
GI: constipation, diarrhea, dyspepsia, flatulence, nausea, vomiting
Musculoskeletal: muscle cramps, myalgia, myositis, rhabdomyolysis

NURSING CONSIDERATIONS
• Have patient follow a diet restricted in saturated fat and cholesterol during therapy.
• Obtain liver function test results at the start of therapy, at 6 and 12 weeks after the start of therapy, and when increasing dose; then monitor results periodically.
• Don't confuse lovastatin with Lotensin, Leustatin, or Livostin. Don't confuse Mevacor with Mivacron.

PATIENT TEACHING
• Instruct patient to take drug with the evening meal.
• Teach patient about proper dietary management of cholesterol and triglycerides. When appropriate, recommend weight control, exercise, and smoking cessation programs.
• Advise patient to have periodic eye examinations; related compounds cause cataracts.
• Instruct patient to store tablets at room temperature in a light-resistant container.
• Advise patient to promptly report unexplained muscle pain, tenderness, or weakness, particularly when accompanied by malaise or fever.
• Advise patient not to crush or chew extended-release tablets.

pravastatin sodium (eptastatin)
prah-va-STA-tin

Pravachol

Pharmacologic class: HMG-CoA reductase inhibitor

INDICATIONS
➤ Primary and secondary prevention of coronary events; hyperlipidemia
➤ Heterozygous familial hypercholesterolemia

ACTION
Inhibits HMG-CoA reductase, an early (and rate-limiting) step in cholesterol biosynthesis.

ADVERSE REACTIONS
CNS: dizziness, fatigue, headache
GI: nausea, constipation, diarrhea, flatulence, heartburn, vomiting
GU: renal failure caused by myoglobinuria, urinary abnormality
Musculoskeletal: localized muscle pain, rhabdomyolysis, myalgia, myopathy, myositis

NURSING CONSIDERATIONS
• Patient should follow a diet restricted in saturated fat and cholesterol during therapy.
• Use in children with heterozygous familial hypercholesterolemia if LDL cholesterol level is at least 190 mg/dl, or if LDL cholesterol is at least 160 mg/dl and patient has either a positive family history of premature CV disease or two or more other CV disease risk factors.
• Obtain liver function test results at start of therapy and then periodically.
• Don't confuse Pravachol with Prevacid or propranolol.

PATIENT TEACHING
• Advise patient who is also taking a bile-acid resin such as cholestyramine to take pravastatin at least 1 hour before or 4 hours after taking resin.
• Tell patient to notify prescriber of adverse reactions, particularly muscle aches and pains.
• Inform patient that it will take up to 4 weeks to achieve full therapeutic effect.

rosuvastatin calcium
row-SUE-va-sta-tin

Crestor

Pharmacologic class: HMG-CoA reductase inhibitor

INDICATIONS
➤ Adjunct to diet to reduce LDL cholesterol, total cholesterol, apolipoprotein B, non-HDL cholesterol, and triglyceride levels and to increase HDL cholesterol level
➤ Risk reduction in patients without clinical evidence of coronary heart disease but with multiple risk factors
➤ Children with heterozygous familial hypercholesterolemia

ACTION
Inhibits HMG-CoA reductase, increases LDL receptors on liver cells, and inhibits hepatic synthesis of very–low-density lipoprotein.

ADVERSE REACTIONS
CNS: anxiety, asthenia, dizziness, headache, insomnia, pain
CV: chest pain, hypertension, palpitations, peripheral edema
GI: constipation, diarrhea, dyspepsia, flatulence, vomiting
Musculoskeletal: arthralgia, arthritis, back pain, hypertonia, myalgia, neck pain, pathologic fracture, pelvic pain
Respiratory: asthma, bronchitis, dyspnea, increased cough

NURSING CONSIDERATIONS
• Test liver function before therapy starts, 12 weeks afterward, 12 weeks after any increase in dosage, and twice a year routinely. If AST or ALT level persists at more than three times the upper limit of normal, decrease dose or stop drug.
• Notify prescriber if CK level becomes markedly elevated or myopathy is suspected, or if routine urinalysis shows persistent proteinuria and patient is taking 40 mg daily.

PATIENT TEACHING
• Instruct patient to take drug exactly as prescribed.
• Tell patient to immediately report unexplained muscle pain, tenderness, or weakness, especially if accompanied by malaise or fever.
• Instruct patient to take drug at least 2 hours before taking aluminum- or magnesium-containing antacids.

simvastatin (synvinolin)
sim-va-STAH-tin

Zocor

Pharmacologic class: HMG-CoA reductase inhibitor

INDICATIONS
➤ To reduce risk of death from CV disease and CV events in patients at high risk for coronary events
➤ To reduce total and LDL cholesterol levels
➤ Heterozygous familial hypercholesterolemia

ACTION
Inhibits HMG-CoA reductase, an early (and rate-limiting) step in cholesterol biosynthesis.

ADVERSE REACTIONS
CNS: asthenia, headache
GI: abdominal pain, constipation, diarrhea, dyspepsia, flatulence, nausea, vomiting
Respiratory: upper respiratory tract infection

NURSING CONSIDERATIONS
• Patient should follow a diet restricted in saturated fat and cholesterol during therapy.
• Obtain liver function test results at start of therapy and then periodically.
• Don't confuse Zocor with Cozaar.

PATIENT TEACHING
• Instruct patient to take drug in the evening.
• Teach patient about proper dietary management of cholesterol and triglycerides. When appropriate, recommend weight control, exercise, and smoking cessation programs.
• Tell patient to inform prescriber if adverse reactions occur, particularly muscle aches and pains or tenderness or weakness with malaise or fever.

Antimigraine drugs

eletriptan hydrobromide
frovatriptan succinate
sumatriptan succinate
zolmitriptan

INDICATIONS
➤ Migraines with or without aura

ACTION
The antimigraine drugs are serotonin $5HT_1$ agonists. These drugs constrict cranial vessels, inhibit neuropeptide release, and reduce transmission in the trigeminal nerve pathway.

ADVERSE REACTIONS
These drugs have a wide range of adverse reactions. These include tingling, warmth or hot sensations, flushing, nasal discomfort, visual disturbances, parasthesias, dizziness, fatigue, somnolence, chest pain, neck, throat or jaw pain, weakness, dry mouth, dyspepsia, nausea, sweating, and injection site reactions. Intranasal sumatriptan can cause nasal or throat discomfort and taste disturbances.

CONTRAINDICATIONS AND CAUTIONS
• Contraindicated in patients hypersensitive to any of the drug components.
• Contraindicated in patients with ischemic heart disease, angina, previous MI, uncontrolled hypertension or other significant underlying CV conditions, cerebrovascular disease, peripheral vascular disease, and ischemic bowel disease.

eletriptan hydrobromide
ell-ah-TRIP-tan

Relpax

Pharmacologic class: Serotonin 5-HT$_1$ receptor agonist

INDICATIONS
➤ Acute migraine with or without aura

ACTION
Binds to 5-HT$_1$ receptors and may constrict intracranial blood vessels and inhibit proinflammatory neuropeptide release.

ADVERSE REACTIONS
CNS: asthenia, dizziness, headache, pain, paresthesia, somnolence
CV: chest tightness, pain, and pressure, flushing, palpitations
EENT: pharyngitis
GI: discomfort or cramps, dry mouth, dyspepsia, dysphagia, nausea
Musculoskeletal: back pain
Skin: increased sweating

NURSING CONSIDERATIONS
• Drug isn't intended for migraine prevention.
• Combining a triptan with an SSRI or an SSNRI may cause serotonin syndrome.
• Serious cardiac events, including acute MI, arrhythmias, and death, occur rarely within a few hours after use of 5-HT$_1$ agonists.
• Ophthalmologic effects may occur with long-term use.
• Older patients may develop higher blood pressure than younger patients after taking drug.

PATIENT TEACHING
• Instruct patient to take dose at the first sign of a migraine headache. If the headache comes back after the first dose, he may take a second dose after 2 hours. Caution patient not to take more than 80 mg in 24 hours.
• Warn patient to avoid driving and operating machinery if he feels dizzy or fatigued after taking the drug.
• Tell patient to immediately report pain, tightness, heaviness, or pressure in the chest, throat, neck, or jaw.
• Tell patient to swallow tablet whole and not to split, crush, or chew.
• Instruct patient to take each dose with a full glass of water.

frovatriptan succinate

frow-vah-TRIP-tan

Frova

Pharmacologic class: Serotonin 5-HT$_1$ receptor agonist

INDICATIONS
➤ Acute migraine with or without aura

ACTION
May inhibit excessive dilation of extracerebral and intracranial arteries during migraine headaches.

ADVERSE REACTIONS
CNS: dizziness, headache, fatigue, paresthesia, insomnia, anxiety, somnolence, dysesthesia, hypoesthesia, hot or cold sensation, pain
CV: coronary artery vasospasm, transient myocardial ischemia, MI, ventricular tachycardia, ventricular fibrillation
EENT: abnormal vision, tinnitus, sinusitis, rhinitis
GI: dry mouth, dyspepsia, vomiting, abdominal pain, diarrhea, nausea

NURSING CONSIDERATIONS
• Serious cardiac events, including acute MI, life-threatening cardiac arrhythmias, and death, may occur within a few hours of taking a triptan.
• Combining a triptan with an SSRI or an SSNRI may cause serotonin syndrome.

PATIENT TEACHING
• Instruct patient to take dose at first sign of migraine headache. If headache comes back after first dose, he may take a second dose after 2 hours. Tell patient not to take more than 3 tablets in 24 hours.
• Caution patient to take extra care or avoid driving and operating machinery if dizziness or fatigue develops after taking drug.
• Stress importance of immediately reporting pain, tightness, heaviness, or pressure in chest, throat, neck, or jaw, or rash or itching after taking drug.
• Instruct patient not to take drug within 24 hours of taking another serotonin-receptor agonist or ergot-type drug.
• Tell patient that dose may be taken with or without food, but to take with a full glass of fluid.

sumatriptan succinate

sue-mah-TRIP-tan

Imitrex

Pharmacologic class: Serotonin 5-HT$_1$ receptor agonist

INDICATIONS
➤ Acute migraine attacks
➤ Cluster headache

ACTION
May act as an agonist at serotonin receptors on extracerebral intracranial blood vessels, which constricts the affected vessels, inhibits neuropeptide release, and reduces pain transmission in the trigeminal pathways.

ADVERSE REACTIONS
CNS: dizziness, vertigo, drowsiness, headache, anxiety, fatigue
CV: atrial fibrillation, ventricular fibrillation, ventricular tachycardia, coronary artery vasospasm, transient myocardial ischemia, MI
EENT: discomfort of throat, nasal cavity or sinus, mouth, jaw, or tongue; altered vision
GI: diarrhea, nausea, vomiting, unusual or bad taste (nasal spray)
Skin: injection site reaction, tingling, diaphoresis, flushing
Other: warm or hot sensation, burning sensation

NURSING CONSIDERATIONS
• Combining drug with an SSRI or an SSNRI may cause serotonin syndrome.
• After subcutaneous injection, most patients experience relief in 1 to 2 hours.
• Don't confuse sumatriptan with somatropin.

PATIENT TEACHING
• Inform patient that drug is intended only to treat migraine attacks, not to prevent them or reduce their occurrence.
• Tell patient that drug may be taken at any time during a migraine attack, as soon as signs or symptoms appear.
• Tell patient to tell prescriber immediately about persistent or severe chest pain. Warn him to stop using drug and to call prescriber if he develops pain or tightness in the throat, wheezing, heart throbbing, rash, lumps, hives, or swollen eyelids, face, or lips.

zolmitriptan

zohl-mah-TRIP-tan

Zomig, Zomig ZMT

Pharmacologic class: Serotonin 5-HT$_1$ receptor agonist

INDICATIONS

➤ Acute migraine headaches

ACTION

May act as an agonist at serotonin receptors on extracerebral intracranial blood vessels, which constricts the affected vessels, inhibits neuropeptide release, and reduces pain transmission in the trigeminal pathways.

ADVERSE REACTIONS

CNS: dizziness, somnolence, vertigo, paresthesia, asthenia, pain
CV: coronary artery vasospasm, transient myocardial ischemia, MI, ventricular tachycardia, ventricular fibrillation
EENT: pain, tightness, or pressure in the neck, throat, or jaw

NURSING CONSIDERATIONS

• Drug isn't intended for preventing migraines or treating hemiplegic or basilar migraines.
• Combining drug with an SSRI or an SSNRI may cause serotonin syndrome.

PATIENT TEACHING

• Tell patient that drug is intended to relieve, not prevent, signs and symptoms of migraine.
• Advise patient to take drug as prescribed and not to take a second dose unless instructed by prescriber. Tell patient if a second dose is indicated and permitted, he should take it 2 hours after first dose.
• Instruct patient to release the ODTs from the blister pack just before taking; tablet should dissolve on tongue.
• Advise patient not to break the ODTs in half.
• Advise patient to immediately report pain or tightness in the chest or throat, heart throbbing, rash, skin lumps, or swelling of the face, lips, or eyelids.

Antineoplastics

letrozole
mercaptopurine
methotrexate/methotrexate sodium
tamoxifen

INDICATIONS
➤ Treatment of various types of cancers' mycosis fungoides, psoriasis, rheumatoid arthritis, polyarticular course JRA (methotrexate), gynecomastia, oligospermia (tamoxifen)

ACTION
Antineoplastic drugs include aromatase inhibitors, purine analogs, folic acid antagonists, and nonsteroidal antiestrogens. Aromatase inhibitors work by lowering the body's production of the female hormone estrogen. Purine analogs inhibit RNA and DNA synthesis. Folic acid antagonists reversibly bind to dihydrofolate reductase, blocking reduction of folic acid to tetrahydrofolate, a cofactor necessary for purine, protein, and DNA synthesis, resulting in cell death. The exact action of nonsteroidal antiestrogens is unknown. However, it is known that they act as estrogen antagonists.

ADVERSE REACTIONS
Nausea, vomiting, anemia, leukopenia, thrombocytopenia, thromboembolism (letrozole, tamoxifen), pancreatitis (mercaptopurine), renal failure (methotrexate), hot flashes (letrozole, tamoxifen).

CONTRAINDICATIONS AND CAUTIONS
• Contraindicated in patients hypersensitive to drug or its components.
• Use cautiously in patients with severe liver impairment (letrozole).
• Contraindicated in patients with psoriasis or rheumatoid arthritis who also have alcoholism, alcoholic liver, chronic liver disease, immunodeficiency syndromes, or blood dyscrasias (methotrexate).
• Contraindicated as therapy to reduce risk of breast cancer in high-risk women who also need anticoagulants or in women with history of deep vein thrombosis or PE (tamoxifen).

letrozole

LE-tro-zol

Femara

Pharmacologic class: Aromatase inhibitor

INDICATIONS
➤ Metastatic breast cancer
➤ Adjuvant treatment of hormone-sensitive early breast cancer
➤ Extended adjuvant treatment of early breast cancer following 5 years of adjuvant tamoxifen therapy

ACTION
Inhibits conversion of androgens to estrogens, which decreases tumor mass or delays progression of tumor growth in some women.

ADVERSE REACTIONS
CNS: headache, somnolence, dizziness, fatigue, mood changes
CV: hot flashes, MI, thromboembolism, chest pain, edema, hypertension
GI: nausea, vomiting, constipation, diarrhea, anorexia
Musculoskeletal: bone pain, limb pain, back pain, arthralgia, fractures
Skin: rash, pruritus, alopecia, diaphoresis

NURSING CONSIDERATIONS
• Dosage adjustment isn't needed in patients with creatinine clearance of 10 ml/minute or more.
• Use drug only in postmenopausal women. Rule out pregnancy before starting drug.
• Don't confuse Femara with FemHRT.

PATIENT TEACHING
• Instruct patient to take drug exactly as prescribed.
• Tell patient to take drug with a small glass of water, with or without food.
• Inform patient about potential adverse effects.
• Advise patient to use caution performing tasks that require alertness, coordination, or dexterity, such as driving, until effects are known.

mercaptopurine (6-mercaptopurine, 6-MP)

mer-kap-toe-PYOOR-een

Purinethol

Pharmacologic class: Purine analog

INDICATIONS
➤ Acute lymphoblastic leukemia

ACTION
Inhibits RNA and DNA synthesis.

ADVERSE REACTIONS
GI: nausea, vomiting, anorexia, painful oral ulcers, diarrhea, pancreatitis, GI ulceration
Hematologic: leukopenia, thrombocytopenia, anemia
Hepatic: jaundice, hepatotoxicity

NURSING CONSIDERATIONS
• Risk of relapse is lower with evening administration than with morning administration.
• Drug may be ordered as "6-mercaptopurine" or as "6-MP." The numeral 6 is part of drug name and doesn't refer to dosage.
• Monitor CBC and transaminase, alkaline phosphatase, and bilirubin levels weekly during induction and monthly during maintenance.
• Leukopenia, thrombocytopenia, or anemia may persist for several days after drug is stopped.
• Watch for signs of bleeding and infection.
• Monitor fluid intake and output. Encourage 3 L fluid intake daily.
• Watch for jaundice, clay-colored stools, and frothy, dark urine. Hepatic dysfunction is reversible when drug is stopped. If right-sided abdominal tenderness occurs, stop drug and notify prescriber.
• Don't confuse Purinethol and propylthiouracil (PTU). Both are available in 50-mg strengths.

PATIENT TEACHING
• Instruct patient to watch for signs and symptoms of infection (fever, sore throat, fatigue) and bleeding (easy bruising, nosebleeds, bleeding gums, tarry stools). Tell patient to take temperature daily.
• Tell patient to take drug on an empty stomach in the evening.

methotrexate (amethopterin, MTX)/methotrexate sodium

meth-oh-TREX-ate

Methotrexate LPF, Rheumatrex, Trexall

Pharmacologic class: Folic acid antagonist

INDICATIONS
➤ Trophoblastic tumors (choriocarcinoma, hydatidiform mole), acute lymphocytic leukemia, meningeal leukemia, Burkitt lymphoma (stage I, II), lymphosarcoma (stage III), osteosarcoma, breast cancer, head and neck carcinomas
➤ Mycosis fungoides, psoriasis, rheumatoid arthritis, polyarticular course JRA

ACTION
Reversibly binds to dihydrofolate reductase, blocking reduction of folic acid to tetrahydrofolate, a cofactor necessary for purine, protein, and DNA synthesis.

ADVERSE REACTIONS
CNS: arachnoiditis within hours of intrathecal use, leukoencephalopathy, seizures
GI: stomatitis, diarrhea, GI ulceration and bleeding, nausea, vomiting
GU: tubular necrosis, renal failure
Hematologic: anemia, leukopenia, thrombocytopenia
Hepatic: acute toxicity, chronic toxicity, hepatic fibrosis
Metabolic: diabetes, hyperuricemia
Respiratory: pulmonary fibrosis, pulmonary interstitial infiltrates
Skin: urticaria
Other: septicemia, sudden death

NURSING CONSIDERATIONS
• Monitor pulmonary function tests periodically and fluid intake and output daily. Encourage fluid intake of 2 to 3 L daily.
• Monitor uric acid level.
• Watch for signs and symptoms of bleeding (especially GI) and infection.

PATIENT TEACHING
• Advise patient to watch for signs and symptoms of infection (fever, sore throat, fatigue) and bleeding (easy bruising, nosebleeds, bleeding gums, tarry stools). Tell patient to take temperature daily.
• Teach and encourage diligent mouth care to reduce risk of superinfection in the mouth.

tamoxifen citrate
ta-MOX-i-fen

Pharmacologic class: Nonsteroidal antiestrogen

INDICATIONS
➤ Advanced breast cancer in women and men; adjunct treatment of breast cancer
➤ To reduce breast cancer occurrence
➤ Ductal carcinoma in situ (DCIS) after breast surgery and radiation

ACTION
Unknown. Drug is selective estrogen-receptor modulator.

ADVERSE REACTIONS
CNS: stroke, confusion, weakness, sleepiness, headache
CV: fluid retention, hot flashes, thromboembolism
GI: nausea, vomiting, diarrhea
GU: amenorrhea, irregular menses, vaginal discharge, endometrial cancer, uterine sarcoma, vaginal bleeding
Hematologic: leukopenia, thrombocytopenia
Hepatic: hepatic necrosis, fatty liver, cholestasis
Metabolic: hypercalcemia, weight gain or loss
Respiratory: pulmonary embolism (PE)
Skin: skin changes, rash, alopecia

NURSING CONSIDERATIONS
• Monitor calcium level. At start of therapy, drug may compound hypercalcemia related to bone metastases.
• Women should have periodic eye exams because of increased risk of cataracts, retinal vein thrombosis, and retinopathy.
• Monitor CBC closely in patients with leukopenia or thrombocytopenia.

PATIENT TEACHING
• Reassure patient that acute worsening of bone pain during therapy usually indicates drug will produce good response. Give analgesics to relieve pain.
• Tell patient to report symptoms of stroke, such as headache, vision changes, confusion, difficulty speaking or walking, and weakness of face, arm, or leg, especially on one side of the body.
• Tell patients to report symptoms of PE, such as chest pain, difficulty breathing, rapid breathing, sweating, and fainting.
• Advise patient to report vision changes.

Antiosteoporotics

alendronate sodium
ibandronate sodium
raloxifene hydrochloride
risedronate sodium

INDICATIONS
➤ Prevention or treatment of osteoporosis; Paget disease (alendronate, risedronate); glucocorticoid-induced osteoporosis (alendronate, risedronate)

ACTION
Antiosteoporotics include bisphosphonates and selective estrogen receptor modulators. Bisphosphonates suppress osteoclast activity on newly formed resorption surfaces, which reduces bone turnover. Bone formation exceeds resorption at remodeling sites, leading to progressive gains in bone mass. Selective estrogen receptor modulators reduce resorption of bone and decreases overall bone turnover. These effects on bone are manifested as reductions in serum and urine levels of bone turnover markers and increases in bone mineral density.

ADVERSE REACTIONS
Headache, dyspepsia, back pain, nausea, diarrhea, abdominal pain, rash (alendronate, ibandronate, risedronate); arthralgia, flu-like symptoms, hot flashes (raloxifene)

CONTRAINDICATIONS AND CAUTIONS
• Contraindicated in patients hypersensitive to drug.
• Contraindicated in hypocalcemic patients, in patients with creatinine clearance less than 30 ml/minute, and in those who can't stand or sit upright for 30 minutes after administration (alendronate, ibandronate, risedronate).
• Use cautiously in patients with upper GI disorders, such as dysphagia, esophagitis, and esophageal or gastric ulcers (alendronate, ibandronate, risedronate).
• Contraindicated in women with a history of, or active, venous thromboembolism. Consider the risk-benefit balance in women at risk for stroke (raloxifene).

alendronate sodium
ah-LEN-dro-nate

Fosamax, Fosamax Plus D

Pharmacologic class: Bisphosphonate

INDICATIONS
➤ Osteoporosis
➤ Paget disease of bone (osteitis deformans)
➤ To prevent osteoporosis in postmenopausal women
➤ Glucocorticoid-induced osteoporosis

ACTION
Suppresses osteoclast activity on newly formed resorption surfaces, which reduces bone turnover. Bone formation exceeds resorption at remodeling sites, leading to progressive gains in bone mass.

ADVERSE REACTIONS
CNS: headache
GI: abdominal pain, nausea, dyspepsia, constipation, diarrhea, flatulence, acid regurgitation, esophageal ulcer, vomiting, dysphagia, abdominal distention, gastritis, taste perversion
Musculoskeletal: pain

NURSING CONSIDERATIONS
• Monitor patient's calcium and phosphate levels.
• Severe musculoskeletal pain has been associated with biophosphate use and may occur within days, months, or years of start of therapy. When drug is stopped, symptoms may resolve partially or completely.
• Don't confuse Fosamax with Flomax.

PATIENT TEACHING
• Stress importance of taking tablet only with 6 to 8 ounces of water at least 30 minutes before ingesting anything else, including food, beverages, and other drugs. Tell patient that waiting longer than 30 minutes improves absorption.
• Warn patient not to lie down for at least 30 minutes after taking drug to facilitate delivery to stomach and to reduce risk of esophageal irritation.
• Advise patient to report adverse effects immediately, especially chest pain or difficulty swallowing.
• Tell patient about benefits of weight-bearing exercises in increasing bone mass. If applicable, explain importance of reducing or eliminating cigarette smoking and alcohol use.

ibandronate sodium

eh-BAN-drow-nate

Boniva

Pharmacologic class: Bisphosphonate

INDICATIONS

➤ To treat or prevent postmenopausal osteoporosis

ACTION

Inhibits bone breakdown and removal to reduce bone loss and increase bone mass.

ADVERSE REACTIONS

GI: dyspepsia, abdominal pain, constipation, diarrhea, gastritis, nausea, vomiting

Musculoskeletal: back pain, arthralgia, arthritis, joint disorder, limb pain, localized osteoarthritis, muscle cramps, myalgia

Respiratory: bronchitis, upper respiratory tract infection, pneumonia

NURSING CONSIDERATIONS

• Drug may lead to osteonecrosis, mainly in the jaw. Dental surgery may worsen condition. Consider stopping drug if patient needs a dental procedure.

PATIENT TEACHING

• Tell patient taking monthly dose to take it on same date each month and to wait at least 7 days between doses if she misses a scheduled dose.

• Instruct patient to take oral drug first thing in the morning 1 hour before eating or drinking and before any other drugs, including OTC drugs, such as calcium, antacids, and vitamins.

• Advise patient to swallow drug whole with a full glass of plain water while standing or sitting and to remain upright for at least 1 hour after taking drug.

• Caution patient to take only with plain water.

• Instruct patient not to chew or suck on the tablet.

• Tell patient to report any bone, joint, or muscle pain.

• Advise patient to stop drug and immediately report to prescriber signs and symptoms of esophageal irritation, such as dysphagia, painful swallowing, retrosternal pain, or heartburn.

raloxifene hydrochloride

rah-LOX-i-feen

Evista

Pharmacologic class: Selective estrogen receptor modulator

INDICATIONS

➤ To prevent or treat osteoporosis; to reduce the risk of invasive breast cancer in postmenopausal women with osteoporosis and postmenopausal women at high risk for invasive breast cancer

ACTION

Reduces resorption of bone and decreases overall bone turnover. These effects on bone are manifested as reductions in serum and urine levels of bone turnover markers and increases in bone mineral density.

ADVERSE REACTIONS

EENT: sinusitis, pharyngitis, laryngitis
GI: nausea, dyspepsia, vomiting, flatulence, abdominal pain
Metabolic: weight gain
Musculoskeletal: arthralgia, myalgia, arthritis, leg cramps
Other: infection, flu-like syndrome, hot flashes, breast pain, peripheral edema

NURSING CONSIDERATIONS

• Watch for signs of blood clots. Greatest risk of thromboembolic events occurs during first 4 months of treatment.

PATIENT TEACHING

• Advise patient to avoid long periods of restricted movement because of increased risk of venous thromboembolic events.
• Inform patient that hot flashes or flushing may occur and that drug doesn't aid in reducing them.
• Instruct patient to practice other bone loss—prevention measures, including taking supplemental calcium and vitamin D if dietary intake is inadequate, performing weight-bearing exercises, and stopping alcohol consumption and smoking.

risedronate sodium

rah-SED-dro-nate

Actonel

Pharmacologic class: Bisphosphonate

INDICATIONS
➤ To prevent and treat postmenopausal osteoporosis
➤ Glucocorticoid-induced osteoporosis in patients taking 7.5 mg or more of prednisone or equivalent glucocorticoid daily
➤ Paget disease

ACTION
Reverses the loss of bone mineral density by reducing bone turnover and bone resorption. In patients with Paget disease, drug causes bone turnover to return to normal.

ADVERSE REACTIONS
CNS: headache, depression, dizziness, insomnia, anxiety, pain
CV: hypertension, chest pain, peripheral edema
GI: nausea, diarrhea, abdominal pain
GU: UTI, cystitis
Musculoskeletal: arthralgia, neck pain, back pain, myalgia, bone pain
Skin: rash, pruritus
Other: infection, tooth disorder

NURSING CONSIDERATIONS
• Monitor patient for symptoms of esophageal disease.
• Severe musculoskeletal pain has been associated with biophosphate use and may occur within days, months, or years of start of therapy. When drug is stopped, symptoms may resolve partially or completely.

PATIENT TEACHING
• Tell patient not to chew or suck the tablet because doing so may irritate her mouth.
• Advise patient to contact prescriber immediately if he develops GI discomfort.
• Tell patient to store drug in a cool, dry place, at room temperature, and away from children.
• Tell patient if he misses a dose of the 35-mg tablet, she should take 1 tablet on the morning after she remembers and return to taking 1 tablet once a week, as originally scheduled on her chosen day.
• Patient shouldn't take 2 tablets on the same day.

Antiparkinsonians

amantadine hydrochloride
levodopa and carbidopa
levodopa, carbidopa, and entacapone
rasagiline mesylate
selegiline/selegiline hydrochloride

INDICATIONS
➤ Parkinson disease and drug-induced extrapyramidal reactions

ACTION
Antiparkinsonians include synthetic anticholinergics, dopaminergics, and the antiviral amantadine. Anticholinergics probably prolong the action of dopamine by blocking its reuptake into presynaptic neurons and by suppressing central cholinergic activity. Dopaminergics act in the brain by increasing dopamine availability, thus improving motor function. Entacapone is a reversible inhibitor of peripheral catechol-O-methyltransferase (commonly known as COMT), which is responsible for elimination of various catecholamines, including dopamine. Blocking this pathway when giving levodopa and carbidopa should result in higher levels of levodopa, thereby allowing greater dopaminergic stimulation in the CNS and leading to a greater effect in treating parkinsonian symptoms. Amantadine is thought to increase dopamine release in the substantia nigra.

ADVERSE REACTIONS
Anticholinergics may cause blurred vision, cycloplegia, constipation, dry mouth, headache, mydriasis, palpitations, tachycardia, and urinary hesitancy and urine retention. Dopaminergics may cause arrhythmias, confusion, hallucinations, headache, muscle cramps, nausea, and vomiting. Amantadine also causes irritability and insomnia.

CONTRAINDICATIONS AND CAUTIONS
• Contraindicated in patients hypersensitive to these drugs.
• Use cautiously in patients with prostatic hyperplasia or tardive dyskinesia and in debilitated patients.
• Neuroleptic malignant-like syndrome involving muscle rigidity, increased body temperature, and mental status changes may occur with abrupt withdrawal of antiparkinsonians.
• In pregnant women, safe use hasn't been established. Antiparkinsonians may appear in breast milk; a decision should be made to stop the drug or stop breast-feeding, taking into account the importance of the drug to the mother. In children, safety and effectiveness haven't been established. Elderly patients have an increased risk of adverse reactions; monitor them closely.

amantadine hydrochloride

a-MAN-ta-deen

Pharmacologic class: Synthetic cyclic primary amine

INDICATIONS
➤ Parkinson disease
➤ To prevent or treat symptoms of influenza type A virus and respiratory tract illnesses
➤ Drug-induced extrapyramidal reactions

ACTION
May exert its antiparkinsonian effect by causing the release of dopamine in the substantia nigra. As an antiviral, may prevent release of viral nucleic acid into the host cell, reducing duration of fever and other systemic symptoms.

ADVERSE REACTIONS
CNS: dizziness, insomnia, irritability, light-headedness, depression, fatigue, confusion, hallucinations, anxiety, ataxia, headache, nervousness, dream abnormalities, agitation
CV: heart failure, peripheral edema, orthostatic hypotension
EENT: blurred vision
GI: nausea, anorexia, constipation, vomiting, dry mouth
Skin: livedo reticularis

NURSING CONSIDERATIONS
• Suicidal ideation and attempts may occur in any patient, regardless of psychiatric history.
• Drug can worsen mental problems in patients with a history of psychiatric disorders or substance abuse.
• Don't confuse amantadine with rimantadine.

PATIENT TEACHING
• Tell patient to take drug exactly as prescribed because not doing so may result in serious adverse reactions or death.
• If insomnia occurs, tell patient to take drug several hours before bedtime.
• If patient gets dizzy when he stands up, instruct him not to stand or change positions too quickly.
• Caution patient to avoid activities that require mental alertness until effects of drug are known.
• Encourage patient with Parkinson disease to gradually increase his physical activity as his symptoms improve.
• Advise patient to avoid alcohol while taking drug.

levodopa and carbidopa

lee-voe-DOE-pa and kar-bih-DOE-pa

Parcopa, Sinemet, Sinemet CR

Pharmacologic class: Decarboxylase inhibitor and dopamine precursor

INDICATIONS
➤ Parkinson disease

ACTION
Levodopa, a dopamine precursor, relieves parkinsonian symptoms by being converted to dopamine in the brain. Carbidopa inhibits the decarboxylation of peripheral levodopa, which allows more intact levodopa to travel to the brain.

ADVERSE REACTIONS
CNS: syncope, agitation, suicidal tendencies, dizziness, insomnia, neuroleptic malignant syndrome, psychotic episodes, somnolence
CV: cardiac irregularities, orthostatic hypotension, MI
GI: dark saliva, diarrhea, dry mouth, GI bleeding, vomiting
GU: dark urine, urinary frequency, UTI
Hematologic: agranulocytosis, leukopenia, thrombocytopenia
Musculoskeletal: back pain, muscle cramps, shoulder pain
Respiratory: dyspnea, upper respiratory tract infection
Skin: alopecia, rash, diaphoresis, dark sweat

NURSING CONSIDERATIONS
• Give drug with food to decrease GI upset, but avoid giving with high-protein meals, which can impair absorption and reduce effectiveness.
• Don't crush or break extended-release form.
• Give orally disintegrating tablet (ODT) immediately after removing from bottle. Place tablet on patient's tongue, where it will dissolve in seconds and be swallowed with saliva. No additional fluid is needed.
• Test patients receiving long-term therapy regularly for diabetes and acromegaly, and periodically for hepatic, renal, and hematopoietic function.

PATIENT TEACHING
• Explain to patient that he may become dizzy if he rises quickly. Urge patient to use caution when rising.

levodopa, carbidopa, and entacapone

lee-voe-DOE-pa, kar-bih-DOE-pa, and en-ta-KAP-own

Stalevo

Pharmacologic class: Dopamine precursor, decarboxylase inhibitor, and catecholamine-O-methyltransferase (COMT) inhibitor

INDICATIONS
➤ Parkinson disease

ACTION
Levodopa, a dopamine precursor, relieves parkinsonian symptoms by converting to dopamine in the brain. Carbidopa inhibits the decarboxylation of peripheral levodopa, which allows more intact levodopa to travel to the brain. Entacapone is a reversible COMT inhibitor that increases levodopa level.

ADVERSE REACTIONS
CNS: dyskinesia, suicidal tendencies, neuroleptic malignant syndrome
CV: cardiac irregularities, orthostatic hypotension, MI
GI: dark saliva, diarrhea, dry mouth, GI bleeding, nausea
GU: dark urine, urinary frequency, UTI
Hematologic: agranulocytosis, leukopenia, thrombocytopenia
Musculoskeletal: back pain, muscle cramps, shoulder pain

NURSING CONSIDERATIONS
• Give drug with food to decrease GI upset, but avoid giving with high-protein meal, which can decrease absorption.
• During extended therapy, periodically monitor hepatic, hematopoietic, CV, and renal function.
• Monitor patient for hallucinations, depression, and suicidal tendencies.

PATIENT TEACHING
• Tell patient that urine, sweat, and saliva may turn dark (red, brown, or black) during treatment.
• Advise patient to notify the prescriber if problems making voluntary movements increase.
• Tell patient that diarrhea is common with this treatment.
• Urge patient to immediately report depression or suicidal thoughts.
• Explain to patient that he may become dizzy if he rises quickly. Urge patient to use caution when rising.
• Tell patient that a high-protein diet, excessive acidity, and iron salts may reduce the drug's effectiveness.

rasagiline mesylate

reh-SAH-jih-leen

Azilect

Pharmacologic class: Irreversible, selective MAO inhibitor type B

INDICATIONS

➤ Parkinson disease

ACTION

Unknown. May increase extracellular dopamine level in the CNS, improving neurotransmission and relieving signs and symptoms of Parkinson disease.

ADVERSE REACTIONS

CNS: dizziness, falls, headache, depression, hallucinations
CV: chest pain, angina pectoris, postural hypotension
GI: anorexia, diarrhea, dyspepsia, gastroenteritis, vomiting
Hematologic: leukopenia
Skin: alopecia, carcinoma, ecchymosis, vesiculobullous rash

NURSING CONSIDERATIONS

• Orthostatic hypotension may occur during first 2 months of therapy; help patient to rise from a reclining position.
• Notify prescriber if patient experiences adverse effects; levodopa dose may need to be reduced.
• Examine the patient's skin periodically for possible melanoma because of drug's associated risk of skin cancer.
• Notify prescriber if patient is having elective surgery; drug should be stopped at least 2 weeks before.

PATIENT TEACHING

• Explain the risk of hypertensive crisis if patient ingests foods containing very high levels of tyramine while taking rasagiline. Give patient a list of these foods and products.
• Tell patient to contact prescriber if hallucinations occur.
• Urge patient to watch for skin changes that could suggest melanoma and to have periodic skin examinations by a health professional.
• Instruct patient to maintain his usual dosage schedule if he misses a dose and not to double the next dose to make up for a missed one.

selegiline/selegiline hydrochloride (l-deprenyl hydrochloride)

se-LEH-ge-leen

Emsam/Eldepryl, Zelapar

Pharmacologic class: MAO inhibitor

INDICATIONS
➤ Adjunctive treatment of Parkinson disease
➤ Major depressive disorder

ACTION
May inhibit MAO type B (mainly found in the brain) and dopamine metabolism. At higher-than-recommended doses, drug nonselectively inhibits MAO, including MAO type A (mainly found in the intestine). May also directly increase dopaminergic activity by decreasing the reuptake of dopamine into nerve cells.

ADVERSE REACTIONS
CNS: headache, insomnia, dizziness
CV: arrhythmias, orthostatic blood pressure
GI: nausea, diarrhea, dry mouth, dyspepsia
Skin: application site reaction, rash

NURSING CONSIDERATIONS
• Don't confuse selegiline with Stelazine or Eldepryl with enalapril.

PATIENT TEACHING
• Warn patient to move cautiously or change positions slowly at start of therapy because he may become dizzy or light-headed.
• Advise patient not to take drug in the evening because doing so may cause insomnia.
• Advise patient not to overindulge in tyramine-rich foods or beverages. If using a 9 mg/day or higher transdermal system, avoid these products all together.
• Advise patient to avoid liquids for 5 minutes before and after taking ODTs.
• Tell patient to avoid exposing transdermal system to direct external heat sources, such as heating pads, electric blankets, hot tubs, heated water beds, and prolonged sunlight.
• Tell patient to stop using the transdermal system 10 days before having surgery requiring general anesthesia.
• Tell patient not to cut the transdermal system into smaller pieces.

Antiplatelet drugs

clopidogrel bisulfate
dipyridamole
prasugrel
ticlopidine hydrochloride

INDICATIONS
➤ Non-ST-segment elevation acute coronary syndrome and ST-segment elevation MI, recent MI, recent stroke or peripheral vascular disease (clopidogrel and ticlopidine)

ACTION
Clopidogrel is an inhibitor of platelet aggregation by inhibiting the binding of adenosine diphosphate (ADP) to its platelet receptor and the subsequent ADP-mediated activation of the glycoprotein (GP) IIb/IIIa complex. Dipyridamole may involve drug's ability to increase adenosine, which is a coronary vasodilator and platelet aggregation inhibitor. Prasugrel inhibits platelet activation and aggregation through irreversible binding of its active metabolite to the P2Y12 class of ADP receptors on platelets. Ticlopidine inhibits the binding of fibrinogen to platelets.

ADVERSE REACTIONS
The I.V. drugs can cause serious bleeding, thrombocytopenia, and anaphylaxis. The most common adverse reactions to the oral agents include anaphylaxis, rash, stomach pain, nausea, and headache. Ticlopidine may cause neutropenia and elevated alkaline phosphatase and serum transaminase levels.

CONTRAINDICATIONS AND CAUTIONS
• Contraindicated in patients hypersensitive to any of the drug components.
• Contraindicated in active bleeding, bleeding disorders, intracranial neoplasm, AV malformation or aneurysm, cerebrovascular accident (within 2 years), recent major surgery or trauma, severe uncontrolled hypertension, or thrombocytopenia.

clopidogrel bisulfate
cloe-PID-oh-grel

Plavix

Pharmacologic class: ADP-induced platelet aggregation inhibitor

INDICATIONS
➤ To reduce thrombotic events in patients with atherosclerosis documented by recent stroke, MI, or peripheral arterial disease and patients with acute coronary syndrome
➤ ST-segment elevation acute MI
➤ Coronary stent placement

ACTION
Inhibits the binding of ADP to its platelet receptor, impeding ADP-mediated activation and subsequent platelet aggregation, and irreversibly modifies the platelet ADP receptor.

ADVERSE REACTIONS
CNS: confusion, fatal intracranial bleeding, hallucinations
GI: hemorrhage, constipation, diarrhea, dyspepsia, gastritis, ulcers
Skin: rash, pruritus, bruising, Stevens-Johnson syndrome, toxic epidermal necrolysis
Other: angioedema, anaphylaxis, serum sickness

NURSING CONSIDERATIONS
• Platelet aggregation won't return to normal for at least 5 days after drug has been stopped.
• Don't confuse Plavix with Paxil.

PATIENT TEACHING
• Advise patient it may take longer than usual to stop bleeding. Tell him to refrain from activities in which trauma and bleeding may occur, and encourage him to wear a seat belt when in a car.
• Instruct patient to notify prescriber if unusual bleeding or bruising occurs.
• Tell patient to inform all health care providers, including dentists, before undergoing procedures or starting new drug therapy, that he is taking drug.
• Inform patient that drug may be taken without regard to meals.

dipyridamole
dye-peer-IH-duh-mohl

Persantine

Pharmacologic class: Pyrimidine analog

INDICATIONS
➤ To inhibit platelet adhesion in prosthetic heart valves
➤ Alternative to exercise in evaluation of coronary artery disease during thallium myocardial perfusion scintigraphy

ACTION
May involve drug's ability to increase adenosine, which is a coronary vasodilator and platelet aggregation inhibitor.

ADVERSE REACTIONS
CNS: dizziness, headache
CV: angina pectoris, chest pain, ECG abnormalities, flushing
GI: nausea, abdominal distress, diarrhea, vomiting
Skin: rash, pruritus

NURSING CONSIDERATIONS
• Observe for adverse reactions, especially with large doses. Monitor blood pressure.
• Observe for signs and symptoms of bleeding; note prolonged bleeding time (especially with large doses or long-term therapy).
• Don't confuse dipyridamole with disopyramide. Don't confuse Persantine with Periactin or Bosentan.

PATIENT TEACHING
• Instruct patient to take drug exactly as prescribed.
• Tell patient to report adverse reactions promptly.
• Tell patient receiving drug I.V. to report discomfort at insertion site.

prasugrel

PRAH-soo-grel

Effient

Pharmacologic class: ADP-induced platelet aggregation inhibitor

INDICATIONS

➤ To reduce thrombotic events in patients with acute coronary syndrome managed with percutaneous coronary intervention

ACTION

Inhibits platelet activation and aggregation through irreversible binding of its active metabolite to the P2Y12 class of ADP receptors on platelets.

ADVERSE REACTIONS

GI: GI bleeding, nausea, diarrhea
EENT: epistaxis
Hematologic: bleeding, leukopenia, thrombotic thrombocytopenic purpura (TTP)

NURSING CONSIDERATIONS

• Monitor patient for unusual bleeding or bruising.
• Drug should be taken with aspirin (75 to 325 mg) daily.
• Drug may cause fatal thrombotic TTP that requires urgent treatment, including plasmapheresis.

PATIENT TEACHING

• Advise patient that drug can be taken without regard to food.
• Inform patient that he will bruise more easily and that it may take longer than usual to stop bleeding.
• Instruct patient to report prolonged or excessive bleeding or blood in his stool or urine.
• Advise patient to inform health care providers that he's taking prasugrel before scheduling surgery or taking new drugs.

ticlopidine hydrochloride

tye-KLOH-pih-deen

Pharmacologic class: Platelet aggregation inhibitor

INDICATIONS

➤ To reduce risk of thrombotic stroke in patients who have had a stroke or stroke precursors

➤ Adjunct to aspirin to prevent subacute stent thrombosis in patients having coronary stent placement

ACTION

Unknown. An antiplatelet that probably blocks ADP induced platelet-to-fibrinogen and platelet-to-platelet binding.

ADVERSE REACTIONS

CNS: intracranial bleeding, dizziness, peripheral neuropathy

GI: diarrhea, bleeding, dyspepsia, flatulence, nausea, vomiting

GU: dark urine, hematuria

Hematologic: agranulocytosis, aplastic anemia, immune thrombocytopenia, neutropenia, pancytopenia

Skin: TTP, ecchymoses, pruritus, rash, urticaria

Other: hypersensitivity reactions, postoperative bleeding

NURSING CONSIDERATIONS

• During first 3 months of treatment, monitor patient for symptoms of neutropenia or thrombotic TTP; discontinue drug immediately if they occur.

• Determine CBC and WBC differentials prior to initiating therapy and repeat every 2 weeks until end of third month.

• Monitor liver function test results.

PATIENT TEACHING

• Tell patient to take drug with meals.

• Warn patient to avoid aspirin and aspirin-containing products unless directed to by prescriber.

• Instruct the patient to report unusual or prolonged bleeding. Advise patient to tell dentists and other health care providers that he takes ticlopidine.

• Because neutropenia can result with increased risk of infection, tell patient to immediately report signs and symptoms of infection, such as fever, chills, or sore throat.

• Tell patient to immediately report to prescriber yellow skin or sclera, severe or persistent diarrhea, rashes, bleeding under the skin, light-colored stools, or dark urine.

Antiprotozoals

metronidazole/metronidazole hydrochloride
tinidazole

INDICATIONS
➤ Protozoal infection (specific drug varies by pathogen)

ACTION
Metronidazole is a direct-acting trichomonacide and amebicide that works inside and outside the intestines. It's thought to enter the cells of microorganisms that contain nitroreductase, forming unstable compounds that bind to DNA and inhibit synthesis, causing cell death. When tinidazole is used to treat trichomonas, the drug reduces the compound's nitro group into a free nitro radical that may be responsible for the antiprotozoal activity. Mechanism of action against *Giardia* and *Entamoeba* is unknown.

ADVERSE REACTIONS
Headache, seizures, dizziness, fatigue, nausea; vaginitis, transient leukopenia, neutropenia (metronidazole).

CONTRAINDICATIONS AND CAUTIONS
• Contraindicated in patients hypersensitive to drug, its components, or other nitroimidazole derivatives.
• Contraindicated in pregnant women during first trimester.
• Use cautiously in patients with CNS disorders, in elderly patients, and in those with blood dyscrasias or hepatic dysfunction.

metronidazole (oral; injection)/metronidazole hydrochloride

me-troe-NI-da-zole

Flagyl, Flagyl ER/Flagyl IV RTU

Pharmacologic class: Nitroimidazole

INDICATIONS
➤ Amebic liver abscess; intestinal amebiasis
➤ Trichomoniasis; bacterial vaginosis
➤ Bacterial infections caused by anaerobic microorganisms
➤ Prevention of postoperative infection in contaminated or potentially contaminated colorectal surgery

ACTION
Direct-acting trichomonacide and amebicide that works inside and outside the intestines. It's thought to enter the cells of microorganisms that contain nitroreductase, forming unstable compounds that bind to DNA and inhibit synthesis, causing cell death.

ADVERSE REACTIONS
CNS: headache, seizures, fever, vertigo, ataxia, dizziness, syncope
GI: nausea, vomiting, anorexia, diarrhea, dry mouth, metallic taste
GU: vaginitis, darkened urine
Hematologic: transient leukopenia, neutropenia

NURSING CONSIDERATIONS
• Monitor liver function test results carefully in elderly patients.
• Observe patient for edema, especially if he's receiving corticosteroids; Flagyl IV RTU may cause sodium retention.
• Sexual partners of patients being treated for *Trichomonas vaginalis* infection, even if asymptomatic, must also be treated to avoid reinfection.

PATIENT TEACHING
• Instruct patient to take extended-release tablets at least 1 hour before or 2 hours after meals but to take all other oral forms with food to minimize GI upset.
• Inform patient of need for sexual partners to be treated simultaneously to avoid reinfection.
• Tell patient to avoid alcohol and alcohol-containing drugs during and for at least 3 days after treatment course.
• Tell patient he may experience a metallic taste and have dark or red-brown urine.

tinidazole
teh-NID-ah-zol

Tindamax

Pharmacologic class: Antiprotozoal

INDICATIONS
➤ Bacterial vaginosis in nonpregnant adult women
➤ Trichomoniasis caused by *Trichomonas vaginalis*
➤ Giardiasis caused by *Giardia lamblia (G. duodenalis)*
➤ Intestinal amebiasis caused by *Entamoeba histolytica*
➤ Amebic liver abscess (amebiasis)

ACTION
For *Trichomonas,* drug reduces the compound's nitro group into a free nitro radical that may be responsible for the antiprotozoal activity. Mechanism of action against *Giardia* and *Entamoeba* is unknown.

ADVERSE REACTIONS
CNS: seizures, dizziness, fatigue, headache, malaise, weakness
GI: anorexia, constipation, dyspepsia, metallic taste, nausea, vomiting

NURSING CONSIDERATIONS
• If therapy exceeds 3 days, monitor children closely.
• If candidiasis develops during therapy, the patient may need an antifungal.
• Women shouldn't breast-feed during therapy and for 3 days after the last dose.

PATIENT TEACHING
• Tell patient to take drug with food.
• Tell patient to report to prescriber seizures and numbness in arms or legs.
• Warn patient not to drink alcohol or use alcohol-containing products while taking drug and for 3 days afterward.
• Advise woman to immediately notify her prescriber if she becomes pregnant.
• Tell woman to stop breast-feeding during therapy and for 3 days after the last dose.
• If patient is being treated for a sexually transmitted infection, explain that his sexual partners should be treated at the same time.

Antipsychotics

aripiprazole
clozapine
haloperidol/haloperidol decanoate
olanzapine/olanzapine pamoate
quetiapine fumarate
risperidone
ziprasidone hydrochloride/ziprasidone mesylate

INDICATIONS

➤ Schizophrenia (aripiprazole, clozapine, olanzapine, quetiapine, risperidone, ziprasidone); bipolar mania (aripiprazole, olanzapine, quetiapine, ziprasidone); psychotic disorders (haloperidol); adjunctive treatment of major depressive disorder (aripiprazole, quetiapine); irritability associated with autistic disorder (aripiprazole, risperidone); Tourette syndrome (haloperidol)

ACTION

Quinolinone derivatives are thought to exert partial agonist activity at D2 and serotonin 1A receptors and antagonist activity at serotonin 2A receptors. Dibenzapine derivatives bind selectively to dopaminergic receptors in the CNS and interfere with adrenergic, cholinergic, histaminergic, and serotonergic receptors. Phenylbutylpiperadine derivatives probably exert antipsychotic effects by blocking postsynaptic dopamine receptors in the brain. Dibenzothiazepine and benzisoxazole derivatives block dopamine and serotonin 5-HT2 receptors.

ADVERSE REACTIONS

Drowsiness; sedation; insomnia; agitation; nervousness; hostility; increased suicide risk (aripiprazole, risperidone, ziprasidone); seizures (clozapine, haloperidol); leukopenia (clozapine, haloperidol, olanzapine, quetiapine); neuroleptic malignant syndrome (haloperidol, olanzapine, quetiapine, risperidone); torsades de pointes (haloperidol).

CONTRAINDICATIONS AND CAUTIONS

• Contraindicated in patients hypersensitive to drug.
• Use in pregnancy only if the potential benefit to the mother justifies the risk to the fetus. Neonates exposed to antipsychotic drugs during the third trimester of pregnancy are at risk for developing extrapyramidal signs and symptoms and withdrawal symptoms following delivery.
• Use cautiously in elderly and debilitated patients and in patients with history of seizures or EEG abnormalities, severe CV disorders, allergies, glaucoma, or urine retention.

aripiprazole
air-eh-PIP-rah-zole

Abilify, Abilify Discmelt

Pharmacologic class: Quinolinone derivative

INDICATIONS
➤ Schizophrenia; bipolar mania
➤ Adjunctive treatment of major depressive disorder
➤ Irritability associated with autistic disorder

ACTION
Thought to exert partial agonist activity at D2 and serotonin 1A receptors and antagonist activity at serotonin 2A receptors.

ADVERSE REACTIONS
CNS: headache, anxiety, insomnia, light-headedness, somnolence, akathisia, increased suicide risk, neuroleptic malignant syndrome, seizures, suicidal thoughts, extrapyramidal disorder (children), restlessness
CV: bradycardia
GI: nausea, vomiting, constipation
Metabolic: weight gain

NURSING CONSIDERATIONS
• Neuroleptic malignant syndrome may occur. Monitor patient for hyperpyrexia, muscle rigidity, altered mental status, irregular pulse or blood pressure, tachycardia, diaphoresis, and cardiac dysrhythmias.
• Hyperglycemia may occur. Monitor patient with diabetes regularly. Patient with risk factors for diabetes should undergo fasting blood glucose testing at baseline and periodically. Monitor all patients for symptoms of hyperglycemia, including increased hunger, thirst, frequent urination, and weakness. Hyperglycemia may resolve when patient stops taking drug.
• Treat patient with the smallest dose for the shortest time and periodically reevaluate for need to continue.

PATIENT TEACHING
• Advise families and caregivers to closely observe patient for clinical worsening, suicidality, or unusual changes in behavior.
• Advise patients that grapefruit juice may interact with aripiprazole and to limit or avoid its use.
• Tell patients to avoid alcohol use while taking drug.

clozapine
KLOE-za-peen

Clozaril, FazaClo

Pharmacologic class: Dibenzapine derivative

INDICATIONS
➤ Schizophrenia

ACTION
Unknown. Binds selectively to dopaminergic receptors in the CNS and may interfere with adrenergic, cholinergic, histaminergic, and serotonergic receptors.

ADVERSE REACTIONS
CNS: drowsiness, sedation, dizziness, vertigo, headache, seizures
CV: tachycardia, cardiomyopathy, myocarditis, pulmonary embolism, cardiac arrest, ECG changes, orthostatic hypotension
GI: constipation, excessive salivation
Hematologic: leukopenia, agranulocytosis, granulocytopenia
Metabolic: hyperglycemia
Respiratory: respiratory arrest

NURSING CONSIDERATIONS
• Monitor WBC and ANCA values.
• Monitor patient for signs and symptoms of cardiomyopathy.
• Don't stop suddenly; withdraw drug gradually over 1 or 2 weeks.
• Don't confuse clozapine with clonidine, clofazimine, or Klonopin.

PATIENT TEACHING
• Tell patient about need for weekly blood tests to check for blood-cell deficiency. Advise him to report flulike symptoms, fever, sore throat, lethargy, malaise, or other signs of infection.
• Warn patient to avoid hazardous activities that require alertness and good coordination while taking drug.
• Advise patient that smoking may decrease drug effectiveness.
• Tell patient to rise slowly to avoid dizziness.

haloperidol/haloperidol decanoate
ha-loe-PER-i-dole

Haldol/Haldol Decanoate

Pharmacologic class: Phenylbutylpiperadine derivative

INDICATIONS
➤ Psychotic disorders
➤ Nonpsychotic behavior disorders
➤ Tourette syndrome

ACTION
A butyrophenone that probably exerts antipsychotic effects by blocking postsynaptic dopamine receptors in the brain.

ADVERSE REACTIONS
CNS: severe extrapyramidal reactions, tardive dyskinesia, neuroleptic malignant syndrome, seizures, sedation
CV: torsades de pointes, with I.V. use
Hematologic: leukopenia, leukocytosis

NURSING CONSIDERATIONS
• Monitor patient for tardive dyskinesia, which may occur after prolonged use.
• Watch for signs and symptoms of neuroleptic malignant syndrome.
• Don't withdraw drug abruptly unless required by severe adverse reactions.
• Don't confuse Haldol with Halcion or Halog.

PATIENT TEACHING
• Although drug is the least sedating of the antipsychotics, warn patient to avoid activities that require alertness and good coordination until effects of drug are known. Drowsiness and dizziness usually subside after a few weeks.
• Warn patient to avoid alcohol during therapy.

olanzapine/olanzapine pamoate
oh-LAN-za-peen

Zyprexa, Zyprexa Zydis/Zyprexa Relprevv

Pharmacologic class: Dibenzapine derivative

INDICATIONS
➤ Schizophrenia
➤ Bipolar I disorder
➤ Treatment-resistant depression

ACTION
May block dopamine and 5-HT$_2$ receptors.

ADVERSE REACTIONS
CNS: somnolence, insomnia, parkinsonism, dizziness, neuroleptic malignant syndrome, suicide attempt, extrapyramidal events (I.M.)
GI: constipation, dry mouth, dyspepsia, increased appetite
Hematologic: leukopenia
Metabolic: hyperglycemia, weight gain

NURSING CONSIDERATIONS
• Obtain baseline and periodic liver function test results.
• Monitor patient for weight gain.
• Watch for evidence of neuroleptic malignant syndrome.
• Drug may cause hyperglycemia. Monitor patients with diabetes regularly.
• Monitor patient for mental status changes, sedation, coma, or delirium.
• Drug may increase the risk of suicidal thinking and behavior in young adults ages 18 to 24 during the first 2 months of treatment.
• Don't confuse olanzapine with olsalazine or Zyprexa with Zyrtec.

PATIENT TEACHING
• Warn patient to avoid hazardous tasks until full effects of drug are known.
• Warn patient against exposure to extreme heat; drug may impair body's ability to reduce temperature.
• Advise patient to avoid alcohol.
• Tell patient to rise slowly to avoid dizziness upon standing up quickly.

quetiapine fumarate

kwe-TIE-ah-peen

Seroquel, Seroquel XR

Pharmacologic class: Dibenzothiazepine derivative

INDICATIONS
➤ Schizophrenia
➤ Bipolar I disorder
➤ Major depressive disorder, adjunctive therapy

ACTION
Blocks dopamine and serotonin 5-HT$_2$ receptors. Its action may be mediated through this antagonism.

ADVERSE REACTIONS
CNS: dizziness, headache, somnolence, neuroleptic malignant syndrome, seizures, hypertonia, dysarthria, asthenia, agitation
Hematologic: leukopenia
Metabolic: weight gain, hyperglycemia

NURSING CONSIDERATIONS
• Watch for evidence of neuroleptic malignant syndrome.
• Drug may cause hyperglycemia. Monitor patients with diabetes regularly.
• Monitor patient for mental status changes, sedation, coma, or delirium.
• Drug may increase the risk of suicidal thinking and behavior in young adults ages 18 to 24 during the first 2 months of treatment.
• Drug use may cause cataract formation. Obtain baseline ophthalmologic examination and reassess every 6 months.

PATIENT TEACHING
• Warn patient about risk of dizziness when standing up quickly.
• Tell patient to avoid becoming overheated or dehydrated.
• Remind patient to have an eye examination at start of therapy and every 6 months during therapy to check for cataracts.
• Advise patient to avoid alcohol while taking drug.
• Tell patient not to crush, chew, or break extended-release tablets.
• Tell patient to take extended-release tablets without food or with a light meal.

risperidone

ris-PEER-i-dohn

Risperdal, Risperdal Consta

Pharmacologic class: Benzisoxazole derivative

INDICATIONS

➤ Schizophrenia
➤ Bipolar I disorder
➤ Irritability associated with an autistic disorder

ACTION

Blocks dopamine and 5-HT$_2$ receptors in the brain.

ADVERSE REACTIONS

CNS: akathisia, somnolence, dystonia, headache, insomnia, agitation, anxiety, pain, parkinsonism, neuroleptic malignant syndrome, suicide attempt, parkinsonism
CV: orthostatic hypotension
EENT: rhinitis
GI: constipation, nausea, vomiting, dyspepsia, abdominal pain
Metabolic: weight gain, hyperglycemia, weight loss

NURSING CONSIDERATIONS

• Watch for orthostatic hypotension, especially during first dosage adjustment.
• Watch for evidence of neuroleptic malignant syndrome.
• Drug may cause hyperglycemia. Monitor patients with diabetes regularly.
• Don't confuse risperidone with reserpine.

PATIENT TEACHING

• Warn patient to rise slowly, avoid hot showers, and use other precautions to avoid fainting when starting therapy.
• Tell patient to use sunblock and wear protective clothing outdoors.
• Advise patient to avoid alcohol during therapy.

ziprasidone hydrochloride/ziprasidone mesylate
zih-PRAZ-i-done

Geodon

Pharmacologic class: Benzisoxazole derivative

INDICATIONS
➤ Schizophrenia
➤ Acute bipolar mania

ACTION
May inhibit dopamine and serotonin-2 receptors, causing reduction in schizophrenia symptoms.

ADVERSE REACTIONS
CNS: dizziness, headache, somnolence, suicide attempt
CV: bradycardia, QT interval prolongation, orthostatic hypotension
GI: nausea, constipation, rectal hemorrhage
GU: dysmenorrhea, priapism (I.M.)

NURSING CONSIDERATIONS
• Watch for evidence of neuroleptic malignant syndrome.
• Drug may cause hyperglycemia. Monitor patients with diabetes regularly.
• Stop drug in patients with a QTc interval more than 500 milliseconds
• Monitor patient for abnormal body temperature regulation, especially if he or she is exercising strenuously, is exposed to extreme heat, is also receiving anticholinergics, or is subject to dehydration.

PATIENT TEACHING
• Tell patient to take drug with food.
• Tell patient to immediately report to prescriber signs or symptoms of dizziness, fainting, irregular heartbeat, or relevant heart problems.
• Advise patient to report any recent episodes of diarrhea, abnormal movements, sudden fever, muscle rigidity, or change in mental status.
• Advise patient that symptoms may not improve for 4 to 6 weeks.

Antispasmodics

darifenacin hydrobromide
hyoscyamine/hyoscyamine sulfate

INDICATIONS

►Urge incontinence, urgency, and frequency from an overactive bladder (darifenacin hydrobromide); acute rhinitis, anticholinesterase poisoning, GI disorders, GU disorders (cystitis, renal colic), parkinsonism (hyoscyamine); preanesthetic medication (hyoscyamine); to reduce drug-induced bradycardia during surgery (hyoscyamine); reversal of neuromuscular blockade (hyoscyamine)

ACTION

Blocks acetylcholine action at muscarinic receptors.

ADVERSE REACTIONS

Constipation; dry mouth; urine retention; abnormal vision; confusion or excitement in elderly patients, palpitations, paralytic ileus (hyoscyamine).

CONTRAINDICATIONS AND CAUTIONS

• Contraindicated in patients hypersensitive to drug or its ingredients.
• Contraindicated in patients who have or who are at risk for urine retention, gastric retention, or uncontrolled narrow-angle glaucoma.

darifenacin hydrobromide

da-ree-FEN-ah-sin

Enablex

Pharmacologic class: Anticholinergic

INDICATIONS

➤ Urge incontinence, urgency, and frequency from an overactive bladder

ACTION

Relaxes smooth muscle of bladder by antagonizing muscarinic receptors, relieving symptoms of overactive bladder.

ADVERSE REACTIONS

CNS: asthenia, dizziness, pain, headache
CV: hypertension, peripheral edema
EENT: abnormal vision, dry eyes, pharyngitis, rhinitis, sinusitis
GI: dry mouth, constipation, abdominal pain, diarrhea, dyspepsia, nausea, vomiting
GU: urinary tract disorder, UTI, vaginitis, urine retention

NURSING CONSIDERATIONS

• Assess bladder function, and monitor drug effects.
• If patient has bladder outlet obstruction, watch for urine retention.
• Assess patient for decreased gastric motility and constipation.

PATIENT TEACHING

• Tell patient to swallow tablet whole with plenty of liquid; caution against crushing or chewing tablet.
• Inform patient that drug may be taken with or without food.
• Tell patient to use caution, especially when performing hazardous tasks, until drug effects are known.
• Tell patient to report blurred vision, constipation, and urine retention.
• Discourage use of other drugs that may cause dry mouth, constipation, urine retention, or blurred vision.
• Tell patient that drug decreases sweating, and advise cautious use in hot environments and during strenuous activity.

hyoscyamine/hyoscyamine sulfate

hye-AH-ska-meen

Cystospaz, Hyospaz/Anaspaz, Cystospaz, Cystospaz-M, HyoMax-FT, IB-Stat, Levbid, Levsin, Levsin Drops, Levsin SL, Levsinex Timecaps, Mar-Spas, Neosol, NuLev, Symax Duotab, Symax FasTab, Symax SL, Symax SR

Pharmacologic class: Belladonna alkaloid, anticholinergic

INDICATIONS

➤ Acute rhinitis, anticholinesterase poisoning, GI disorders, GU disorders (cystitis, renal colic), parkinsonism
➤ Preanesthetic medication
➤ To reduce drug-induced bradycardia during surgery
➤ Reversal of neuromuscular blockade

ACTION

Blocks acetylcholine action at muscarinic receptors, which decreases GI motility and inhibits gastric acid secretion.

ADVERSE REACTIONS

CNS: confusion or excitement in elderly patients, fever
CV: palpitations, tachycardia
EENT: blurred vision, mydriasis, increased intraocular pressure, cycloplegia, photophobia
GI: constipation, dry mouth, paralytic ileus, dysphagia, heartburn, loss of taste, nausea, vomiting
GU: urinary hesitancy, urine retention, impotence

NURSING CONSIDERATIONS

• Give drug 30 minutes to 1 hour before meals and at bedtime. Bedtime dose can be larger; give at least 2 hours after last meal of day.
• Extended-release tablets are scored and may be broken to allow for dosage titration. Don't crush or allow patient to chew tablets.
• Monitor patient's vital signs and urine output carefully.
• Don't confuse Anaspaz with Anaprox or Antispas.

PATIENT TEACHING

• Caution patient not to crush or chew extended-release tablets.
• Advise patient to avoid driving and other hazardous activities if drowsiness, dizziness, or blurred vision occurs; to drink plenty of fluids to help prevent constipation and heat stroke; and to report rash or other skin eruption.

Antituberculotics

ethambutol hydrochloride
isoniazid
rifampin

INDICATIONS
➤ Acute pulmonary and extrapulmonary tuberculosis, acute UTIs

ACTION
Inhibits cell wall synthesis in susceptible strains of gram-positive and gram-negative bacteria and if *Mycobacterium* tuberculosis is identified.

ADVERSE REACTIONS
Adverse reactions primarily affect the GI tract, peripheral nervous system, and hepatic system. Isoniazid may precipitate seizures in patients with a seizure disorder and produce optic or peripheral neuritis, as well as elevated liver enzymes. Optic neuritis is the only significant reaction to ethambutol. The most common adverse reactions to rifampin include epigastric pain, nausea, vomiting, flatulence, abdominal cramps, anorexia, and diarrhea.

CONTRAINDICATIONS AND CAUTIONS
• Contraindicated in patients hypersensitive to any of the drug components.
• Drugs should be discontinued or dosage reduced if patients develop signs of CNS toxicity, including convulsions, psychosis, somnolence, depression, confusion, hyperreflexia, headache, tremor, vertigo, paresis, or dysarthria.

ethambutol hydrochloride

e-THAM-byoo-tole

Myambutol

Pharmacologic class: Synthetic antituberculotic

INDICATIONS
➤ Adjunctive treatment for pulmonary tuberculosis

ACTION
May inhibit synthesis of one or more metabolites of susceptible bacteria, changing cell metabolism during cell division; bacteriostatic.

ADVERSE REACTIONS
CNS: dizziness, fever, hallucinations, headache, malaise, mental confusion, peripheral neuritis
EENT: optic neuritis, irreversible blindness
GI: abdominal pain, anorexia, GI upset, nausea, vomiting
Hematologic: thrombocytopenia, leukopenia, neutropenia
Metabolic: hyperuricemia
Musculoskeletal: joint pain
Skin: toxic epidermal necrolysis, dermatitis, pruritus
Other: anaphylactoid reactions, precipitation of acute gout

NURSING CONSIDERATIONS
• Perform visual acuity and color discrimination tests before and during therapy.
• Ensure that any changes in vision don't result from an underlying condition.
• Obtain AST and ALT levels before therapy, and monitor these levels every 3 to 4 weeks.
• In patients with impaired renal function, base dosage on drug level.
• Monitor uric acid level; observe patient for signs and symptoms of gout.

PATIENT TEACHING
• Reassure patient that visual disturbances usually disappear several weeks to months after drug is stopped. Inflammation of the optic nerve is related to dosage and duration of treatment.
• Inform patient that drug is given with other antituberculotics.
• Stress importance of compliance with drug therapy.
• Advise patient to report adverse reactions to prescriber.

isoniazid (INH, isonicotinic acid hydrazide)
eye-soe-NYE-a-zid

Pharmacologic class: Isonicotinic acid hydrazine

INDICATIONS
➤ Actively growing tubercle bacilli
➤ To prevent tubercle bacilli in those exposed to tuberculosis

ACTION
May inhibit cell-wall biosynthesis by interfering with lipid and DNA synthesis; bactericidal.

ADVERSE REACTIONS
CNS: peripheral neuropathy, seizures, toxic encephalopathy, memory impairment, toxic psychosis
EENT: optic neuritis and atrophy
GI: epigastric distress, nausea, vomiting
Hematologic: agranulocytosis, aplastic anemia, thrombocytopenia
Hepatic: hepatitis, bilirubinemia, jaundice
Metabolic: hyperglycemia, hypocalcemia, metabolic acidosis

NURSING CONSIDERATIONS
• Peripheral neuropathy is more common in patients who are slow acetylators, malnourished, alcoholic, or diabetic. Give pyridoxine to prevent peripheral neuropathy.
• Monitor hepatic function closely for changes. Monitor patients older than age 35 monthly and measure hepatic enzyme levels before starting treatment.

PATIENT TEACHING
• Instruct patient to take drug exactly as prescribed; warn against stopping drug without prescriber's consent.
• Advise patient to take drug 1 hour before or 2 hours after meals.
• Tell patient to notify prescriber immediately if signs and symptoms of liver impairment occur, such as appetite loss, fatigue, malaise, yellow skin or eye discoloration, and dark urine.
• Advise patient to avoid alcoholic beverages while taking drug. Also tell him to avoid certain foods: fish, such as skipjack and tuna, and products containing tyramine, such as aged cheese, beer, and chocolate, because drug has some MAO inhibitor activity.

rifampin (rifampicin)

RIF-am-pin

Rifadin, Rimactane

Pharmacologic class: Semisynthetic rifamycin

INDICATIONS
➤ Pulmonary tuberculosis, with other antituberculotics
➤ Meningococcal carriers

ACTION
Inhibits DNA-dependent RNA polymerase, which impairs RNA synthesis; bactericidal.

ADVERSE REACTIONS
CNS: headache, dizziness, mental confusion, generalized numbness
CV: shock
GI: pancreatitis, pseudomembranous colitis, epigastric distress, anorexia, nausea, vomiting, abdominal pain, diarrhea, flatulence, sore mouth and tongue
GU: acute renal failure
Hematologic: thrombocytopenia, transient leukopenia
Hepatic: hepatotoxicity

NURSING CONSIDERATIONS
• Monitor hepatic function, hematopoietic studies, and uric acid levels. Drug's systemic effects may asymptomatically raise liver function test results and uric acid level.
• Don't confuse rifampin with rifabutin or rifapentine.

PATIENT TEACHING
• Instruct patient who can't tolerate capsules on an empty stomach to take drug with meals and a full glass of water.
• Advise patient who is unable to swallow capsules whole that an oral suspension can be prepared by the pharmacist.
• Warn patient that he or she may feel drowsy and that drug can turn body fluids red-orange and permanently stain contact lenses.
• Advise patient to contact prescriber if he or she experiences fever, loss of appetite, malaise, nausea, vomiting, dark urine, or yellow discoloration of the eyes or skin.
• Advise patient to avoid alcohol during drug therapy.

Antivirals

acyclovir/acyclovir sodium
interferon beta-1a
interferon beta-1b, recombinant
oseltamivir phosphate
valacyclovir hydrochloride

INDICATIONS
➤Herpes, varicella zoster infection (acyclovir, valacyclovir hydrochloride); to slow progression of multiple sclerosis (interferon beta-1a, interferon beta-1b); and influenza (oseltamivir phosphate)

ACTION
Acyclovir interferes with DNA synthesis and inhibits viral multiplication. The action of interferon beta-1a is not completely understood. Interferon beta-1b attaches to the membrane receptors and causes cellular changes. Oseltamivir phosphate interferes with viral replication. Valacyclovir hydrochloride converts to acyclovir to interfere with DNA synthesis and inhibits viral multiplication.

ADVERSE REACTIONS
Antivirals may cause anorexia, chills, confusion, depression, diarrhea, dizziness, dry mouth, edema, fatigue, hallucinations, headache, insomnia, nausea, and vomiting.

CONTRAINDICATIONS AND CAUTIONS
• Contraindicated in patients hypersensitive to the drug.
• In breast-feeding women, some antivirals are contraindicated, but others require cautious use. For infants and children, recommendations vary according to the antiviral prescribed. Geriatric patients have a higher risk of adverse reaction.
• Use cautiously in patients with depression, seizure disorders, or severe cardiac conditions.

acyclovir/acyclovir sodium
ay-SYE-kloe-ver

Zovirax

Pharmacologic class: Synthetic purine nucleoside

INDICATIONS
➤ Herpes simplex virus (HSV-1 and HSV-2) infection
➤ Varicella zoster infections in immunocompromised patients

ACTION
Interferes with DNA synthesis and inhibits viral multiplication.

ADVERSE REACTIONS
CNS: headache, malaise, encephalopathic changes (including lethargy, obtundation, tremor, confusion, hallucinations, agitation, seizures, coma)
GI: nausea, vomiting, diarrhea
GU: acute renal failure, hematuria
Hematologic: leukopenia, thrombocytopenia, thrombocytosis
Skin: inflammation or phlebitis at injection site, rash, urticaria

NURSING CONSIDERATIONS
• In patients with renal disease or dehydration and in those taking other nephrotoxic drugs, monitor renal function.
• If signs and symptoms of extravasation occur, stop I.V. infusion immediately and notify prescriber. Hyaluronidase may need to be injected subcutaneously at extravasation site as an antidote.
• Don't confuse acyclovir sodium (Zovirax) with acetazolamide sodium (Diamox) vials, which may look alike. Don't confuse Zovirax with Zyvox.

PATIENT TEACHING
• Tell patient to take drug as prescribed, even after he or she feels better.
• Tell patient that drug is effective in managing herpes infection but doesn't eliminate or cure it. Warn patient that drug won't prevent spread of infection to others.
• Tell patient to avoid sexual contact while visible lesions are present.
• Teach patient about early signs and symptoms of herpes infection (such as tingling, itching, or pain). Tell him or her to notify prescriber and get a prescription for drug before the infection fully develops. Early treatment is most effective.

interferon beta-1a
in-ter-FEER-on

Avonex, Rebif

Pharmacologic class: Biologic response modifier

INDICATIONS
➤ Relapsing forms of multiple sclerosis

ACTION
Unknown. Interacts with specific cell receptors found on the surface of cells. Binding of these receptors causes the expression of a number of interferon-induced gene products believed to mediate the biological actions of interferon beta-1a.

ADVERSE REACTIONS
CNS: asthenia, dizziness, fatigue, fever, headache, pain, sleep difficulty, depression, seizures, suicidal ideation or attempt
EENT: abnormal vision, sinusitis, decreased hearing
GI: abdominal pain, diarrhea, dyspepsia, nausea, dry mouth
Hematologic: lymphadenopathy, leukopenia, pancytopenia, thrombocytopenia, anemia
Hepatic: autoimmune hepatitis, bilirubinemia, hepatitis
Musculoskeletal: back pain, muscle ache, skeletal pain
Respiratory: upper respiratory tract infection, dyspnea
Skin: injection site reaction
Other: chills, flulike syndrome, infection

NURSING CONSIDERATIONS
• Monitor patient closely for depression and suicidal ideation.
• Monitor WBC count, platelet count, and blood chemistries, including liver function tests.
• Give analgesics or antipyretics to decrease flulike symptoms.

PATIENT TEACHING
• Advise patient to read medication guide that comes with drug.
• Teach patient and family member how to reconstitute drug and give I.M.
• If a dose is missed, tell patient to take it as soon as he or she remembers. The patient may then resume his or her regular schedule. Tell patient not to take two injections within 48 hours of each other.
• Advise patient to report depression, suicidal thoughts, or other adverse reactions.

interferon beta-1b, recombinant
in-ter-FEER-on

Betaseron, Extavia
Pharmacologic class: Biologic response modifier

INDICATIONS
➤ Relapsing forms of multiple sclerosis

ACTION
Drug attaches to membrane receptors and causes cellular changes, including increased protein synthesis.

ADVERSE REACTIONS
CNS: suicidal tendencies, confusion, hypertonia, asthenia, migraine, seizures, headache, pain, dizziness, malaise, fever, chills, insomnia
CV: chest pain, peripheral edema, palpitations, hypertension
EENT: laryngitis, sinusitis, conjunctivitis, abnormal vision
GI: diarrhea, constipation, abdominal pain, vomiting, dyspepsia
GU: menstrual bleeding or spotting, early or delayed menses, fewer days of menstrual flow, menorrhagia, urgency, impotence
Hematologic: leukopenia, lymphadenopathy
Musculoskeletal: myasthenia, arthralgia, myalgia, leg cramps
Skin: inflammation, pain, necrosis at injection site, diaphoresis, alopecia, rash, skin disorder
Other: breast pain, flulike syndrome, pelvic pain, generalized edema

NURSING CONSIDERATIONS
• Serious liver damage, including hepatic failure requiring transplant, can occur. Monitor liver function at 1, 3, and 6 months after therapy starts and periodically thereafter.
• Monitor patient for signs of depression.

PATIENT TEACHING
• Tell patient to take drug at bedtime to minimize mild flulike signs and symptoms that commonly occur.
• Advise patient to report suicidal thoughts or depression.
• Urge patient to immediately report signs or symptoms of tissue death at injection site.
• Advise patient of importance of obtaining routine blood tests.

oseltamivir phosphate
oz-el-TAM-ah-ver

Tamiflu

Pharmacologic class: Selective neuraminidase inhibitor

INDICATIONS
➤ To prevent and treat influenza during a community outbreak

ACTION
Inhibits influenza A and B virus enzyme neuraminidase, which is thought to play a role in viral particle aggregation and release from the host cell and appears to interfere with viral replication.

ADVERSE REACTIONS
CNS: dizziness, fatigue, headache, insomnia, vertigo
GI: abdominal pain, diarrhea, nausea, vomiting
Respiratory: bronchitis, cough

NURSING CONSIDERATIONS
• Drug must be given within 2 days of onset of symptoms.
• Closely monitor patients with influenza for neuropsychiatric symptoms, such as hallucinations, delirium, and abnormal behavior. Risks and benefits of continuing drug should be evaluated.

PATIENT TEACHING
• Instruct patient to begin treatment as soon as possible after appearance of flu symptoms.
• Inform patient that drug may be taken with or without meals. If nausea or vomiting occurs, he or she can take drug with food or milk.
• Tell patient that, if a dose is missed, he or she should take it as soon as possible. However, if next dose is due within 2 hours, tell him or her to skip the missed dose and take the next dose on schedule.
• Advise patient to complete the full course of treatment, even if symptoms resolve.
• Alert patient that drug isn't a replacement for the annual influenza vaccination. Patients for whom vaccine is indicated should continue to receive the vaccine each fall.

valacyclovir hydrochloride
val-ah-SYE-kloe-ver

Valtrex
Pharmacologic class: Synthetic purine nucleoside

INDICATIONS
➤ Herpes zoster infection (shingles)
➤ Genital herpes
➤ Cold sores (herpes labialis)
➤ Chickenpox

ACTION
Rapidly converts to acyclovir, which in turn becomes incorporated into viral DNA, thereby terminating growth of the DNA chain; inhibits viral DNA polymerase, causing inhibition of viral replication.

ADVERSE REACTIONS
CNS: headache, depression, dizziness
GI: nausea, abdominal pain, diarrhea, vomiting
GU: dysmenorrhea
Musculoskeletal: arthralgia

NURSING CONSIDERATIONS
• Start treatment for herpes zoster infection at earliest signs or symptoms. It's most effective when started within 48 hours of onset of rash.
• Don't confuse valacyclovir (Valtrex) with valganciclovir (Valcyte).

PATIENT TEACHING
• Inform patient that drug may be taken without regard for meals.
• Teach patient the signs and symptoms of herpes infection (rash, tingling, itching, and pain), and advise him or her to notify prescriber immediately if they occur. Treatment should begin as soon as possible after symptoms appear, preferably within 48 hours of the onset of zoster rash.
• Tell patient that drug isn't a cure for herpes but may decrease the length and severity of symptoms.

Anxiolytics

busPIRone hydrochloride
hydrOXYzine hydrochloride/hydrOXYzine pamoate

INDICATIONS
➤Anxiety; adjunctive therapy for preoperative and preprocedure sedation, pruritis (hydrOXYzine)

ACTION
BusPIRone may inhibit neuronal firing and reduce serotonin turnover in cortical, amygdaloid, and septohippocampal tissue, although it's exact action isn't completely understood. HydrOXYzine suppresses activity in certain essential regions of the subcortical area of the CNS.

ADVERSE REACTIONS
Dizziness, drowsiness, dry mouth.

CONTRAINDICATIONS AND CAUTIONS
• Contraindicated in patients hypersensitive to drug.
• Contraindicated within 14 days of MAO inhibitor therapy (busPIRone).
• Not recommended for patients with severe hepatic or renal impairment (busPIRone).
• In pregnant and breast-feeding women, safety hasn't been established; use cautiously. Elderly patients are more sensitive to adverse effects.

busPIRone hydrochloride
byoo-SPYE-rone

BuSpar

Pharmacologic class: Azaspirodecanedione derivative

INDICATIONS
➤ Anxiety disorders

ACTION
May inhibit neuronal firing and reduce serotonin turnover in cortical, amygdaloid, and septohippocampal tissue.

ADVERSE REACTIONS
CNS: dizziness, drowsiness, headache, nervousness, insomnia, light-headedness, fatigue, numbness, excitement, confusion, depression, anger, decreased concentration
CV: tachycardia, nonspecific chest pain
EENT: blurred vision
GI: dry mouth, nausea, diarrhea, abdominal distress

NURSING CONSIDERATIONS
• Don't give drug with grapefruit juice.
• Give drug at the same times each day, and always with or always without food.
• Monitor patient closely for adverse CNS reactions. Drug is less sedating than other anxiolytics, but CNS effects may be unpredictable.
• Before starting therapy, don't stop a previous benzodiazepine regimen abruptly because a withdrawal reaction may occur.
• Drug shows no potential for abuse and isn't classified as a controlled substance.
• Don't confuse buspirone with bupropion or risperidone.

PATIENT TEACHING
• Warn patient to avoid hazardous activities that require alertness and good coordination until effects of drug are known.
• Remind patient that drug effects may not be noticeable for several weeks.
• Warn patient not to abruptly stop a benzodiazepine because of risk of withdrawal symptoms.
• Tell patient to avoid use of alcohol during therapy.

hydrOXYzine hydrochloride/hydrOXYzine pamoate
hye-DROX-i-zeen

Vistaril

Pharmacologic class: Piperazine derivative

INDICATIONS
➤ Anxiety
➤ Preoperative and postoperative adjunctive therapy for sedation
➤ Pruritus

ACTION
Suppresses activity in certain essential regions of the subcortical area of the CNS.

ADVERSE REACTIONS
CNS: drowsiness, involuntary motor activity
GI: dry mouth, constipation
Skin: pain at I.M. injection site
Other: hypersensitivity reactions

NURSING CONSIDERATIONS
• If patient takes other CNS drugs, watch for oversedation.
• Elderly patients may be more sensitive to adverse anticholinergic effects; monitor these patients for dizziness, excessive sedation, confusion, hypotension, and syncope.
• Don't confuse hydrOXYzine with hydroxyurea, Hydrogesic, or hydralazine. Don't confuse Vistaril with Restoril.

PATIENT TEACHING
• Warn patient to avoid hazardous activities that require alertness and good coordination until effects of drug are known.
• Tell patient to avoid use of alcohol while taking drug.

Benign prostatic hyperplasia drugs

finasteride
tamsulosin hydrochloride

INDICATIONS
➤ Benign prostatic hyperplasia; male pattern hair loss (finasteride)

ACTION
Finasteride inhibits the conversion of testosterone to dihydrotestosterone (DHT). Tamsulosin hydrochloride selectively blocks alpha receptors in the prostate, and relaxes smooth muscles in the bladder neck and prostate, improving urine flow and reducing symptoms of BPH.

ADVERSE REACTIONS
Dizziness, headache, rhinitis, infection, orthostatic hypotension, impotence

CONTRAINDICATIONS AND CAUTIONS
• Contraindicated in patients hypersensitive to drug or its components.
• Use cautiously in patients with liver dysfunction (finasteride).
• Finasteride is a potential teratogen. Follow safe handling procedures when preparing, administering, or dispensing drug.
• Use cautiously in patients with serious or life-threatening sulfa allergy (tamsulosin hydrochloride).

finasteride
fin-AS-teh-ride

Propecia, Proscar
Pharmacologic class: 5-alpha-reductase enzyme inhibitor

INDICATIONS
➤ Benign prostatic hyperplasia
➤ Male pattern hair loss (androgenetic alopecia) in men only

ACTION
Inhibits conversion of testosterone to dihydrotestosterone (DHT), the androgen primarily responsible for the initial development and subsequent enlargement of the prostate gland. In male pattern baldness, the scalp contains increased DHT level; drug decreases scalp DHT level in such cases.

ADVERSE REACTIONS
CNS: dizziness, asthenia, headache
CV: hypotension, orthostatic hypotension
GU: impotence, decreased volume of ejaculate, decreased libido
Other: gynecomastia

NURSING CONSIDERATIONS
• Carefully monitor patients who have a large residual urine volume or severely diminished urine flow.
• Sustained increase in PSA level could indicate noncompliance with therapy.
• A minimum of 6 months of therapy may be needed for treatment of BPH.

PATIENT TEACHING
• Tell patient that drug may be taken with or without meals.
• Warn woman who is or may become pregnant not to handle crushed tablets because of risk of adverse effects on male fetus.
• Reassure patient that drug may decrease volume of ejaculate without impairing normal sexual function.
• Instruct patient to report breast changes, such as lumps, pain, or nipple discharge.

tamsulosin hydrochloride

tam-soo-LOE-sin

Flomax

Pharmacologic class: Alpha blocker

INDICATIONS

➤ BPH

ACTION

Selectively blocks alpha receptors in the prostate, leading to relaxation of smooth muscles in the bladder neck and prostate, improving urine flow and reducing symptoms of BPH.

ADVERSE REACTIONS

CNS: dizziness, headache, asthenia, insomnia, somnolence, syncope, vertigo

CV: chest pain, orthostatic hypotension

EENT: rhinitis, amblyopia, pharyngitis, sinusitis

GI: diarrhea, nausea

GU: decreased libido, abnormal ejaculation, priapism

Musculoskeletal: back pain

Respiratory: increased cough

Other: infection, tooth disorder

NURSING CONSIDERATIONS

• Monitor patient for decreases in blood pressure.
• Don't confuse Flomax with Fosamax or Volmax.

PATIENT TEACHING

• Instruct patient not to crush, chew, or open capsules.
• Tell patient to rise slowly from chair or bed when starting therapy and to avoid situations in which injury could occur as a result of fainting. Advise him or her that drug may cause sudden drop in blood pressure, especially after first dose or when changing doses.
• Instruct patient not to drive or perform hazardous tasks for 12 hours after first dose or changes in dose until response can be monitored.
• Tell patient to take drug about 30 minutes after same meal each day.
• Advise patient considering cataract surgery to inform the ophthalmologist that he or she is taking the drug. Floppy iris syndrome may occur during surgery.

Benzodiazepines

alprazolam
chlordiazepoxide hydrochloride
diazepam
lorazepam
midazolam hydrochloride
oxazepam

INDICATIONS
➤ Seizure disorders (diazepam, midazolam, parenteral lorazepam); anxiety, tension, and insomnia (chlordiazepoxide, diazepam, oxazepam); conscious sedation or amnesia in surgery (diazepam, lorazepam, midazolam); skeletal muscle spasm and tremor (oral forms of chlordiazepoxide and diazepam); delirium

ACTION
Benzodiazepines act selectively on polysynaptic neuronal pathways throughout the CNS. Precise sites and mechanisms of action aren't fully known. Benzodiazepines enhance or facilitate the action of GABA, an inhibitory neurotransmitter in the CNS. These drugs appear to act at the limbic, thalamic, and hypothalamic levels of the CNS to produce anxiolytic, sedative, hypnotic, skeletal muscle relaxant, and anticonvulsant effects.

ADVERSE REACTIONS
Therapeutic dose may cause drowsiness, impaired motor function, constipation, diarrhea, vomiting, altered appetite, urinary changes, visual disturbances, and CV irregularities.

CONTRAINDICATIONS AND CAUTIONS
• Contraindicated in patients hypersensitive to these drugs and in those with acute angle-closure glaucoma.
• Avoid use in patients with suicidal tendencies and patients with a history of drug abuse.
• In pregnant patients, benzodiazepines increase the risk of congenital malformation if taken in the first trimester. Use during labor may cause neonatal flaccidity. A neonate whose mother took a benzodiazepine during pregnancy may have withdrawal symptoms. In breast-feeding women, benzodiazepines may cause sedation, feeding difficulties, and weight loss in the infant. In children, use caution; they're especially sensitive to CNS depressant effects. In elderly patients, benzodiazepine elimination may be prolonged; consider a lower dosage.

alprazolam
al-PRAH-zoe-lam

Niravam, Xanax, Xanax XR

Pharmacologic class: Benzodiazepine

INDICATIONS
➤ Anxiety
➤ Panic disorders

ACTION
Unknown. Probably potentiates the effects of GABA, depresses the CNS, and suppresses the spread of seizure activity.

ADVERSE REACTIONS
CNS: insomnia, irritability, dizziness, headache, anxiety, confusion, drowsiness, light-headedness, sedation, somnolence, difficulty speaking, impaired coordination, memory impairment, fatigue, depression, suicide, mental impairment, ataxia
EENT: allergic rhinitis, blurred vision, nasal congestion
GI: diarrhea, dry mouth, constipation, nausea

NURSING CONSIDERATIONS
• Don't withdraw drug abruptly; withdrawal symptoms, including seizures, may occur. Abuse or addiction is possible.
• Monitor hepatic, renal, and hematopoietic function periodically in patients receiving repeated or prolonged therapy.
• Closely monitor addiction-prone patients.
• Don't confuse alprazolam with alprostadil or lorazepam. Don't confuse Xanax with Zantac, Xopenex, or Tenex.

PATIENT TEACHING
• Warn patient to avoid hazardous activities that require alertness and good coordination until effects of drug are known.
• Tell patient to avoid use of alcohol while taking drug.
• Tell patient to swallow extended-release tablets whole.
• Tell patient using ODT to remove it from bottle using dry hands and to immediately place it on his tongue, where it will dissolve and can be swallowed with saliva.
• Tell patient taking half a scored ODT to discard the unused half.

chlordiazepoxide hydrochloride

klor-dye-az-e-POX-ide

Librium

Pharmacologic class: Benzodiazepine

INDICATIONS

➤ Anxiety

➤ Withdrawal symptoms of acute alcoholism

ACTION

A benzodiazepine that may potentiate the effects of GABA, depress the CNS, and suppress the spread of seizure activity.

ADVERSE REACTIONS

CNS: drowsiness, lethargy, ataxia, confusion, extrapyramidal reactions

GI: nausea, constipation

Hematologic: agranulocytosis

Skin: swelling and pain at injection site, skin eruptions

NURSING CONSIDERATIONS

• May increase digoxin level and risk of toxicity. Monitor patient and digoxin level closely.

• Watch for paradoxical reaction in psychiatric patients and hyperactive, aggressive children.

• Use of this drug may lead to abuse and addiction. Don't withdraw drug abruptly after long-term use because withdrawal symptoms may occur.

• Don't confuse Librium with Librax.

PATIENT TEACHING

• Warn patient to avoid hazardous activities that require alertness and coordination until effects of drug are known.

• Tell patient to avoid use of alcohol while taking drug.

• Warn patient drug may cause psychological and physical dependence. Tell patient not to increase dose or abruptly stop the drug because withdrawal symptoms may occur.

diazepam
dye-AZ-e-pam

Diastat, Diastat Acudial, Diazepam Intensol, Valium
Pharmacologic class: Benzodiazepine

INDICATIONS
➤ Anxiety
➤ Acute alcohol withdrawal
➤ Muscle spasm; tetanus
➤ Preoperative and preprocedure sedation
➤ Status epilepticus; seizures

ACTION
A benzodiazepine that probably potentiates the effects of GABA, depresses the CNS, and suppresses the spread of seizure activity.

ADVERSE REACTIONS
CNS: drowsiness, dysarthria, slurred speech, tremor, transient amnesia, fatigue, ataxia, headache, insomnia, pain
CV: CV collapse, bradycardia, hypotension
EENT: diplopia, blurred vision, nystagmus
GI: nausea, constipation, diarrhea with rectal form
GU: incontinence, urine retention
Hematologic: neutropenia
Respiratory: respiratory depression, apnea
Skin: rash, phlebitis at injection site

NURSING CONSIDERATIONS
• May increase digoxin level and risk of toxicity. Monitor patient and digoxin level closely.
• Monitor elderly patients for dizziness, ataxia, and mental status changes. Patients are at an increased risk for falls.
• Use of drug may lead to abuse and addiction. Don't withdraw drug abruptly after long-term use; withdrawal symptoms may occur.
• Don't confuse diazepam with diazoxide or Ditropan. Don't confuse Valium with Valcyte.

PATIENT TEACHING
• Warn patient to avoid activities that require alertness and good coordination until effects of drug are known.
• Tell patient to avoid alcohol while taking drug.

lorazepam

lor-AZ-e-pam

Ativan, Lorazepam Intensol
Pharmacologic class: Benzodiazepine

INDICATIONS
➤ Anxiety; insomnia from anxiety
➤ Preoperative sedation
➤ Status epilepticus

ACTION
May potentiate the effects of GABA, depress the CNS, and suppress the spread of seizure activity.

ADVERSE REACTIONS
CNS: drowsiness, sedation, amnesia, insomnia, agitation, dizziness, weakness, unsteadiness, disorientation, depression, headache
CV: hypotension
EENT: visual disturbances, nasal congestion
GI: abdominal discomfort, nausea, change in appetite

NURSING CONSIDERATIONS
• Monitor hepatic, renal, and hematopoietic function periodically in patients receiving repeated or prolonged therapy.
• Use of this drug may lead to abuse and addiction. Don't stop drug abruptly after long-term use because withdrawal symptoms may occur.
• Don't confuse lorazepam with alprazolam or clonazepam. Don't confuse Ativan with Atgam.

PATIENT TEACHING
• When used before surgery, drug causes substantial preoperative amnesia. Patient teaching requires extra care to ensure adequate recall. Provide written materials or inform a family member, if possible.
• Warn patient to avoid hazardous activities that require alertness or good coordination until effects of drug are known.
• Tell patient to avoid use of alcohol while taking drug.

midazolam hydrochloride

mid-AY-zoh-lam

Pharmacologic class: Benzodiazepine

INDICATIONS
➤ Preoperative and preprocedure sedation
➤ To induce general anesthesia
➤ To sedate intubated patients in critical care unit

ACTION
May potentiate the effects of GABA, depress the CNS, and suppress the spread of seizure activity.

ADVERSE REACTIONS
CNS: oversedation, drowsiness, amnesia, headache, involuntary movements, nystagmus, paradoxical behavior or excitement
CV: variations in blood pressure and pulse rate
GI: nausea, vomiting
Respiratory: apnea, decreased respiratory rate, hiccups
Other: pain at injection site

NURSING CONSIDERATIONS
• A qualified individual, other than the practitioner performing the procedure, should monitor patient throughout procedure. Have oxygen and resuscitation equipment available in case of severe respiratory depression.
• Give slowly over at least 2 minutes, and wait at least 2 minutes when titrating doses to produce therapeutic effect.
• Monitor blood pressure, heart rate and rhythm, respirations, airway integrity, and arterial oxygen saturation during procedure.

PATIENT TEACHING
• Because drug diminishes patient's recall of events around the time of surgery, provide written information, family member instructions, and follow-up contact.
• Warn patient to avoid hazardous activities that require alertness or good coordination until effects of drug are known.

oxazepam
ox-AZ-e-pam

Pharmacologic class: Benzodiazepine

INDICATIONS
➤ Alcohol withdrawal
➤ Anxiety

ACTION
May stimulate GABA receptors in the ascending reticular activating system.

ADVERSE REACTIONS
CNS: drowsiness, lethargy, dizziness, vertigo, headache, syncope, tremor, slurred speech, changes in EEG patterns
CV: edema
GI: nausea
Hepatic: hepatic dysfunction
Skin: rash
Other: altered libido

NURSING CONSIDERATIONS
• May increase digoxin level and risk of toxicity. Monitor patient closely.
• Monitor hepatic, renal, and hematopoietic function periodically in patients receiving repeated or prolonged therapy.
• Use of this drug may lead to abuse and addiction. Don't stop drug abruptly because withdrawal symptoms may occur.
• Don't confuse oxazepam with oxaprozin.

PATIENT TEACHING
• Warn patient to avoid hazardous activities that require alertness or good coordination until effects of drug are known.
• Tell patient to avoid use of alcohol while taking drug.

Beta blockers

atenolol
carvedilol
labetalol hydrochloride
metoprolol succinate/metoprolol tartrate
nadolol
propranolol hydrochloride
sotalol hydrochloride

INDICATIONS

➤ Hypertension (most drugs), angina pectoris (atenolol, metoprolol, nadolol, and propranolol), arrhythmias (propranolol and sotalol), prevention of MI (atenolol, metoprolol, and propranolol), prevention of recurrent migraine and other vascular headaches (propranolol), heart failure (atenolol, carvedilol, metoprolol)

ACTION

Beta blockers compete with beta agonists for available beta receptors; individual drugs differ in their ability to affect beta receptors. Some drugs are nonselective: they block $beta_1$ receptors in cardiac muscle and $beta_2$ receptors in bronchial and vascular smooth muscle. Several drugs are cardioselective and, in lower doses, inhibit mainly $beta_1$ receptors. Some beta blockers have intrinsic sympathomimetic activity and stimulate and block beta receptors, thereby slowing heart rate less.

ADVERSE REACTIONS

Therapeutic dose may cause bradycardia, dizziness, and fatigue; some may cause other CNS disturbances, such as depression, hallucinations, memory loss, and nightmares.

CONTRAINDICATIONS AND CAUTIONS

• Contraindicated in patients hypersensitive to these drugs and in patients with cardiogenic shock, sinus bradycardia, heart block greater than first degree, and bronchial asthma.
• Use caution in discontinuing drug; suddenly stopping can worsen angina or precipitate MI.
• In pregnant women, use cautiously. Drugs appear in breast milk. In children, safety and effectiveness haven't been established; use only if the benefits outweigh the risks. In elderly patients, use cautiously; these patients may need reduced maintenance doses because of increased bioavailability, delayed metabolism, and increased adverse effects.

atenolol

a-TEN-o-lol

Tenormin

Pharmacologic class: Beta blocker

INDICATIONS
➤ Hypertension
➤ Angina pectoris

ACTION
Selectively blocks beta$_1$ receptors, decreases cardiac output and cardiac oxygen consumption, and depresses renin secretion.

ADVERSE REACTIONS
CNS: dizziness, fatigue, lethargy, vertigo, drowsiness, fever
CV: hypotension, bradycardia, heart failure
GI: nausea, diarrhea
Respiratory: bronchospasm, dyspnea

NURSING CONSIDERATIONS
• Monitor patient's blood pressure.
• Drug may mask signs and symptoms of hypoglycemia in diabetic patients.
• Avoid abrupt discontinuation of therapy. Withdraw drug gradually over 1 to 2 weeks to avoid serious adverse reactions, such as severe exacerbations of angina, MI, and ventricular arrhythmias.
• Don't confuse atenolol with timolol or albuterol.

PATIENT TEACHING
• Instruct patient to take drug exactly as prescribed, at the same time every day.
• Caution patient not to stop drug suddenly, but to notify prescriber if unpleasant adverse reactions occur.
• Teach patient how to take his pulse. Tell him to withhold drug and call prescriber if pulse rate is below 60 beats/minute.

carvedilol/carvedilol phosphate

kar-VAH-da-lol

Coreg/Coreg CR

Pharmacologic class: Alpha-nonselective beta blocker

INDICATIONS

➤ Hypertension

➤ Left ventricular dysfunction after MI

➤ Mild to severe heart failure

ACTION

Nonselective beta blocker with alpha-blocking activity

ADVERSE REACTIONS

CNS: asthenia, dizziness, fatigue, stroke, pain, headache

CV: hypotension, postural hypotension, AV block, bradycardia, edema, syncope, palpitations, chest pain

EENT: abnormal vision, blurred vision, periodontitis

GI: diarrhea, vomiting, nausea, abdominal pain, dyspepsia

GU: impotence, abnormal renal function

Hematologic: thrombocytopenia, purpura

Metabolic: hyperglycemia, hyperkalemia, hypoglycemia

Respiratory: lung edema, cough, rales

NURSING CONSIDERATIONS

• If drug must be stopped, do so gradually over 1 to 2 weeks, if possible.

• Monitor diabetic patient closely; drug may mask signs of hypoglycemia, or hyperglycemia may be worsened.

PATIENT TEACHING

• Inform patient that he may experience low blood pressure when standing. If dizziness or fainting occurs (rare), advise him to sit or lie down and to notify prescriber if symptoms persist.

• Inform patient who wears contact lenses that his eyes may feel dry.

• Tell patient to take drug with food. Extended-release capsule may be opened and contents mixed with cool applesauce and taken immediately; don't store.

• Advise patient that capsules shouldn't be crushed, chewed, or contents divided.

labetalol hydrochloride
la-BET-ah-loll

Trandate

Pharmacologic class: Alpha and beta blocker

INDICATIONS
➤ Hypertension

ACTION
May be related to reduced peripheral vascular resistance, as a result of alpha and beta blockade.

ADVERSE REACTIONS
CNS: dizziness, vivid dreams, fatigue, headache, paresthesia, transient scalp tingling, syncope, vertigo, asthenia
CV: orthostatic hypotension, ventricular arrhythmias
GI: nausea, vomiting
GU: sexual dysfunction, urine retention
Respiratory: bronchospasm, dyspnea
Skin: rash

NURSING CONSIDERATIONS
• Monitor blood pressure frequently. Drug masks common signs and symptoms of shock.
• In diabetic patients, monitor glucose level closely because drug may mask certain signs and symptoms of hypoglycemia.
• Don't confuse Trandate with Trental or Tridrate.

PATIENT TEACHING
• Tell patient that stopping drug abruptly can worsen chest pain and trigger a heart attack.
• Advise patient that dizziness is the most troublesome adverse reaction and tends to occur in the early stages of treatment, in patients taking diuretics, and with higher dosages. Inform patient that dizziness can be minimized by rising slowly and avoiding sudden position changes.
• Warn patient that occasional, harmless scalp tingling may occur, especially when therapy begins.

metoprolol succinate/metoprolol tartrate

meh-TOH-pruh-lol

Toprol-XL/Lopressor

Pharmacologic class: Selective beta blocker

INDICATIONS

➤ Hypertension
➤ Early intervention in acute MI
➤ Angina pectoris
➤ Stable symptomatic heart failure

ACTION

Unknown. A selective beta blocker that selectively blocks beta$_1$ receptors; decreases cardiac output, peripheral resistance, and cardiac oxygen consumption; and depresses renin secretion.

ADVERSE REACTIONS

CNS: fatigue, dizziness, depression
CV: hypotension, bradycardia, heart failure, AV block, edema
Respiratory: dyspnea, wheezing

NURSING CONSIDERATIONS

• Always check patient's apical pulse rate before giving drug. If it's slower than 60 beats/minute, withhold drug and call prescriber immediately.
• In diabetic patients, monitor glucose level closely because drug masks common signs and symptoms of hypoglycemia.
• Avoid abrupt discontinuation of therapy. Withdraw drug gradually over 1 to 2 weeks to avoid serious adverse reactions, such as severe exacerbations of angina, MI, and ventricular arrhythmias.
• Don't confuse metoprolol with metaproterenol, misoprostol, or metolazone. Don't confuse Toprol-XL with Topamax, Tegretol, or Tegretol-XR.

PATIENT TEACHING

• Instruct patient to take drug exactly as prescribed and with meals.
• Advise patient to inform dentist or prescriber about use of this drug before procedures or surgery.
• Tell patient to alert prescriber if shortness of breath occurs.

nadolol

nay-DOE-lol

Corgard

Pharmacologic class: Nonselective beta blocker

INDICATIONS

➤ Angina pectoris
➤ Hypertension

ACTION

Reduces cardiac oxygen demand by blocking catecholamine-induced increases in heart rate, blood pressure, and force of myocardial contraction. Depresses renin secretion.

ADVERSE REACTIONS

CNS: fatigue, dizziness, fever
CV: bradycardia, heart failure, hypotension, peripheral vascular disease, rhythm and conduction disturbances
GI: nausea, vomiting, diarrhea, constipation, anorexia
Respiratory: increased airway resistance

NURSING CONSIDERATIONS

• Monitor blood pressure frequently. If patient develops severe hypotension, give a vasopressor, as prescribed.
• Drug masks signs and symptoms of shock and hyperthyroidism.
• Avoid abrupt discontinuation of therapy. Withdraw drug gradually over 1 to 2 weeks to avoid serious adverse reactions, such as severe exacerbations of angina, MI, and ventricular arrhythmias.

PATIENT TEACHING

• Explain importance of taking drug as prescribed, even when patient feels well.
• Teach patient how to check pulse rate and tell him to check it before each dose. If pulse rate is below 60 beats/minute, tell patient to notify prescriber.

propranolol hydrochloride
proe-PRAN-oh-lol

Inderal, Inderal LA, InnoPran XL

Pharmacologic class: Nonselective beta blocker

INDICATIONS
➤ Angina pectoris; hypertrophic subaortic stenosis
➤ To decrease risk of death after MI
➤ Hypertension; prevention of migraine
➤ Essential tremor; adjunct therapy in pheochromocytoma

ACTION
Reduces cardiac oxygen demand by blocking catecholamine-induced increases in heart rate, blood pressure, and force of myocardial contraction. Drug depresses renin secretion and prevents vasodilation of cerebral arteries.

ADVERSE REACTIONS
CNS: fatigue, lethargy, fever, vivid dreams, hallucinations
CV: hypotension, bradycardia, heart failure, AV block
GI: abdominal cramping, constipation, diarrhea, nausea
Hematologic: agranulocytosis
Respiratory: bronchospasm

NURSING CONSIDERATIONS
• Give drug consistently with meals.
• For direct injection, give into a large vessel or into the tubing of a free-flowing, compatible I.V. solution; don't give by continuous I.V. infusion.
• Monitor blood pressure, ECG, central venous pressure, and heart rate and rhythm frequently, especially during I.V. administration. If patient develops severe hypotension, notify prescriber; a vasopressor may be prescribed.
• Drug masks signs and symptoms of shock and hypoglycemia.
• Don't confuse propranolol with Pravachol. Don't confuse Inderal with Inderide, Isordil, Adderall, or Imuran.

PATIENT TEACHING
• Caution patient to continue taking this drug as prescribed, even when he's feeling well.
• Instruct patient to take drug with food. Food may increase absorption of propranolol.

sotalol hydrochloride
SOH-ta-lol

Betapace, Betapace AF
Pharmacologic class: Nonselective beta blocker

INDICATIONS
➤ Documented, life-threatening ventricular arrhythmias
➤ To maintain normal sinus rhythm or to delay recurrence of atrial fibrillation or atrial flutter in patients with symptomatic atrial fibrillation or flutter who are currently in sinus rhythm

ACTION
Depresses sinus heart rate, slows AV conduction, decreases cardiac output, and lowers systolic and diastolic blood pressure. Drug also has class III antiarrhythmic action potential's duration and prolongation.

ADVERSE REACTIONS
CNS: asthenia, headache, dizziness, weakness, fatigue, light-headedness, sleep problems
CV: chest pain, palpitations, bradycardia, arrhythmias, heart failure, AV block, proarrhythmic events (including polymorphic ventricular tachycardia, PVCs, ventricular fibrillation)
GI: nausea, vomiting, diarrhea, dyspepsia
Respiratory: dyspnea, bronchospasm

NURSING CONSIDERATIONS
• Monitor QTc interval. If QT interval is 500 milliseconds or more, dosage or frequency must be decreased or drug discontinued.
• Assess patient for new or worsened symptoms of heart failure.
• Monitor electrolytes regularly, especially if patient is receiving diuretics. Electrolyte imbalances, such as hypokalemia or hypomagnesemia, may enhance QT-interval prolongation and increase the risk of serious arrhythmias such as torsades de pointes.
• Don't confuse sotalol with Stadol.

PATIENT TEACHING
• Stress need to take drug as prescribed, even when he is feeling well. Caution patient against stopping drug suddenly.
• Because food and antacids can interfere with absorption, tell patient to take drug on an empty stomach, 1 hour before or 2 hours after meals or antacids.

Bronchodilators

albuterol sulfate
ipratropium bromide
salmeterol
terbutaline sulfate
theophylline

INDICATIONS
➤ To prevent or treat bronchospasm (albuterol sulfate, ipratropium bromide, salmeterol, terbutaline sulfate, theophylline), rhinorrhea (ipratropium bromide), COPD (salmeterol)

ACTION
Albuterol sulfate, salmeterol, and terbutaline sulfate relax bronchial and vascular smooth muscle by stimulating beta$_2$ receptors. Ipratropium bromide inhibits vagally mediated reflexes by antagonizing acetylcholine at muscarinic receptors on bronchial smooth muscle. Theophylline inhibits phosphodiesterase, the enzyme that degrades cAMP, resulting in relaxation of smooth muscle of the bronchial airways and pulmonary blood vessels.

ADVERSE REACTIONS
Bronchodilators may cause headaches, nausea and vomiting, restlessness (theophylline), tachycardia, palpitations, drowsiness, nervousness, or upper respiratory tract infection (ipratropium bromide, salmeterol).

CONTRAINDICATIONS AND CAUTIONS
• Contraindicated in patients hypersensitive to drug or its components.
• Use cautiously in patients with CV disorders, hyperthyroidism or diabetes (albuterol sulfate, terbutaline sulfate), angle-closure glaucoma, prostatic hyperplasia or bladder-neck obstruction (ipratropium bromide), hepatic impairment, seizure disorders (salmeterol), young children, infants, neonates and elderly patients, and those with COPD, cardiac failure, cor pulmonale, renal or hepatic disease, peptic ulceration, hyperthyroidism, diabetes mellitus, glaucoma, severe hypoxemia, hypertension, compromised cardiac or circulatory function, angina, acute MI, or sulfite sensitivity (theophylline).
• Use extended-release tablets cautiously in patients with GI narrowing (albuterol sulfate).

albuterol sulfate
al-BYOO-ter-ole

AccuNeb, ProAir HFA, Proventil HFA, Ventolin HFA, VoSpire ER
Pharmacologic class: Adrenergic

INDICATIONS
➤ Bronchospasm

ACTION
Relaxes bronchial and vascular smooth muscle by stimulating beta$_2$ receptors.

ADVERSE REACTIONS
CNS: tremor, nervousness, headache, hyperactivity, insomnia, dizziness, weakness, CNS stimulation, malaise
CV: tachycardia, palpitations, hypertension
EENT: dry and irritated nose and throat with inhaled form, nasal congestion, epistaxis, hoarseness, conjunctivitis
GI: nausea, vomiting, heartburn, anorexia, altered taste
Respiratory: bronchospasm, cough, wheezing, dyspnea

NURSING CONSIDERATIONS
• Syrup contains no alcohol or sugar and may be taken by children as young as age 2.
• In children, syrup may rarely cause erythema multiforme or Stevens-Johnson syndrome.
• Patient may use tablets and aerosol together. Monitor these patients closely for signs and symptoms of toxicity.
• Don't confuse albuterol with atenolol or Albutein.

PATIENT TEACHING
• Warn patient about risk of paradoxical bronchospasm and to stop drug immediately if it occurs.
• If prescriber orders more than one inhalation, tell patient to wait at least 2 minutes before repeating procedure.
• If patient is also using a corticosteroid inhaler, instruct him to use the bronchodilator first and then to wait about 5 minutes before using the corticosteroid. This lets the bronchodilator open the air passages for maximal effectiveness of the corticosteroid.
• Advise patient not to chew or crush extended-release tablets or mix them with food.

ipratropium bromide
ih-pra-TROE-pee-um

Atrovent, Atrovent HFA
Pharmacologic class: Anticholinergic

INDICATIONS
➤ Bronchospasm
➤ Rhinorrhea

ACTION
Inhibits vagally mediated reflexes by antagonizing acetylcholine at muscarinic receptors on bronchial smooth muscle.

ADVERSE REACTIONS
CNS: dizziness, pain, headache
CV: palpitations, chest pain
EENT: blurred vision, rhinitis, pharyngitis, sinusitis, epistaxis
GI: nausea, GI distress, dry mouth
Respiratory: upper respiratory tract infection, bronchitis, bronchospasm, cough, dyspnea, increased sputum

NURSING CONSIDERATIONS
• If patient uses a face mask for a nebulizer, take care to prevent leakage around the mask because eye pain or temporary blurring of vision may occur.
• Don't confuse Atrovent with Alupent.

PATIENT TEACHING
• Warn patient that drug isn't effective for treating acute episodes of bronchospasm when rapid response is needed.
• If more than one inhalation is prescribed, tell patient to wait at least 2 minutes before repeating procedure.
• Instruct patient to remove canister and wash inhaler in warm, soapy water at least once weekly.
• If patient is also using a corticosteroid inhaler, instruct him to use ipratropium first and then to wait about 5 minutes before using the corticosteroid. This lets the bronchodilator open air passages for maximal effectiveness of the corticosteroid.
• Instruct patient to prime nasal spray by pumping seven times before first use or after unused for 1 week. Prime with two pumps after unused for 1 day.
• Instruct patient to sniff deeply after each spray and to breathe out through mouth. Tell patient to tilt head backward to allow drug to spread to back of nose.

salmeterol xinafoate
sal-MEE-ter-ol

Serevent Diskus

Pharmacologic class: Long-acting selective beta$_2$ agonist

INDICATIONS
➤ To prevent bronchospasm
➤ COPD or emphysema

ACTION
Unclear. Selectively activates beta$_2$ receptors, which results in bronchodilation; also, blocks the release of allergic mediators from mast cells lining the respiratory tract.

ADVERSE REACTIONS
CNS: headache, sinus headache, tremor, nervousness
CV: ventricular arrhythmias, tachycardia, palpitations
EENT: nasopharyngitis, pharyngitis, hoarseness
GI: nausea, vomiting, diarrhea, heartburn
Respiratory: upper respiratory tract infection, bronchospasm

NURSING CONSIDERATIONS
• Interacts with diuretics. May worsen hypokalemia and ECG changes. Use cautiously together.
• Drug may increase the risk of asthma-related death. Only use salmeterol as additional therapy for patients whose condition is not adequately controlled on other medications or patients whose disease severity warrants initiation of treatment with two maintenance therapies.
• Drug isn't indicated for acute bronchospasm.
• Don't confuse Serevent with Serentil.

PATIENT TEACHING
• If patient is taking drug to prevent exercise-induced bronchospasm, tell him or her to take it 30 to 60 minutes before exercise.
• Tell patient drug shouldn't be used to treat acute bronchospasm. The patient must use a short-acting beta agonist, such as albuterol, to treat worsening symptoms.
• Instruct patient never to wash the mouthpiece or any part of the dry-powder multidose inhaler; it must be kept dry.

terbutaline sulfate

ter-BYOO-ta-leen

Pharmacologic class: Beta$_2$ agonist

INDICATIONS
➤ Bronchospasm
➤ Preterm labor

ACTION
Relaxes bronchial smooth muscle by stimulating beta$_2$ receptors.

ADVERSE REACTIONS
CNS: nervousness, tremor, drowsiness, dizziness, headache, weakness
CV: palpitations, arrhythmias, tachycardia, flushing
GI: vomiting, nausea, heartburn
Metabolic: hypokalemia
Respiratory: paradoxical bronchospasm with prolonged use, dyspnea
Skin: diaphoresis

NURSING CONSIDERATIONS
• Drug may reduce the sensitivity of spirometry for the diagnosis of bronchospasm.
• Withhold drug and notify prescriber if patient's heart rate is greater than 120 beats/minute.
• Monitor patient for circulatory overload.
• Don't confuse terbutaline with tolbutamide or terbinafine.

PATIENT TEACHING
• Make sure patient and caregivers understand why patient needs drug.
• Remind patient to separate oral doses by 6 hours.

theophylline
thee-OFF-i-lin

Pharmacologic class: Xanthine derivative

INDICATIONS
➤ Parenteral theophylline (preferred route) for acute bronchospasm in patients not currently receiving theophylline
➤ Oral theophylline for acute bronchospasm in patients not currently receiving theophylline
➤ Chronic bronchospasm using 8- to 12-hour extended-release preparations

ACTION
Inhibits phosphodiesterase, the enzyme that degrades cAMP, resulting in relaxation of smooth muscle of the bronchial airways and pulmonary blood vessels.

ADVERSE REACTIONS
CNS: restlessness, dizziness, insomnia, seizures, headache, irritability, muscle twitching
CV: palpitations, sinus tachycardia, arrhythmias, extrasystoles, flushing, marked hypotension
GI: nausea, vomiting, diarrhea, epigastric pain
Respiratory: respiratory arrest, tachypnea

NURSING CONSIDERATIONS
• Monitor vital signs; measure and record fluid intake and output. Expect improved quality of pulse and respirations.
• Patients metabolize xanthines at different rates; dosage is determined by monitoring response, tolerance, pulmonary function, and drug level. Drug levels range from 10 to 20 mcg/ml; toxicity may occur at levels above 20 mcg/ml.

PATIENT TEACHING
• Warn patient not to dissolve, crush, or chew extended-release products. Small children unable to swallow these can ingest (without chewing) the contents of capsules sprinkled over soft food.
• Tell patient to relieve GI symptoms by taking oral drug with full glass of water after meals, although food in stomach delays absorption.
• Inform elderly patient that dizziness is common at start of therapy.

Calcium channel blockers

amlodipine besylate
diltiazem hydrochloride
felodipine
NIFEdipine
verapamil hydrochloride

INDICATIONS
➤ Prinzmetal variant angina, chronic stable angina, unstable angina, mild to moderate hypertension, arrhythmias

ACTION
Calcium channel blockers inhibit calcium influx across the slow channels of myocardial and vascular smooth-muscle cells. By inhibiting calcium flow into these cells, calcium channel blockers reduce intracellular calcium levels. This, in turn, dilates coronary arteries, peripheral arteries, and arterioles and slows cardiac conduction.

ADVERSE REACTIONS
Verapamil may cause bradycardia, hypotension, various degrees of heart block, and worsening of heart failure after rapid IV delivery. Prolonged oral verapamil therapy may cause constipation. Nifedipine may cause flushing, headache, heartburn, hypotension, light-headedness, and peripheral edema. The most common adverse reactions with diltiazem are anorexia and nausea.

CONTRAINDICATIONS AND CAUTIONS
• Contraindicated in patients hypersensitive to these drugs and in those with second- or third-degree heart block (except those with a pacemaker) and cardiogenic shock.
• Some patients, especially those with severe obstructive coronary artery disease, have developed increased frequency, duration, or severity of angina or acute MI after initiation of calcium channel blocker therapy or at time of dosage increase.
• In pregnant women, use cautiously. Calcium channel blockers may appear in breast milk; instruct patient to stop breast-feeding during therapy. In neonates and infants, adverse hemodynamic effects of parenteral verapamil are possible, but safety and effectiveness of other calcium channel blockers haven't been established; avoid use, if possible. In elderly patients, the half-life of calcium channel blockers may be increased as a result of decreased clearance; use cautiously.

amlodipine besylate
am-LOE-di-peen

Norvasc

Pharmacologic class: Calcium channel blocker

INDICATIONS
➤ Chronic stable angina, vasospastic angina
➤ Hypertension

ACTION
Inhibits calcium ion influx across cardiac and smooth-muscle cells, dilates coronary arteries and arterioles, and decreases blood pressure and myocardial oxygen demand.

ADVERSE REACTIONS
CNS: headache, somnolence, fatigue, dizziness, light-headedness, asthenia, paresthesia
CV: edema, flushing, palpitations
GI: dyspepsia, nausea, abdominal pain
Respiratory: dyspnea
Skin: rash, pruritus

NURSING CONSIDERATIONS
• Monitor blood pressure frequently during initiation of therapy. Because drug-induced vasodilation has a gradual onset, acute hypotension is rare.
• Notify prescriber if signs of heart failure occur, such as swelling of hands and feet or shortness of breath.
• Abrupt withdrawal of drug may increase frequency and duration of chest pain. Taper dose gradually under medical supervision.
• Don't confuse amlodipine with amiloride.

PATIENT TEACHING
• Caution patient to continue taking drug, even when he feels better.
• Tell patient S.L. nitroglycerin may be taken as needed when angina symptoms are acute. If patient continues nitrate therapy during adjustment of amlodipine dosage, urge continued compliance.

diltiazem hydrochloride
dil-TYE-a-zem

Cardizem, Cardizem CD, Cardizem LA, Cartia XT, Dilacor XR, Dilt-CD, Dilt-XR, Diltzac, Taztia XT, Tiazac

Pharmacologic class: Calcium channel blocker

INDICATIONS
➤ Chronic stable angina, vasospastic angina
➤ Hypertension
➤ Atrial fibrillation or flutter; paroxysmal supraventricular tachycardia

ACTION
A calcium channel blocker that inhibits calcium ion influx across cardiac and smooth-muscle cells, decreasing myocardial contractility and oxygen demand. Drug also dilates coronary arteries and arterioles.

ADVERSE REACTIONS
CNS: headache, dizziness, asthenia, somnolence
CV: edema, arrhythmias, AV block, bradycardia, heart failure
GI: nausea, constipation, abdominal discomfort
Hepatic: acute hepatic injury

NURSING CONSIDERATIONS
• For direct injection or continuous infusion; give slowly while monitoring ECG and blood pressure continuously.
• If systolic blood pressure is below 90 mm Hg or heart rate is below 60 beats/minute, withhold dose and notify prescriber.
• Don't confuse Tiazac with Ziac.

PATIENT TEACHING
• Advise patient to avoid hazardous activities during start of therapy.
• Tell patient that S.L. nitroglycerin may be taken with drug, as needed, when angina symptoms are acute.
• Tell patient to swallow extended-release tablets whole, and not to crush or chew them.
• If patient is taking Tiazac extended-release capsules, inform him that these capsules can be opened and the contents sprinkled onto a spoonful of applesauce. He must eat the applesauce immediately and without chewing, and then drink a glass of cool water.

felodipine
fell-OH-di-peen
Pharmacologic class: Calcium channel blocker

INDICATIONS
➤ Hypertension
➤ Pediatric hypertension

ACTION
Unknown. A dihydropyridine-derivative calcium channel blocker that prevents entry of calcium ions into vascular smooth-muscle and cardiac cells; shows some selectivity for smooth muscle compared with cardiac muscle.

ADVERSE REACTIONS
CNS: headache, dizziness, paresthesia, asthenia
CV: peripheral edema, chest pain, palpitations, flushing
EENT: rhinorrhea, pharyngitis
GI: abdominal pain, nausea, constipation, diarrhea
Musculoskeletal: muscle cramps, back pain
Respiratory: upper respiratory tract infection, cough
Skin: rash

NURSING CONSIDERATIONS
• Monitor blood pressure for response.
• Monitor patient for peripheral edema, which appears to be both dose and age related. It's more common in patients taking higher doses, especially those older than age 60.

PATIENT TEACHING
• Tell patient to swallow tablets whole and not to crush or chew them.
• Tell patient to take drug without food or with a light meal.
• Advise patient not to take drug with grapefruit juice.
• Advise patient to continue taking drug even when he feels better, to watch his diet, and to check with prescriber or pharmacist before taking other drugs, including OTC drugs, nutritional supplements, or herbal remedies.
• Advise patient to observe good oral hygiene and to see a dentist regularly; use of drug may cause mild gum problems.

NIFEdipine

nye-FED-i-peen

Adalat CC, Afeditab CR, Procardia, Procardia XL
Pharmacologic class: Calcium channel blocker

INDICATIONS
➤ Vasospastic angina, chronic stable angina pectoris
➤ Hypertension

ACTION
Thought to inhibit calcium ion influx across cardiac and smooth-muscle cells, decreasing contractility and oxygen demand. Drug may also dilate coronary arteries and arterioles.

ADVERSE REACTIONS
CNS: dizziness, light-headedness, headache, weakness, somnolence, syncope, nervousness
CV: flushing, peripheral edema, heart failure, MI, hypotension, palpitations
GI: nausea, diarrhea, constipation, abdominal discomfort
Respiratory: dyspnea, pulmonary edema, cough

NURSING CONSIDERATIONS
• Monitor blood pressure and heart rate regularly, especially in patients who take beta blockers or antihypertensives.
• Watch for symptoms of heart failure.
• Don't confuse nifedipine with nimodipine or nicardipine.

PATIENT TEACHING
• If patient is kept on nitrate therapy while nifedipine dosage is being adjusted, urge continued compliance. Patient may take S.L. nitroglycerin, as needed, for acute chest pain.
• Tell patient that chest pain may worsen briefly as therapy starts or dosage increases.
• Instruct patient to swallow extended-release tablets without breaking, crushing, or chewing them.
• Advise patient to avoid taking drug with grapefruit juice.
• Reassure patient taking the extended-release tablet that the wax mold may be passed in the stools. Assure him that drug has already been completely absorbed.
• Tell patient to protect capsules from direct light and moisture and to store at room temperature.

verapamil hydrochloride
ver-AP-a-mill

Calan, Covera-HS, Isoptin SR, Verelan, Verelan PM
Pharmacologic class: Calcium channel blocker

INDICATIONS
➤ Vasospastic angina; unstable angina; classic chronic, stable angina pectoris; chronic atrial fibrillation
➤ Supraventricular arrhythmias
➤ Digitalized patients with chronic atrial fibrillation or flutter
➤ Hypertension

ACTION
Not clearly defined. A calcium channel blocker that inhibits calcium ion influx across cardiac and smooth-muscle cells, thus decreasing myocardial contractility and oxygen demand; it also dilates coronary arteries and arterioles.

ADVERSE REACTIONS
CNS: dizziness, headache, asthenia, fatigue, sleep disturbances
CV: transient hypotension, heart failure, bradycardia, AV block, ventricular asystole, ventricular fibrillation, peripheral edema
GI: constipation, nausea, diarrhea, dyspepsia
Respiratory: dyspnea, pharyngitis, pulmonary edema, rhinitis, sinusitis, upper respiratory infection

NURSING CONSIDERATIONS
• Patients receiving beta blockers should receive lower doses of this drug. Monitor these patients closely.
• Monitor blood pressure at the start of therapy and during dosage adjustments.
• If signs and symptoms of heart failure occur, notify prescriber.
• Monitor liver function test results during prolonged treatment.
• Don't confuse Verelan with Vivarin, Voltaren, or Virilon.

PATIENT TEACHING
• Tell patient that long-acting forms shouldn't be crushed or chewed.
• Caution patient against abruptly stopping drug.
• Encourage patient to increase fluid and fiber intake to combat constipation. Give a stool softener.
• Drug significantly inhibits alcohol elimination. Advise patient to avoid or severely limit alcohol use.

Cephalosporins

cefadroxil
cefdinir
cefepime hydrochloride
cefotaxime sodium
cefoxitin sodium
cefprozil
cefuroxime axetil/cefuroxime sodium
cephalexin

INDICATIONS

➤ Infections of the lungs, skin, soft tissue, bones, joints, urinary and respiratory tracts, blood, abdomen, and heart; CNS infections caused by susceptible strains of *Neisseria meningitidis*, *Haemophilus influenzae*, and *Streptococcus pneumoniae*; meningitis caused by *Escherichia coli* or *Klebsiella*; infections that develop after surgical procedures classified as contaminated or potentially contaminated; penicillinase-producing *Neisseria gonorrhoeae*; otitis media and ampicillin-resistant middle ear infection caused by *H. influenzae*.

ACTION

Cephalosporins are chemically and pharmacologically similar to penicillin; they act by inhibiting bacterial cell-wall synthesis, causing rapid cell destruction. Their sites of action are enzymes known as penicillin-binding proteins. The affinity of certain cephalosporins for these proteins in various microorganisms helps explain the differing actions of these drugs.

ADVERSE REACTIONS

Hypersensitivity reactions range from mild rashes, fever, and eosinophilia to fatal anaphylaxis and are more common in patients with penicillin allergy.

CONTRAINDICATIONS AND CAUTIONS

• Contraindicated in patients hypersensitive to these drugs.
• Use cautiously in patients with renal or hepatic impairment, history of GI disease, or allergy to penicillins.
• In pregnant women, use cautiously; safety hasn't been definitively established. In breast-feeding women, use cautiously because drugs appear in breast milk. In neonates and infants, half-life is prolonged; use cautiously. Elderly patients are susceptible to superinfection and coagulopathies, commonly have renal impairment, and may need a lower dosage; use cautiously.

cefadroxil
sef-a-DROX-ill

Pharmacologic class: First-generation cephalosporin

INDICATIONS
➤ UTIs caused by *Escherichia coli, Proteus mirabilis,* and *Klebsiella* species
➤ Skin and soft-tissue infections caused by staphylococci and streptococci
➤ Pharyngitis or tonsillitis caused by group A beta-hemolytic streptococci

ACTION
Inhibits cell-wall synthesis, promoting osmotic instability; usually bactericidal.

ADVERSE REACTIONS
CNS: seizures, fever
GI: pseudomembranous colitis, glossitis, abdominal cramps
GU: genital pruritus, candidiasis, vaginitis, renal dysfunction
Hematologic: transient neutropenia, leukopenia, agranulocytosis, thrombocytopenia, anemia, eosinophilia
Skin: maculopapular and erythematous rashes, urticaria
Other: anaphylaxis, angioedema, hypersensitivity reactions

NURSING CONSIDERATIONS
• If creatinine clearance is less than 50 ml/minute, lengthen dosage interval so drug doesn't accumulate. Monitor renal function in patients with renal dysfunction.
• If large doses are given, therapy is prolonged, or patient is at high risk, monitor patient for superinfection.
• Don't confuse drug with other cephalosporins that sound alike.

PATIENT TEACHING
• Instruct patient to take drug with food or milk to lessen GI discomfort.
• Tell patient to take entire amount of drug exactly as prescribed, even after he feels better.
• Advise patient to notify prescriber if rash develops or if signs and symptoms of superinfection appear, such as recurring fever, chills, and malaise.

cefdinir
sef-DIN-er

Omnicef

Pharmacologic class: Third-generation cephalosporin

INDICATIONS
➤ Mild to moderate infections caused by susceptible strains of microorganisms in community-acquired pneumonia, acute worsening of chronic bronchitis, acute maxillary sinusitis, acute bacterial otitis media, and uncomplicated skin and skin-structure infections
➤ Pharyngitis, tonsillitis

ACTION
Inhibits cell-wall synthesis, promoting osmotic instability; usually bactericidal.

ADVERSE REACTIONS
CNS: headache
GI: diarrhea, pseudomembranous colitis, abdominal pain, nausea
GU: vaginitis; increased urine proteins, WBCs, and RBCs
Other: hypersensitivity reactions, anaphylaxis

NURSING CONSIDERATIONS
• Prolonged drug treatment may result in emergence and overgrowth of resistant organisms. Monitor patient for signs and symptoms of superinfection.
• Pseudomembranous colitis has been reported with cefdinir and should be considered in patients with diarrhea after antibiotic therapy and in those with history of colitis.
• Don't confuse drug with other cephalosporins that sound alike.

PATIENT TEACHING
• Instruct patient to take antacids and iron supplements 2 hours before or after a dose of cefdinir.
• Advise patient to report severe diarrhea or diarrhea with abdominal pain.
• Tell patient to report adverse reactions or signs and symptoms of superinfection promptly.

cefepime hydrochloride
SEF-ah-peem

Maxipime

Pharmacologic class: Fourth-generation cephalosporin

INDICATIONS
➤ UTI, pyelonephritis, skin infection and skin-structure infection, intra-abdominal infection, pneumonia
➤ Empirical therapy for febrile neutropenia

ACTION
Inhibits bacterial cell-wall synthesis, promotes osmotic instability, and destroys bacteria.

ADVERSE REACTIONS
CNS: fever, headache
CV: phlebitis
GI: diarrhea, nausea, vomiting
Skin: rash, pruritus
Other: anaphylaxis, pain, inflammation, hypersensitivity reactions

NURSING CONSIDERATIONS
• Monitor patient for superinfection. Drug may cause overgrowth of nonsusceptible bacteria or fungi.
• Drug may reduce PT activity. Patients at risk include those with renal or hepatic impairment or poor nutrition and those receiving prolonged therapy. Monitor PT and INR in these patients. Give vitamin K, as indicated.
• Obtain specimen for culture and sensitivity tests before giving. Begin therapy while awaiting results.
• Follow manufacturer's guidelines closely when reconstituting drug. The type of diluent varies with the product used. Use only recommended solutions.
• Infuse over about 30 minutes.
• Don't confuse drug with other cephalosporins that sound alike.

PATIENT TEACHING
• Advise patient to notify prescriber if a rash develops or if signs and symptoms of superinfection appear, such as recurring fever, chills, and malaise.
• Instruct patient to report adverse reactions promptly.

cefotaxime sodium

sef-oh-TAKS-eem

Claforan

Pharmacologic class: Third-generation cephalosporin

INDICATIONS
➤ Perioperative prevention in contaminated surgery
➤ Gonorrhea
➤ Serious infection of the lower respiratory and urinary tract, CNS, skin, bone, and joints; gynecologic and intra-abdominal infection; bacteremia; septicemia caused by susceptible microorganisms

ACTION
Inhibits cell-wall synthesis, promoting osmotic instability; usually bactericidal.

ADVERSE REACTIONS
CNS: fever, headache
CV: phlebitis, thrombophlebitis
GI: diarrhea, pseudomembranous colitis, nausea, vomiting
Hematologic: agranulocytosis, thrombocytopenia, transient neutropenia, eosinophilia, hemolytic anemia
Skin: maculopapular and erythematous rashes, urticaria, pain, induration, sterile abscesses, temperature elevation, tissue sloughing at I.M. injection site
Other: anaphylaxis, hypersensitivity reactions, serum sickness

NURSING CONSIDERATIONS
• If large doses are given, therapy is prolonged, or patient is at high risk, monitor patient for superinfection.
• For direct I.V. injection, inject the drug over 3 to 5 minutes into a large vein or into the tubing of a free-flowing I.V. solution.
• For I.V. infusion, reconstitute with 50 or 100 ml of D_5W or NSS and infuse over 20 to 30 minutes.
• Don't confuse drug with other cephalosporins that sound alike.

PATIENT TEACHING
• Tell patient to report adverse reactions and signs and symptoms of superinfection promptly.
• Instruct patient to report discomfort at I.V. insertion site.

cefoxitin sodium
se-FOX-i-tin

Pharmacologic class: Second-generation cephalosporin

INDICATIONS
➤ Serious infection of the respiratory and GU tracts; skin, soft-tissue, bone, or joint infection; bloodstream or intra-abdominal infection caused by susceptible organisms (such as *Escherichia coli* and other coliform bacteria, penicillinase- and non–penicillinase-producing *Staphylococcus aureus*, *Staphylococcus epidermidis*, streptococci, *Klebsiella*, *Haemophilus influenzae*, and *Bacteroides*, including *B. fragilis*)
➤ Perioperative prevention
➤ Uncomplicated gonorrhea

ACTION
Inhibits cell-wall synthesis, promoting osmotic instability; usually bactericidal.

ADVERSE REACTIONS
CV: phlebitis, thrombophlebitis, hypotension
GI: diarrhea, pseudomembranous colitis, nausea, vomiting
GU: acute renal failure
Hematologic: thrombocytopenia, transient neutropenia
Skin: maculopapular and erythematous rashes, urticaria, pain, induration, sterile abscesses, tissue sloughing at injection site
Other: anaphylaxis, hypersensitivity reactions, serum sickness

NURSING CONSIDERATIONS
• Reconstitute 1 g with at least 10 ml of sterile water for injection and 2 g with 10 to 20 ml of sterile water for injection.
• For direct injection, give drug over 3 to 5 minutes into a large vein or into the tubing of a free-flowing I.V. solution.
• For intermittent infusion, add reconstituted drug to 50 or 100 ml of D₅W or normal saline solution for injection.
• Don't confuse drug with other cephalosporins that sound alike.

PATIENT TEACHING
• Tell patient to report adverse reactions and signs and symptoms of superinfection promptly.
• Instruct patient to report discomfort at I.V. site.
• Advise patient to notify prescriber about loose stools or diarrhea.

cefprozil
sef-PRO-zil

Pharmacologic class: Second-generation cephalosporin

INDICATIONS

➤ Pharyngitis or tonsillitis caused by *Streptococcus pyrogenes*

➤ Otitis media caused by *Streptococcus pneumoniae, Haemophilus influenzae,* and *Moraxella catarrhalis*

➤ Bronchitis caused by *S. pneumoniae, H. influenzae,* and *M. catarrhalis*

➤ Uncomplicated skin and skin-structure infections caused by *Staphylococcus aureus* and *S. pyrogenes*

➤ Acute sinusitis caused by *S. pneumoniae, H. influenzae* (beta-lactamase–positive and –negative strains), and *M. catarrhalis*

ACTION

Inhibits cell-wall synthesis, promoting osmotic instability; usually bactericidal.

ADVERSE REACTIONS

CNS: dizziness
GI: diarrhea, nausea, vomiting, abdominal pain
GU: genital pruritus, vaginitis
Hematologic: eosinophilia
Skin: diaper rash
Other: anaphylaxis, superinfection, hypersensitivity reactions, serum sickness

NURSING CONSIDERATIONS

• Monitor renal function and liver function test results.
• Monitor patient for superinfection. May cause overgrowth of nonsusceptible bacteria or fungi.
• Don't confuse drug with other cephalosporins that sound alike.

PATIENT TEACHING

• Tell patient to shake suspension well before measuring dose.
• Inform patient or parent that oral suspension is bubble gum–flavored to improve palatability and promote compliance in children. Tell him to refrigerate reconstituted suspension and to discard unused drug after 14 days.
• Instruct patient to notify prescriber if rash or signs and symptoms of superinfection occur.

cefuroxime axetil/cefuroxime sodium

se-fyoor-OX-eem

Ceftin/Zinacef

Pharmacologic class: Second-generation cephalosporin

INDICATIONS

➤ Serious lower respiratory tract infection, UTI, skin or skin-structure infections, bone or joint infection, septicemia, meningitis, and gonorrhea

➤ Perioperative prevention

➤ Acute bacterial maxillary sinusitis; pharyngitis and tonsillitis; otitis media

➤ Early Lyme disease

ACTION

Inhibits cell-wall synthesis, promoting osmotic instability; usually bactericidal.

ADVERSE REACTIONS

CV: phlebitis, thrombophlebitis

GI: diarrhea, pseudomembranous colitis, nausea, vomiting

Hematologic: hemolytic anemia, thrombocytopenia, transient neutropenia, eosinophilia

Skin: maculopapular and erythematous rashes, urticaria, pain, induration, sterile abscesses, temperature elevation, tissue sloughing at I.M. injection site

Other: anaphylaxis, hypersensitivity reactions, serum sickness

NURSING CONSIDERATIONS

• Monitor patient for signs and symptoms of superinfection.

• Don't confuse drug with other cephalosporins that sound alike.

PATIENT TEACHING

• If patient has difficulty swallowing tablets, show him how to dissolve or crush tablets but warn him that the bitter taste is hard to mask, even with food.

• Tell parent to shake suspension well before measuring dose. Suspension may be stored at room temperature or refrigerated, but must be discarded after 10 days.

• Instruct caregiver to give oral suspension with food.

• Instruct patient to notify prescriber about rash, loose stools, diarrhea, or evidence of superinfection.

cephalexin
sef-a-LEX-in

Pharmacologic class: First-generation cephalosporin

INDICATIONS
➤ Respiratory tract, GI tract, skin, soft-tissue, bone, and joint infections and otitis media caused by *Escherichia coli* and other coliform bacteria, group A beta-hemolytic streptococci, *Klebsiella* species, *Proteus mirabilis*, *Streptococcus pneumoniae*, and staphylococci

ACTION
Inhibits cell-wall synthesis, promoting osmotic instability; usually bactericidal.

NURSING CONSIDERATIONS
• If large doses are given or if therapy is prolonged, monitor patient for superinfection, especially if patient is at high risk.
• Treat group A beta-hemolytic streptococcal infections for a minimum of 10 days.
• Don't confuse drug with other cephalosporins that sound alike.

PATIENT TEACHING
• Instruct patient to take drug with food or milk to lessen GI discomfort. If patient is taking suspension form, instruct him to shake container well before measuring dose and to store in refrigerator.
• Tell patient to notify prescriber if rash or signs and symptoms of superinfection develop.

CNS stimulants

dextroamphetamine sulfate
methylphenidate hydrochloride
phentermine hydrochloride

INDICATIONS
➤ Obesity (phentermine); ADHD, narcolepsy (methylphenidate)

ACTION
Dextroamphetamine probably promotes nerve impulse transmission by releasing stored dopamine and norepinephrine from nerve terminals in the brain. Methylphenidate releases nerve terminal stores of norepinephrine, promoting nerve impulse transmission. At high doses, effects are mediated by dopamine. Phentermine is a sympathomimetic amine. The exact mechanism of action in treating obesity isn't established.

ADVERSE REACTIONS
Adverse reactions include hypertension, palpitations, tachyarrhythmias, urticaria, constipation, diarrhea, dizziness, excitement, insomnia, tremor, and restlessness.

CONTRAINDICATIONS AND CAUTIONS
• Contraindicated in patients hypersensitive to any of the drug components.
• Phentermine is contraindicated in agitated states, CV disease, history of drug abuse, severe hypertension, hyperthyroidism, glaucoma, and during or within 14 days following use of MAO inhibitors.
• Use methylphenidate cautiously in patients who have a history of drug dependence or alcoholism. Long-term abusive use can lead to tolerance and psychological dependence. Psychotic episodes can occur. Monitor patient for severe depression during drug withdrawal.

dextroamphetamine sulfate
dex-troe-am-FET-a-meen

Dexedrine, Dexedrine Spansule, DextroStat, Liquadd
Pharmacologic class: Amphetamine

INDICATIONS
➤ Narcolepsy
➤ ADHD

ACTION
Unknown. Probably promotes nerve impulse transmission by releasing stored dopamine and norepinephrine from nerve terminals in the brain. Main sites of activity appear to be the cerebral cortex and the reticular activating system.

ADVERSE REACTIONS
CNS: insomnia, nervousness, restlessness, tremor, dizziness, headache, chills, overstimulation, dysphoria, euphoria
CV: tachycardia, palpitations, arrhythmias, hypertension
GI: dry mouth, taste perversion, diarrhea, constipation
Skin: urticaria

NURSING CONSIDERATIONS
• Obtain a detailed patient history, including a family history for mental disorders, family suicide, ventricular arrhythmias, or sudden death.
• Drug has a high abuse potential and may cause dependence. Monitor patient closely.
• Monitor for growth retardation in children.
• Don't confuse Dexedrine with dextran or Excedrin.

PATIENT TEACHING
• Warn patient to avoid activities that require alertness, a clear visual field, or good coordination until CNS effects of drug are known.
• Inform parents that children may show increased aggression or hostility and to report worsening of behavior.
• Advise patient to consume caffeine-containing products cautiously.
• Tell patient not to drink fruit juice at same time as oral solution.
• Warn patient with a seizure disorder that drug may decrease seizure threshold. Instruct him to notify prescriber if seizures occur.

methylphenidate hydrochloride/methylphenidate transdermal system
meth-ill-FEN-i-date

Concerta, Metadate CD, Metadate ER, Methylin, Methylin ER, Ritalin, Ritalin LA, Ritalin-SR/Daytrana
Pharmacologic class: Piperidine derivative

INDICATIONS
➤ ADHD
➤ Narcolepsy

ACTION
Releases nerve terminal stores of norepinephrine, promoting nerve impulse transmission. At high doses, effects are mediated by dopamine.

ADVERSE REACTIONS
CNS: nervousness, headache, insomnia, seizures, mood swings
CV: palpitations, tachycardia, arrhythmias, hypertension
GI: nausea, abdominal pain, decreased appetite, vomiting
Hematologic: thrombocytopenia, thrombocytopenic purpura, leukopenia, anemia
Skin: exfoliative dermatitis, erythema multiforme, rash
Other: viral infection

NURSING CONSIDERATIONS
• Observe patient for signs of excessive stimulation. Monitor blood pressure.
• Check CBC and platelet counts with long-term use.
• Monitor height and weight in children on long-term therapy.

PATIENT TEACHING
• Tell patient to take last daily dose at least 6 hours before bedtime to prevent insomnia.
• Tell patient to take after meals to reduce appetite-suppressant effects.
• Warn patient to take chewable tablet with at least 8 oz of water. Not using enough water may cause choking.
• Tell parent if patch comes off, apply a new one on a different site, but the total wear time for that day should be 9 hours.
• Teach child that patch shouldn't be shared or removed except by parent or health care provider.
• Tell parent the effects of the patch lasts for several hours after its removal.

phentermine hydrochloride
FEN-ter-meen

Adipex-P
Pharmacologic class: Sympathomimetic amine

INDICATIONS
➤ Short-term adjunct in exogenous obesity

ACTION
Unknown. Probably promotes nerve impulse transmission by releasing stored norepinephrine from nerve terminals in the brain, especially in the cerebral cortex and reticular activating system.

ADVERSE REACTIONS
CNS: insomnia, overstimulation, headache, euphoria, dysphoria, dizziness
CV: palpitations, tachycardia, increased blood pressure
GI: dry mouth, dysgeusia, constipation, diarrhea, unpleasant taste, other GI disturbances
GU: impotence
Skin: urticaria
Other: altered libido

NURSING CONSIDERATIONS
• Use drug with a weight-reduction program.
• Monitor patient for tolerance or dependence.
• Don't confuse phentermine with phentolamine.

PATIENT TEACHING
• Tell patient to take sustained-release drug at least 10 hours before bedtime or last dose of immediate-release drug at least 4 to 6 hours before bedtime to avoid sleep interference.
• Advise patient to avoid products that contain caffeine. Tell him to report evidence of excessive stimulation.
• Warn patient that fatigue may result as drug effects wear off and that he'll need more rest.
• Warn patient that drug may lose its effectiveness over time.
• Tell patient to take sustained-release capsule whole and not to chew, crush, or open it.

Contraceptives

ethinyl estradiol/desogestrel
ethinyl estradiol/ethynodiol diacetate
ethinyl estradiol/levonorgestrel
ethinyl estradiol/norethindrone
ethinyl estradiol/norgestimate
ethinyl estradiol/norgestrel
mestranol/norethindrone

INDICATIONS
➤ Contraception; moderate acne vulgaris

ACTION
Contraceptives inhibit ovulation by suppressing follicle-stimulating hormone. Progestin suppresses luteinizing hormone so that ovulation can't occur even if the follicle does develop. It also thickens the cervical mucus, which interferes with sperm migration and prevents implantation of the fertilized ovum. Contraceptives may prevent ovum transport (if ovulation does occur) through the fallopian tubes.

ADVERSE REACTIONS
Headache, dizziness, nausea, breakthrough bleeding, spotting.

CONTRAINDICATIONS AND CAUTIONS
• Contraindicated in patients with thromboembolic disorders, cerebrovascular or coronary artery disease, diplopia or ocular lesions arising from ophthalmic vascular disease, classic migraine, MI, known or suspected breast cancer, known or suspected estrogen-dependent neoplasia, benign or malignant liver tumors, active liver disease or history of cholestatic jaundice with pregnancy or previous use of hormonal contraceptives, and undiagnosed abnormal vaginal bleeding.
• Contraindicated in woman who may be pregnant or breast-feeding.
• Use cautiously in patients with hyperlipidemia; hypertension; migraines; seizure disorders; asthma; cardiac, renal, or hepatic insufficiency; bleeding irregularities; gallbladder disease; ocular disease; diabetes; and emotional disorders.

ethinyl estradiol and desogestrel
monophasic/biphasic/triphasic

Apri, Desogen, Ortho-Cept/Kariva, Mircette/Caziant, Cesia, Cyclessa, Velivet

ethinyl estradiol and ethynodiol diacetate
monophasic

Zovia 1/35E, Zovia 1/50E

ethinyl estradiol and levonorgestrel
monophasic/biphasic/triphasic

Aviane, Lessina, Levlen, Levora-28, Lybrel, Nordette-28, Portia-28, Seasonale/Lo Seasonique, Seasonique/Enpresse, Trivora-28

ethinyl estradiol and norethindrone
monophasic/biphasic/triphasic

Brevicon, Modicon, Necon 1/35, Necon 0.5/35, Norethin 1/35E, Norinyl 1+35, Nortrel 0.5/35, Nortrel 1/35, Ortho-Novum 1/35, Ovcon-35, Ovcon-50/Necon 10/11/Aranelle, Leena, Necon 7/7/7, Nortrel 7/7/7, Ortho-Novum 7/7/7, Tri-Norinyl

ethinyl estradiol and norethindrone acetate
monophasic

Junel 21 Day 1/20, Junel 21 Day 1.5/30, Junel Fe 1/20, Loestrin 21 1.5/30, Loestrin 21 1/20, Microgestin 1.5/30, Microgestin 1/20

ethinyl estradiol and norgestimate
monophasic/triphasic

MonoNessa, Ortho-Cyclen, Sprintec/Ortho Tri-Cyclen, Ortho Tri-Cyclen Lo, Tri-Lo-Sprintec, Tri-Previfem, Tri-Sprintec

ethinyl estradiol and norgestrel
monophasic

Cryselle, Lo/Ovral, Low-Ogestrel, Ogestrel

ethinyl estradiol, norethindrone acetate, and ferrous fumarate
monophasic/triphasic

Femcon Fe, Loestrin 24 Fe, Loestrin Fe 1/20, Loestrin Fe 1.5/30, Microgestin Fe 1/20, Microgestin Fe 1.5/30/Estrostep Fe, Tilia Fe, Tri-Legest Fe

mestranol and norethindrone
monophasic

Necon 1/50, Norinyl 1+50, Ortho-Novum 1/50-28
Pharmacologic class: Estrogenic and progestinic steroids

INDICATIONS
➤ Contraception
➤ Moderate acne vulgaris in women aged 15 and older

ACTION
Inhibit ovulation and may prevent transport of the ovum (if ovulation should occur) through the fallopian tubes. Estrogen suppresses follicle-stimulating hormone, blocking follicular development and ovulation. Progestin suppresses luteinizing hormone so that ovulation can't occur even if the follicle develops; it also thickens cervical mucus, interfering with sperm migration, and prevents implantation of the fertilized ovum.

ADVERSE REACTIONS
CNS: headache, dizziness, stroke, cerebral hemorrhage
CV: thromboembolism, edema, pulmonary embolism, MI
GI: nausea, vomiting, abdominal cramps, bloating, anorexia
GU: breakthrough bleeding, spotting
Hepatic: cholestatic jaundice, liver tumors, gallbladder disease
Metabolic: weight change
Skin: rash, acne, erythema multiforme, melasma, hirsutism
Other: anaphylaxis, hemolytic uremic syndrome

NURSING CONSIDERATIONS
• Monitor lipid levels, blood pressure, body weight, and hepatic function.
• Stop drug at least 1 week before surgery to decrease risk of thromboembolism.

PATIENT TEACHING
• Tell patient to take tablets at same time each day; nighttime doses may reduce nausea and headaches.
• Advise the patient not to smoke. Smoking may increase risk of adverse CV effects.
• Tell patient that hormonal contraceptives don't protect against HIV or other sexually transmitted diseases.
• Warn patient to immediately report abdominal pain; numbness, stiffness, or pain in legs or buttocks; pressure or pain in chest; shortness of breath; severe headache; visual disturbances, such as blind spots, blurriness, or flashing lights; undiagnosed vaginal bleeding or discharge; two consecutive missed menstrual periods; lumps in the breast; swelling of hands or feet; or severe pain in the abdomen.

Corticosteroids

beclomethasone dipropionate
budesonide
dexamethasone/dexamethasone sodium phosphate
flunisolide/flunisolide hemihydrate
fluocinonide
fluticasone furoate/fluticasone propionate
hydrocortisone/hydrocortisone acetate/hydrocortisone
    cypionate/hydrocortisone sodium succinate
methylprednisolone/methylprednisolone
    acetate/methylprednisolone sodium succinate
prednisolone/prednisolone acetate/prednisolone sodium
    phosphate
prednisone
triamcinolone acetonide

INDICATIONS
➤ Hypersensitivity; inflammation; to initiate immunosuppression;
replacement therapy in adrenocortical insufficiency; dermatologic
diseases; respiratory disorders; rheumatic disorders

ACTION
Corticosteroids suppress cell-mediated and humoral immunity. They
reduce inflammation disrupting inflammatory processes.

ADVERSE REACTIONS
Excessive use may cause cushingoid symptoms and various systemic
disorders, such as diabetes and osteoporosis.

CONTRAINDICATIONS AND CAUTIONS
• Contraindicated in patients hypersensitive to these drugs or any of
their components and in those with systemic fungal infection.
• In pregnant women, avoid use, if possible, because of risk to the fetus.
Women should stop breast-feeding because these drugs appear in breast
milk and could cause serious adverse effects in infants. In children,
long-term use should be avoided whenever possible because stunted
growth may result.
• Elderly patients may have an increased risk of adverse reactions;
monitor them closely.

beclomethasone dipropionate (intranasal)
be-kloe-METH-a-sone

Beconase AQ
Pharmacologic class: Corticosteroid

INDICATIONS
➤ To relieve symptoms of seasonal or perennial rhinitis; to prevent nasal polyp recurrence after surgical removal

ACTION
May reduce nasal inflammation by inhibiting mediators of inflammation.

ADVERSE REACTIONS
CNS: headache, light-headedness
EENT: mild, transient nasal burning and stinging, dryness, epistaxis, nasal congestion, nasopharyngeal fungal infections, rhinorrhea, sneezing, watery eyes
GI: nausea
Metabolic: growth velocity reduction in children and adolescents

NURSING CONSIDERATIONS
• Observe patient for fungal infections.
• Stop drug if no significant symptom improvement occurs after 3 weeks.

PATIENT TEACHING
• Advise patient to pump nasal spray six times until a fine mist is produced before first use.
• To instill, instruct patient to blow nose to clear nasal passages, shake container, tilt head slightly forward, and insert nozzle into nostril, pointing away from septum. Tell him to hold other nostril closed and inhale gently while spraying, hold breath for a few seconds, and exhale through the mouth. Next, have him shake container and repeat in other nostril.
• Tell patient to pump nasal spray once or twice before first use each day. He should clean the cap and nosepiece of the activator in warm water every day, and then allow them to air-dry.
• Explain that unlike decongestants, drug doesn't work right away. Most patients notice improvement within a few days, but some may need 2 to 3 weeks.

budesonide (inhalation)
byoo-DES-oh-nide

Pulmicort Flexhaler, Pulmicort, Respules
Pharmacologic class: Corticosteroid

INDICATIONS
➤ Asthma

ACTION
Exhibits potent glucocorticoid activity and weak mineralocorticoid activity. Drug inhibits mast cells, macrophages, and mediators (such as leukotrienes) involved in inflammation.

ADVERSE REACTIONS
CNS: headache, asthenia, fever, insomnia, pain, syncope
EENT: sinusitis, pharyngitis, otitis media, voice alteration
GI: abdominal pain, dry mouth, dyspepsia, diarrhea, gastroenteritis, nausea, oral candidiasis, taste perversion
Respiratory: respiratory tract infection, bronchospasm

NURSING CONSIDERATIONS
• Use cautiously, in patients with active or inactive tuberculosis, ocular herpes simplex, or untreated systemic fungal, bacterial, viral, or parasitic infections.
• Watch for *Candida* infections of the mouth or pharynx.

PATIENT TEACHING
• Instruct patient to use the inhaler at regular intervals because effectiveness depends on twice-daily use on a regular basis.
• Tell patient that improvement in asthma control may be seen within 24 hours, although the maximum benefit may not appear for 1 to 2 weeks. If signs or symptoms worsen during this time, instruct patient to contact prescriber.
• Advise patient to avoid exposure to chickenpox or measles and to contact prescriber if exposure occurs.
• Instruct patient to carry or wear medical identification indicating need for supplementary corticosteroids during periods of stress or an asthma attack.

dexamethasone/dexamethasone sodium phosphate

dex-a-METH-a-sone

Dexamethasone Intensol, Dexpak Taperpak
Pharmacologic class: Glucocorticoid

INDICATIONS
➤ Cerebral edema; shock
➤ Adrenocortical insufficiency
➤ Acute exacerbation of multiple sclerosis

ACTION
Unclear. Decreases inflammation, mainly by stabilizing leukocyte lysosomal membranes; suppresses immune response.

ADVERSE REACTIONS
CNS: euphoria, insomnia, psychotic behavior, pseudotumor cerebri, seizures, depression
CV: heart failure, hypertension, edema, arrhythmias, thrombophlebitis, thromboembolism
GI: peptic ulceration, increased appetite, pancreatitis
Musculoskeletal: growth suppression in children
Skin: hirsutism, delayed wound healing, acne

NURSING CONSIDERATIONS
• Most adverse reactions to corticosteroids are dose or duration dependent.
• Monitor patient for cushingoid effects.
• Diabetic patient may need increased insulin; monitor glucose levels.
• Drug may mask or worsen infections.
• Don't confuse dexamethasone with desoximetasone.

PATIENT TEACHING
• Tell patient not to stop drug abruptly or without prescriber's consent.
• Instruct patient to take drug with food or milk.
• Teach patient signs and symptoms of early adrenal insufficiency: fatigue, muscle weakness, joint pain, fever, anorexia, nausea, shortness of breath, dizziness, and fainting.
• Tell patient to avoid alcohol.

flunisolide/flunisolide hemihydrate
floo-NISS-oh-lide

Nasarel/AeroSpan HFA

Pharmacologic class: Glucocorticoid

INDICATIONS
➤ Chronic asthma
➤ Seasonal or perennial rhinitis

ACTION
A corticosteroid that may decrease inflammation of asthma by inhibiting macrophages, T cells, eosinophils, and mediators such as leukotrienes, while reducing the number of mast cells within the airway.

ADVERSE REACTIONS
CNS: headache, dizziness, fever, irritability, nervousness
CV: chest pain, edema, palpitations
EENT: nasal congestion, sore throat, altered taste, nasal irritation, nasopharyngeal fungal infections, throat irritation
GI: diarrhea, nausea, unpleasant taste, upset stomach, vomiting, abdominal pain, decreased appetite, dry mouth
Respiratory: cold symptoms, upper respiratory tract infection
Other: influenza

NURSING CONSIDERATIONS
• Store drug at room temperature.
• Don't confuse flunisolide with fluocinonide.
• Stop nasal spray after 3 weeks if symptoms don't improve.

PATIENT TEACHING
• Tell patient who also uses a bronchodilator to use it several minutes before beginning flunisolide treatment.
• Instruct patient to allow 1 minute to elapse before repeating inhalations and to hold his breath for a few seconds to enhance drug action.
• Advise patient to prevent oral fungal infections by gargling or rinsing mouth with water after each inhaler use. Caution him not to swallow the water.

fluocinonide

floo-oh-SIN-oh-nide

Lidex, Lidex-E, Vanos

Pharmacologic class: Corticosteroid

INDICATIONS
➤ Inflammation from corticosteroid-responsive dermatoses

ACTION
Unclear. Diffuses across cell membranes to form complexes with cytoplasmic receptors, showing anti-inflammatory, antipruritic, vasoconstrictive, and antiproliferative activity.

ADVERSE REACTIONS
Skin: burning, pruritus, irritation, dryness, erythema, folliculitis, hypertrichosis, hypopigmentation, acneiform eruptions, perioral dermatitis, allergic contact dermatitis, maceration, secondary infection, atrophy, striae, miliaria with occlusive dressings
Other: hypothalamic-pituitary-adrenal axis suppression, Cushing syndrome

NURSING CONSIDERATIONS
• If an occlusive dressing has been applied and a fever develops, notify prescriber and remove dressing.
• If antifungal or antibiotic combined with corticosteroid fails to provide prompt improvement, stop corticosteroid until infection is controlled.
• Systemic absorption is likely with use of occlusive dressings, prolonged treatment, or extensive body surface treatment. Watch for such symptoms as hyperglycemia, glycosuria, and hypothalamic-pituitary-adrenal axis suppression.
• Children may absorb larger amounts of drug and be more susceptible to systemic toxicity.
• Don't confuse fluocinonide with fluocinolone or fluticasone.

PATIENT TEACHING
• If an occlusive dressing is ordered, advise patient to leave it in place no more than 12 hours each day and not to use the dressing on infected or weeping lesions.
• Tell patient to stop drug and report signs of systemic absorption, skin irritation or ulceration, hypersensitivity, or infection.

fluticasone furoate/fluticasone propionate
FLOO-tih-ka-sone

Veramyst/Flonase, Flovent Diskus, Flovent HFA
Pharmacologic class: Corticosteroid

INDICATIONS
➤ Chronic asthma
➤ Nasal symptoms of seasonal and perennial allergic and nonallergic rhinitis

ACTION
Anti-inflammatory and vasoconstrictor that may decrease inflammation by inhibiting mast cells, macrophages, and mediators such as leukotrienes.

ADVERSE REACTIONS
CNS: headache, dizziness, fever, migraine, nervousness
EENT: pharyngitis, cataracts, conjunctivitis, dry eye, dysphonia, epistaxis, hoarseness, laryngitis, rhinitis, sinusitis
GI: oral candidiasis, abdominal discomfort, diarrhea, mouth irritation, nausea, viral gastroenteritis, vomiting
Metabolic: cushingoid features, growth retardation in children, hyperglycemia, weight gain
Respiratory: upper respiratory tract infection, bronchospasm, asthma symptoms, bronchitis, cough, dyspnea
Other: angioedema, influenza, viral infections

NURSING CONSIDERATIONS
• Observe patient carefully for evidence of systemic corticosteroid effects.
• Bronchospasm may occur with an immediate increase in wheezing after a dose. If bronchospasm occurs after a dose of inhalation aerosol, treat immediately with a fast-acting inhaled bronchodilator.

PATIENT TEACHING
• Tell patient that drug isn't indicated for the relief of acute bronchospasm.
• Instruct patient to contact prescriber if nasal spray doesn't improve condition after 4 days of treatment.
• Instruct patient to immediately contact prescriber if asthma episodes unresponsive to bronchodilators occur during treatment with fluticasone. During such episodes, patient may need therapy with oral corticosteroids.

hydrocortisone/hydrocortisone acetate/ hydrocortisone cypionate/hydrocortisone sodium succinate

hye-droe-KOR-ti-sone

Cortef, Cortenema/Anucort-HC, Anusol-HC, Cortifoam, Proctocort/A-Hydrocort, Solu-Cortef

Pharmacologic class: Glucocorticoid

INDICATIONS
➤ Severe inflammation, adrenal insufficiency
➤ Shock
➤ Adjunct treatment for ulcerative colitis and proctitis

ACTION
Unclear. Decreases inflammation, mainly by stabilizing leukocyte lysosomal membranes; suppresses immune response.

ADVERSE REACTIONS
CNS: euphoria, insomnia, psychotic behavior, pseudotumor cerebri, vertigo, headache, paresthesia, seizures
CV: heart failure, hypertension, edema, arrhythmias, thrombophlebitis, thromboembolism
GI: peptic ulceration, GI irritation, increased appetite, pancreatitis, nausea, vomiting
Musculoskeletal: growth suppression in children
Other: cushingoid state

NURSING CONSIDERATIONS
• Monitor patient's weight, blood pressure, and electrolyte level.
• Monitor patient for cushingoid effects.
• Drug may mask or worsen infections
• Watch for depression or psychotic episodes.
• Periodic measurement of growth and development may be needed during high-dose or prolonged therapy in children.

PATIENT TEACHING
• Tell patient not to stop drug abruptly or without prescriber's consent.
• Instruct patient to take oral form of drug with milk or food.
• Warn patient to notify prescriber about sudden weight gain or swelling.
• Teach patient signs and symptoms of early adrenal insufficiency: fatigue, muscle weakness, joint pain, fever, anorexia, nausea, shortness of breath, dizziness, and fainting.

methylPREDNISolone/methylPREDNISolone acetate/methylPREDNISolone sodium succinate

meth-ill-pred-NISS-oh-lone

Medrol, Medrol Dosepak/Depo-Medrol/A-Methapred, Solu-Medrol

Pharmacologic class: Glucocorticoid

INDICATIONS
➤ Severe inflammation or immunosuppression
➤ Shock

ACTION
Unclear. Decreases inflammation, mainly by stabilizing leukocyte lysosomal membranes; suppresses immune response.

ADVERSE REACTIONS
CNS: euphoria, insomnia, psychotic behavior, pseudotumor cerebri, vertigo, headache, paresthesia, seizures
CV: arrhythmias, heart failure, hypertension, edema, thromboembolism, cardiac arrest, circulatory collapse
GI: peptic ulceration, GI irritation, increased appetite, pancreatitis, nausea, vomiting
Musculoskeletal: growth suppression in children
Other: cushingoid state

NURSING CONSIDERATIONS
• Medrol may contain tartrazine. Watch for allergic reaction to tartrazine in patients with sensitivity to aspirin.
• Don't give Solu-Medrol intrathecally because severe adverse reactions may occur.
• Monitor patient's weight, blood pressure, electrolyte level, and sleep patterns.
• Monitor patient for cushingoid effects.
• Measure growth and development periodically in children during high-dose or prolonged treatment.
• Watch for depression or psychotic episodes.

PATIENT TEACHING
• Tell patient not to stop drug abruptly or without prescriber's consent.
• Instruct patient to take oral form of drug with milk or food.
• Teach patient signs and symptoms of early adrenal insufficiency: fatigue, muscle weakness, joint pain, fever, anorexia, nausea, shortness of breath, dizziness, and fainting.

prednisoLONE/prednisoLONE acetate/ prednisoLONE sodium phosphate

pred-NISS-oh-lone

Prelone/Flo-Pred/Orapred, Orapred ODT, Pediapred
Pharmacologic class: Glucocorticoid, mineralocorticoid

INDICATIONS
➤ Severe inflammation, immunosuppression
➤ Uncontrolled asthma
➤ Acute exacerbations of multiple sclerosis
➤ Nephrotic syndrome

ACTION
Unclear. Decreases inflammation, mainly by stabilizing leukocyte lysosomal membranes; suppresses immune response.

ADVERSE REACTIONS
CNS: euphoria, insomnia, pseudotumor cerebri, seizures, psychotic behavior, vertigo, headache, paresthesia
CV: arrhythmias, heart failure, thromboembolism, edema
GI: peptic ulceration, pancreatitis, increased appetite, nausea
Musculoskeletal: growth suppression in children
Other: acute adrenal insufficiency, susceptibility to infections, cushingoid state

NURSING CONSIDERATIONS
• Monitor patient's weight, blood pressure, and electrolyte level.
• Monitor patient for cushingoid effects.
• Watch for depression or psychotic episodes.
• Diabetic patient may need increased insulin; monitor glucose level.
• Drug may mask or worsen infections.
• Gradually reduce dosage after long-term therapy.
• Don't confuse prednisolone with prednisone.

PATIENT TEACHING
• Tell patient not to stop drug abruptly or without prescriber's consent.
• Instruct patient to take oral form of drug with food or milk.
• Teach patient signs and symptoms of early adrenal insufficiency: fatigue, muscle weakness, joint pain, fever, anorexia, nausea, shortness of breath, dizziness, and fainting.
• Tell patient to report slow healing.
• Tell patient to avoid immunizations while taking drug.

predniSONE
PRED-ni-sone

Prednisone Intensol
Pharmacologic class: Adrenocorticoid

INDICATIONS
➤ Severe inflammation, immunosuppression
➤ Contact dermatitis, poison ivy
➤ Acute exacerbations of multiple sclerosis
➤ Advanced pulmonary tuberculosis, tuberculosis meningitis

ACTION
Unclear. Decreases inflammation, mainly by stabilizing leukocyte lysosomal membranes; suppresses immune response.

ADVERSE REACTIONS
CNS: euphoria, insomnia, psychotic behavior, pseudotumor cerebri, vertigo, headache, paresthesia, seizures
CV: heart failure, hypertension, edema, arrhythmias, thrombophlebitis, thromboembolism
GI: peptic ulceration, pancreatitis, GI irritation, increased appetite, nausea, vomiting
Musculoskeletal: growth suppression in children
Other: cushingoid state, susceptibility to infections

NURSING CONSIDERATIONS
• Monitor patient's blood pressure, sleep patterns, and potassium level.
• Weigh patient daily; report sudden weight gain to prescriber.
• Monitor patient for cushingoid effects.
• Watch for depression or psychotic episodes.
• Drug may mask or worsen infections.
• Gradually reduce dosage after long-term therapy.
• Don't confuse prednisone with prednisolone or primidone.

PATIENT TEACHING
• Tell patient not to stop drug abruptly or without prescriber's consent.
• Instruct patient to take drug with food or milk.
• Teach patient signs and symptoms of early adrenal insufficiency: fatigue, muscle weakness, joint pain, fever, anorexia, nausea, shortness of breath, dizziness, and fainting.
• Warn patient to notify prescriber about sudden weight gain or swelling.

triamcinolone acetonide (topical)

trye-am-SIN-oh-lone

Kenalog, Triacet, Triderm

Pharmacologic class: Corticosteroid

INDICATIONS

➤ Inflammation and pruritus from corticosteroid-responsive dermatoses

➤ Inflammation from oral lesions

ACTION

Unclear. Diffuses across cell membranes to form complexes with cytoplasmic receptors, showing anti-inflammatory, antipruritic, vasoconstrictive, and antiproliferative activity. Considered a medium-potency (0.025% and 0.1% cream, ointment, lotion) and high-potency (0.5% cream, ointment) drug, according to vasoconstrictive properties.

ADVERSE REACTIONS

Skin: burning, pruritus, irritation, dryness, erythema, folliculitis, hypertrichosis, hypopigmentation, acneiform eruptions, dermatitis, secondary infection, atrophy, striae

Other: hypothalamic-pituitary-adrenal axis suppression, Cushing syndrome

NURSING CONSIDERATIONS

• Stop drug and tell prescriber if skin infection, striae, or atrophy occur.
• If antifungal or antibiotic combined with corticosteroid fails to provide prompt improvement, stop corticosteroid until infection is controlled.
• Systemic absorption is likely with the use of occlusive dressings, prolonged treatment, or extensive body surface treatment.
• Children may absorb larger amounts of drug and be more susceptible to systemic toxicity.

PATIENT TEACHING

• If an occlusive dressing is ordered, advise patient to leave it in place for no longer than 12 hours each day and not to use the dressing on infected or weeping lesions.
• Tell patient to stop drug and report signs of systemic absorption, skin irritation or ulceration, hypersensitivity, infection, or lack of improvement.

Digestive enzymes

Pancreatin
Pancrelipase

INDICATIONS
➤ Exocrine pancreatic secretion insufficiency; digestive aid in diseases related to deficiency of pancreatic enzymes, such as cystic fibrosis

ACTION
Replaces endogenous exocrine pancreatic enzymes and aids digestion of starches, fats, and proteins.

ADVERSE REACTIONS
Diarrhea, nausea, abdominal cramping

CONTRAINDICATIONS AND CAUTIONS
• Contraindicated in patients hypersensitive to drug, pork protein, or pork enzymes and in those with acute pancreatitis or acute worsening of chronic pancreatitis.
• Use with caution in pregnant or breast-feeding women.

pancreatin

PAN-kree-a-tin

Kutrase

Pharmacologic class: Pancreatic enzyme

INDICATIONS

➤ Exocrine pancreatic secretion insufficiency; digestive aid in diseases related to deficiency of pancreatic enzymes, such as cystic fibrosis

ACTION

Replaces endogenous exocrine pancreatic enzymes and aids digestion of starches, fats, and proteins.

ADVERSE REACTIONS

GI: diarrhea with high doses, nausea
Skin: perianal irritation
Other: allergic reactions

NURSING CONSIDERATIONS

• Antacids may counteract pancreatin's beneficial effect. Avoid using together.
• Oral iron supplement may reduce oral iron supplement level. Separate doses.
• To avoid indigestion, monitor patient's diet to ensure proper balance of fat, protein, and starch.
• Fewer bowel movements and improved stool consistency indicate effective therapy.

PATIENT TEACHING

• Instruct patient to take drug before or with meals and snacks.
• Tell patient not to crush or chew enteric-coated forms. Capsules containing enteric-coated microspheres may be opened and sprinkled on a small quantity of cool, soft food. Stress importance of swallowing immediately, without chewing, and following with a glass of water or juice.
• Warn patient not to inhale powder form or powder from capsules; it may irritate skin or mucous membranes.
• Tell patient to store drug in airtight container at room temperature.

pancrelipase

pan-kre-LYE-pase

Creon 5, Creon 10, Creon 20, Ku-Zyme HP, Lipram 4500, Lipram-CR5, Lipram-CR10, Lipram-CR20, Lipram-PN10, Lipram-PN16, Lipram-PN20, Lipram-UL12, Lipram-UL18, Lipram-L20, Pancrease, Pancrease MT4, Pancrease MT10, Pancrease MT16, Pancrease MT20, Pancrease MT4, Pancreaze MT10, Pancreaze MT16, Pancreaze MT20, Pancrecarb MS4, Pancrecarb MS8, Panokase, Plaretase 8000, Ultrase, Ultrase MT12, Ultrase MT18, Ultrase MT20, Viokase, Viokase 8, Viokase 16, Viokase Tablets

Pharmacologic class: Pancreatic enzyme

INDICATIONS

➤ Exocrine pancreatic secretion insufficiency; cystic fibrosis in adults and children; steatorrhea and other disorders of fat metabolism caused by insufficient pancreatic enzymes

ACTION

Replaces endogenous exocrine pancreatic enzymes and aids digestion of starches, fats, and proteins.

ADVERSE REACTIONS

GI: nausea, cramping, diarrhea with high doses

NURSING CONSIDERATIONS

• Antacids may counteract pancreatin's beneficial effect. Avoid using together.

• Oral iron supplement may reduce oral iron supplement level. Separate doses.

• Monitor patient's stools. Adequate replacement decreases number of bowel movements and improves stool consistency.

PATIENT TEACHING

• Instruct patient to take drug before or with meals and snacks, but always with food.

• Advise patient not to crush or chew enteric-coated forms. Capsules containing enteric-coated microspheres may be opened and sprinkled on a small quantity of cool, soft food. Stress importance of swallowing immediately, without chewing, and following with glass of water or juice.

• Warn patient not to inhale powder form or powder from capsules; it may irritate skin or mucous membranes.

Diuretics, loop

bumetanide
furosemide
torsemide

INDICATIONS
➤ Edema from heart failure, hepatic cirrhosis, or nephrotic syndrome; mild to moderate hypertension; adjunct treatment in acute pulmonary edema or hypertensive crisis

ACTION
Loop diuretics inhibit sodium and chloride reabsorption in the ascending loop of Henle, thus increasing excretion of sodium, chloride, and water. Like thiazide diuretics, loop diuretics increase excretion of potassium. Loop diuretics produce more diuresis and electrolyte loss than thiazide diuretics.

ADVERSE REACTIONS
Therapeutic dose commonly causes metabolic and electrolyte disturbances, particularly potassium depletion. It also may cause hyperglycemia, hyperuricemia, hypochloremic alkalosis, and hypomagnesemia. Rapid parenteral administration may cause hearing loss (including deafness) and tinnitus. High doses can produce profound diuresis, leading to hypovolemia and CV collapse. Photosensitivity also may occur.

CONTRAINDICATIONS AND CAUTIONS
• Contraindicated in patients hypersensitive to these drugs and in patients with anuria, hepatic coma, or severe electrolyte depletion.
• Use cautiously in patients with severe renal disease. Also use cautiously in patients with severe hypersensitivity to sulfonamides because allergic reaction may occur.
• In pregnant women, use cautiously. In breast-feeding women, don't use. In neonates, use cautiously; the usual pediatric dose can be used, but dosage intervals should be extended. In elderly patients, use a lower dose, if needed, and monitor patient closely; these patients are more susceptible to drug-induced diuresis.

bumetanide

byoo-MET-a-nide

Pharmacologic class: Loop diuretic

INDICATIONS

➤ Edema caused by heart failure or hepatic or renal disease

ACTION

Inhibits sodium and chloride reabsorption in the ascending loop of Henle.

ADVERSE REACTIONS

CNS: dizziness, headache, vertigo
CV: orthostatic hypotension
GU: oliguria
Metabolic: volume depletion and dehydration, hypokalemia, hypochloremic alkalosis, hypomagnesemia, hyperuricemia
Skin: rash, pruritus

NURSING CONSIDERATIONS

• May increase risk of digoxin toxicity from bumetanide-induced hypokalemia. Monitor potassium and digoxin levels.
• Licorice may cause unexpected, rapid potassium loss. Discourage use together.
• Monitor fluid intake and output, weight, and electrolyte, BUN, creatinine, and carbon dioxide levels frequently.
• Watch for evidence of hypokalemia, such as muscle weakness and cramps. Instruct patient to report these symptoms.

PATIENT TEACHING

• Instruct patient to take drug with food to minimize GI upset.
• Advise patient to take drug in morning to avoid need to urinate at night; if patient needs second dose, have him take it in early afternoon.
• Advise patient to avoid sudden posture changes and to rise slowly to avoid dizziness upon standing quickly.
• Instruct patient to notify prescriber about extreme thirst, muscle weakness, cramps, nausea, or dizziness.
• Instruct patient to weigh himself daily to monitor fluid status.

furosemide
fur-OH-se-mide

Lasix

Pharmacologic class: Loop diuretic

INDICATIONS
➤ Acute pulmonary edema; edema
➤ Hypertension

ACTION
Inhibits sodium and chloride reabsorption at the proximal and distal tubules and the ascending loop of Henle.

ADVERSE REACTIONS
CNS: vertigo, headache, dizziness, paresthesia
CV: orthostatic hypotension
EENT: transient deafness, blurred or yellowed vision, tinnitus
GI: abdominal discomfort and pain, pancreatitis
GU: azotemia, nocturia, polyuria, frequent urination, oliguria
Hematologic: agranulocytosis, aplastic anemia, leukopenia, thrombocytopenia, anemia
Metabolic: volume depletion and dehydration, hypokalemia, dilutional hyponatremia, hypocalcemia, hypomagnesemia
Musculoskeletal: muscle spasm
Other: gout

NURSING CONSIDERATIONS
• To avoid ototoxicity, infuse no more than 4 mg/minute.
• Monitor fluid intake and output and electrolyte, BUN, uric acid, and carbon dioxide levels frequently.
• Don't confuse furosemide with torsemide, or Lasix with Lonox, Lidex, or Luvox.

PATIENT TEACHING
• Advise patient to take drug with food to prevent GI upset, and to take drug in morning to prevent need to urinate at night.
• Instruct patient to stand slowly to prevent dizziness and to limit alcohol intake and strenuous exercise in hot weather to avoid worsening dizziness upon standing quickly.
• Advise patient to immediately report ringing in ears, severe abdominal pain, or sore throat and fever; these symptoms may indicate toxicity.

torsemide
TOR-seh-mide

Demadex
Pharmacologic class: Loop diuretic

INDICATIONS
➤ Diuresis in patients with heart failure, chronic renal failure, or hepatic cirrhosis
➤ Hypertension

ACTION
Enhances excretion of sodium, chloride, and water by acting on the ascending loop of Henle.

ADVERSE REACTIONS
CNS: asthenia, dizziness, headache, nervousness, insomnia
CV: ECG abnormalities, chest pain, orthostatic hypotension
GI: excessive thirst, diarrhea, constipation, nausea, dyspepsia
GU: excessive urination, impotence
Metabolic: electrolyte imbalances, including hypokalemia and hypomagnesemia; dehydration

NURSING CONSIDERATIONS
• Monitor fluid intake and output, electrolyte levels, blood pressure, weight, and pulse rate during rapid diuresis and routinely with long-term use. Drug can cause profound diuresis and water and electrolyte depletion.
• Watch for signs of hypokalemia, such as muscle weakness and cramps.
• Don't confuse torsemide with furosemide.

PATIENT TEACHING
• Tell patient to take drug in morning to prevent the need to urinate at night.
• Advise patient to change positions slowly to prevent dizziness and to limit alcohol intake and strenuous exercise in hot weather to prevent dizziness.
• Advise patient to immediately report ringing in ears because it may indicate toxicity.
• Tell patient to report weakness, cramping, nausea, and dizziness.

Diuretics, potassium-sparing

spironolactone

INDICATIONS
➤ Edema from hepatic cirrhosis, nephrotic syndrome, and heart failure; mild or moderate hypertension; diagnosis of primary hyperaldosteronism; metabolic alkalosis produced by thiazide and other kaliuretic diuretics; recurrent calcium nephrolithiasis; lithium-induced polyuria secondary to lithium-induced nephrogenic diabetes insipidus; aid in the treatment of hypokalemia; prophylaxis of hypokalemia in patients taking cardiac glycosides; precocious puberty and female hirsutism; adjunct to treatment of myasthenia gravis and familial periodic paralysis

ACTION
Spironolactone competitively inhibits aldosterone at the distal renal tubules, also promoting sodium excretion and potassium retention.

ADVERSE REACTIONS
Hyperkalemia is the most serious adverse reaction; it could lead to arrhythmias. Other adverse reactions include nausea, vomiting, headache, weakness, fatigue, bowel disturbances, cough, and dyspnea.

CONTRAINDICATIONS AND CAUTIONS
• Contraindicated in patients hypersensitive to spironolactone, those with a potassium level above 5.5 mEq/L, those taking other potassium-sparing diuretics or potassium supplements, and those with anuria, acute or chronic renal insufficiency, or diabetic nephropathy.
• Use cautiously in patients with severe hepatic insufficiency, because electrolyte imbalance may lead to hepatic encephalopathy, and in patients with diabetes, who are at increased risk for hyperkalemia.
• In pregnant women, no controlled studies exist. Women who wish to breast-feed should consult prescriber because drug may appear in breast milk. In children, use cautiously; they're more susceptible to hyperkalemia. In elderly and debilitated patients, observe closely and reduce dosage, if needed; they're more susceptible to drug-induced diuresis and hyperkalemia.

spironolactone

speer-on-oh-LAK-tone

Aldactone

Pharmacologic class: Potassium-sparing diuretic; aldosterone receptor antagonist

INDICATIONS
➤ Edema due to heart failure, hepatic cirrhosis, or nephrotic syndrome
➤ Hypertension
➤ Diuretic-induced hypokalemia
➤ Primary hyperaldosteronism
➤ Severe heart failure (Class III or IV)
➤ Hirsutism

ACTION
Antagonizes aldosterone in the distal tubules, increasing sodium and water excretion.

ADVERSE REACTIONS
CNS: headache, drowsiness, lethargy, confusion, ataxia
GI: diarrhea, gastric bleeding, ulceration, cramping, gastritis
Hematologic: agranulocytosis
Metabolic: hyperkalemia, dehydration, hyponatremia
Other: anaphylaxis, gynecomastia, breast soreness, drug fever

NURSING CONSIDERATIONS
• Monitor electrolyte levels, fluid intake and output, weight, and blood pressure.
• Monitor elderly patients closely, who are more susceptible to excessive diuresis.
• Maximum antihypertensive response may be delayed for up to 2 weeks.
• Don't confuse Aldactone with Aldactazide.

PATIENT TEACHING
• Instruct patient to take drug in morning to prevent need to urinate at night.
• To prevent serious hyperkalemia, warn patient to avoid excessive ingestion of potassium-rich foods (such as citrus fruits, tomatoes, bananas, dates, and apricots), salt substitutes containing potassium, and potassium supplements.
• Caution patient not to perform hazardous activities if adverse CNS reactions occur.

Diuretics, thiazide, and thiazide-like

hydrochlorothiazide
indapamide
metolazone

INDICATIONS
➤ Edema from right-sided heart failure, mild to moderate left-sided heart failure, or nephrotic syndrome; edema and ascites caused by hepatic cirrhosis; hypertension; diabetes insipidus, particularly nephrogenic diabetes insipidus

ACTION
Thiazide and thiazide-like diuretics interfere with sodium transport across the tubules of the cortical diluting segment in the nephron, thereby increasing renal excretion of sodium, chloride, water, potassium, and calcium. Thiazide diuretics also exert an antihypertensive effect. Although the exact mechanism is unknown, direct arteriolar dilation may be partially responsible. In diabetes insipidus, thiazides cause a paradoxical decrease in urine volume and an increase in renal concentration of urine, possibly because of sodium depletion and decreased plasma volume. This increases water and sodium reabsorption in the kidneys.

ADVERSE REACTIONS
Therapeutic doses cause electrolyte and metabolic disturbances, most commonly potassium depletion. Other abnormalities include elevated cholesterol levels, hypercalcemia, hyperglycemia, hyperuricemia, hypochloremic alkalosis, hypomagnesemia, and hyponatremia. Photosensitivity also may occur.

CONTRAINDICATIONS AND CAUTIONS
• Contraindicated in patients hypersensitive to these drugs and in those with anuria.
• Use cautiously in patients with severe renal disease, impaired hepatic function, or progressive liver disease.
• In pregnant women, use cautiously. In breast-feeding women, thiazides are contraindicated because they appear in breast milk. In children, safety and effectiveness haven't been established. In elderly patients, reduce dosage, if needed, and monitor patient closely; these patients are more susceptible to drug-induced diuresis.

hydrochlorothiazide

hye-droe-klor-oh-THYE-a-zide

Microzide, Oretic

Pharmacologic class: Thiazide diuretic

INDICATIONS

➤ Edema

➤ Hypertension

ACTION

Increases sodium and water excretion by inhibiting sodium and chloride reabsorption in distal segment of the nephron.

ADVERSE REACTIONS

CNS: dizziness, vertigo, headache, paresthesia, weakness

CV: orthostatic hypotension, allergic myocarditis, vasculitis

GI: pancreatitis, anorexia, nausea, vomiting, abdominal pain

GU: renal failure, polyuria, frequent urination

Hematologic: aplastic anemia, agranulocytosis, leukopenia, thrombocytopenia, hemolytic anemia

Metabolic: fluid and electrolyte imbalances

Respiratory: respiratory distress, pneumonitis

Skin: photosensitivity reactions, rash, purpura, alopecia

Other: anaphylactic reactions, hypersensitivity reactions, gout

NURSING CONSIDERATIONS

• Monitor fluid intake and output, weight, blood pressure, and electrolyte levels.

• Watch for signs and symptoms of hypokalemia, such as muscle weakness and cramps.

• Monitor creatinine and BUN levels regularly. Cumulative effects of drug may occur with impaired renal function.

• Stop thiazides and thiazide-like diuretics before parathyroid function tests.

• In patients with hypertension, therapeutic response may be delayed several weeks.

PATIENT TEACHING

• Instruct patient to take drug with food to minimize GI upset.

• Advise patient to take drug in morning to avoid need to urinate at night.

• Advise patient to avoid sudden posture changes and to rise slowly to avoid dizziness upon standing quickly.

indapamide
in-DAP-a-mide

Pharmacologic class: Thiazide-like diuretic

INDICATIONS
➤ Edema of heart failure
➤ Hypertension

ACTION
Enhances excretion of sodium chloride and water by interfering with sodium transport in the distal tubule.

ADVERSE REACTIONS
CNS: headache, nervousness, dizziness, light-headedness, numbness of limbs, irritability, agitation, lethargy
CV: orthostatic hypotension, palpitations, PVCs
GI: anorexia, nausea, vomiting, abdominal pain or cramps
GU: nocturia, polyuria, frequent urination, erectile dysfunction
Metabolic: fluid and electrolyte imbalances
Musculoskeletal: muscle cramps and spasms
Other: gout, infection

NURSING CONSIDERATIONS
• Monitor fluid intake and output, weight, blood pressure, and electrolyte levels.
• Watch for signs of hypokalemia, such as muscle weakness and cramps. Drug may be used with potassium-sparing diuretic to prevent potassium loss.
• Monitor creatinine and BUN levels regularly. Cumulative effects of drug may occur in patients with impaired renal function. Monitor uric acid level.
• Stop thiazides and thiazide-like diuretics before parathyroid function tests.
• Therapeutic response may be delayed several weeks in hypertensive patients.

PATIENT TEACHING
• Instruct patient to take drug in morning to prevent need to urinate at night.
• Tell patient to take drug with food to minimize GI upset.
• Advise patient to avoid sudden posture changes and to rise slowly to avoid dizziness upon standing quickly.

metolazone
me-TOLE-a-zone

Zaroxolyn

Pharmacologic class: Thiazide-like diuretic

INDICATIONS
➤ Edema in heart failure or renal disease
➤ Hypertension

ACTION
Increases sodium and water excretion by inhibiting sodium reabsorption in ascending loop of Henle.

ADVERSE REACTIONS
CNS: dizziness, headache, fatigue, vertigo, paresthesia, weakness, drowsiness, nervousness, blurred vision

CV: orthostatic hypotension, palpitations, vasculitis

GI: pancreatitis, anorexia, nausea, vomiting, dry mouth

GU: nocturia, polyuria, impotence

Hematologic: aplastic anemia, agranulocytosis, leukopenia

Hepatic: jaundice, hepatitis

Metabolic: fluid and electrolyte imbalances

NURSING CONSIDERATIONS
• Monitor fluid intake and output, weight, blood pressure, and electrolyte levels.

• Watch for signs and symptoms of hypokalemia, such as muscle weakness and cramps. Drug may be used with potassium-sparing diuretic to prevent potassium loss.

• Monitor blood pressure. If response is inadequate, another antihypertensive may be added.

• Unlike thiazide diuretics, metolazone is effective in patients with decreased renal function.

• Stop thiazides and thiazide-like diuretics before parathyroid function tests.

• Don't confuse Zaroxolyn with Zarontin.

PATIENT TEACHING
• Tell patient to take drug in morning to prevent need to urinate at night.

• Advise patient to avoid sudden posture changes and to rise slowly to avoid effects of dizziness upon standing quickly.

Erectile dysfunction drugs

sildenafil citrate
tadalafil
vardenafil

INDICATIONS
➤ Erectile dysfunction; pulmonary arterial hypertension (tadalafil)

ACTION
Increases CGMP levels, prolongs smooth-muscle relaxation, and promotes blood flow into the corpus cavernosum.

ADVERSE REACTIONS
Headache, dyspepsia (sildenafil citrate, tadalafil), nausea, back pain (tadalafil), flushing (vardenafil)

CONTRAINDICATIONS AND CAUTIONS
• Contraindicated in patients hypersensitive to drug or its components.
• Contraindicated in those taking nitrates and alpha blockers (tadalafil).
• Not recommended for patients with Child-Pugh category C, angina, heart failure, uncontrolled arrhythmias, hypotension, uncontrolled hypertension, stroke within the last 6 months, or MI in the last 90 days.
• Tadalafil isn't recommended for patients whose cardiac status makes sexual activity inadvisable.
• Use cautiously in patients taking potent cytochrome P-450 inhibitors (tadalafil), and with bleeding disorders, peptic ulcers, renal or hepatic impairments, or conditions that predispose them to priapism.
• Use cautiously in elderly patients who may be more sensitive to the drug. Drug isn't indicated for use in neonates, children, or women.

sildenafil citrate
sill-DEN-ah-fill

Revatio, Viagra

Pharmacologic class: Phosphodiesterase type-5 inhibitor

INDICATIONS
➤ Erectile dysfunction

ACTION
Increases cGMP levels, prolongs smooth-muscle relaxation, and promotes blood flow into the corpus cavernosum.

ADVERSE REACTIONS
CNS: headache, seizures, anxiety, dizziness, vertigo

CV: MI, sudden cardiac death, ventricular arrhythmias, cerebrovascular hemorrhage, transient ischemic attack, hypotension, flushing

EENT: diplopia, temporary vision loss, decrease or loss of hearing, tinnitus, photophobia, nasal congestion

GI: dyspepsia, diarrhea

GU: hematuria, prolonged erection, priapism, UTI

NURSING CONSIDERATIONS
• Sexual activity may increase cardiac risk. Evaluate patient's cardiac risk before he starts taking drug.

• Systemic vasodilatory properties cause transient decreases in supine blood pressure and cardiac output.

PATIENT TEACHING
• Advise patient that drug shouldn't be used with nitrates under any circumstances.

• Warn patient that erections lasting longer than 4 hours and priapism (painful erections lasting longer than 6 hours) may occur, and tell him to seek immediate medical attention.

• Inform patient that drug doesn't protect against sexually transmitted diseases.

• Instruct patient to take drug 30 minutes to 4 hours before sexual activity; maximum benefit can be expected less than 2 hours after ingestion.

• Advise patient that drug is most rapidly absorbed if taken on an empty stomach.

tadalafil
tah-DAL-ah-fill

Cialis

Pharmacologic class: Phosphodiesterase type-5 inhibitor

INDICATIONS
➤ Erectile dysfunction

ACTION
Increases cGMP levels, prolongs smooth-muscle relaxation, and promotes blood flow into the corpus cavernosum.

ADVERSE REACTIONS
CNS: dizziness, headache
CV: flushing, hypertension
EENT: decrease or loss of hearing, nasal congestion, tinnitus, nasopharyngitis
GI: dyspepsia, abdominal pain, diarrhea, gastroesophageal reflux, gastroenteritis, nausea
Musculoskeletal: back pain, limb pain, myalgia
Respiratory: bronchitis, cough, upper respiratory tract infection

NURSING CONSIDERATIONS
• Sexual activity may increase cardiac risk. Evaluate patient's cardiac risk before he starts taking drug.
• Transient decreases in supine blood pressure may occur.
• Prolonged erections and priapism may occur.

PATIENT TEACHING
• Warn patient that taking drug with nitrates could cause a serious drop in blood pressure, which increases the risk of heart attack or stroke.
• Tell patient to seek immediate medical attention if chest pain develops after taking the drug.
• Tell patient that drug doesn't protect against sexually transmitted diseases.
• Urge patient to seek emergency medical care if his erection lasts more than 4 hours.
• Tell patient to take drug about 60 minutes before anticipated sexual activity.
• Caution patient against drinking large amounts of alcohol while taking drug.
• Instruct patient to notify prescriber of vision or hearing changes.

vardenafil hydrochloride
var-DEN-ah-fill

Levitra, Staxyn
Pharmacologic class: Phosphodiesterase type-5 inhibitor

INDICATIONS
➤ Erectile dysfunction

ACTION
Increases cGMP levels, prolongs smooth-muscle relaxation, and promotes blood flow into the corpus cavernosum.

ADVERSE REACTIONS
CNS: headache, dizziness
CV: flushing
EENT: decrease or loss of hearing, tinnitus, rhinitis, sinusitis
GI: dyspepsia, nausea

NURSING CONSIDERATIONS
• Sexual activity may increase cardiac risk. Evaluate patient's cardiac risk before he starts taking drug.
• Transient decreases in supine blood pressure may occur.
• Prolonged erections and priapism may occur.

PATIENT TEACHING
• Tell patient that drug doesn't protect against sexually transmitted diseases.
• Advise patient that drug is absorbed most rapidly if taken on an empty stomach.
• Tell patient to notify prescriber about vision or hearing changes.
• Urge patient to seek immediate medical care if erection lasts more than 4 hours.
• Tell patient to take drug 60 minutes before anticipated sexual activity.
• Tell patient to stop drug and seek medical attention if he experiences sudden vision loss in one or both eyes or sudden decrease in or loss of hearing.

Estrogens

estradiol/estradiol cypionate/estradiol hemihydrate/estradiol valerate
estrogen, conjugated

INDICATIONS
➤ Prevention of moderate to severe vasomotor symptoms linked to menopause, such as hot flashes and dizziness; stimulation of vaginal tissue development, cornification, and secretory activity; inhibition of hormone-sensitive cancer growth; female hypogonadism; primary ovulation failure; ovulation control; prevention of conception

ACTION
Estrogens promote the development and maintenance of the female reproductive system and secondary sexual characteristics. They inhibit the release of pituitary gonadotropins and have various metabolic effects, including retention of fluid and electrolytes and retention and deposition in bone of calcium and phosphorus. Estrogens and estrogenic substances given as drugs can mimic the action of endogenous estrogen when used as replacement therapy and can inhibit ovulation or the growth of certain hormone-sensitive cancers.

ADVERSE REACTIONS
Adverse reactions include abdominal cramps, bloating, breast swelling and tenderness, changes in menstrual bleeding patterns, headache, loss of appetite, swollen feet or ankles, and weight gain.

CONTRAINDICATIONS AND CAUTIONS
• Contraindicated in women with thrombophlebitis or thromboembolic disorders, unexplained abnormal genital bleeding, or estrogen-dependent neoplasia.
• Use cautiously in patients with hypertension; metabolic bone disease; migraines; seizures; asthma; cardiac, renal, or hepatic impairment; or family history of breast cancer.
• In pregnant or breast-feeding women, use is contraindicated. In adolescents whose bone growth isn't complete, use cautiously because of effects on epiphyseal closure. Postmenopausal women with a history of long-term estrogen use have an increased risk of endometrial cancer and stroke. Postmenopausal women also have increased risk for breast cancer, MI, stroke, and blood clots with long-term use of estrogen plus progestin.

estradiol /estradiol cypionate/estradiol hemihydrate/estradiol valerate

ess-tra-DYE-ole

Alora, Climara, Estrace, Estrace Vaginal Cream, Estraderm, Estring Vaginal Ring, Evamist, Menostar, Vivelle, Vivelle-Dot/ Depo-Estradiol/Estrasorb, Vagifem/Delestrogen

Pharmacologic class: Estrogen

INDICATIONS

➤ Vasomotor menopausal symptoms; female hypogonadism; female castration; ovarian failure; vulvar and vaginal atrophy

➤ Palliative treatment of advanced, inoperable breast cancer or prostate cancer

ACTION

Increases synthesis of DNA, RNA, and protein in responsive tissues; reduces release of follicle-stimulating and luteinizing hormones from the pituitary gland.

ADVERSE REACTIONS

CNS: stroke, headache, dizziness, depression, seizures

CV: thromboembolism, edema, PE, MI

GI: nausea, vomiting, bloating, increased appetite, pancreatitis

GU: breakthrough bleeding, altered menstrual flow, increased risk of endometrial cancer, abnormal Pap smear, impotence

Other: gynecomastia, increased risk of breast cancer, hot flashes, breast tenderness, flu-like syndrome

NURSING CONSIDERATIONS

• Monitor lipid levels, blood pressure, body weight, and hepatic function.

• Stop therapy at least 1 month before high-risk procedures or those that cause prolonged immobilization, such as knee or hip surgery.

PATIENT TEACHING

• Warn patient to immediately report abdominal pain, pressure or pain in chest, shortness of breath, severe headaches, visual disturbances, vaginal bleeding or discharge, breast lumps, swelling of hands or feet, yellow skin or sclera, dark urine, light-colored stools, and pain, numbness, or stiffness in legs or buttocks.

• Encourage patient to stop or reduce smoking because of the risk of CV complications.

estrogens, conjugated

ESS-troe-jenz

Enjuvia, Premarin, Premarin Intravenous

Pharmacologic class: Estrogen

INDICATIONS

➤ Abnormal uterine bleeding (hormonal imbalance); vulvar or vaginal atrophy; castration and primary ovarian failure; female hypogonadism; vasomotor symptoms of menopause

➤ Palliative treatment of breast cancer or inoperable prostatic cancer

ACTION

Increases synthesis of DNA, RNA, and protein in responsive tissues. Also reduces release of follicle-stimulating and luteinizing hormones from the pituitary gland.

ADVERSE REACTIONS

CNS: headache, dizziness, chorea, depression, stroke, seizures

CV: thrombophlebitis, thromboembolism, edema, PE, MI

GI: nausea, vomiting, bloating, increased appetite, pancreatitis

GU: breakthrough bleeding, altered menstrual flow, increased risk of endometrial cancer, abnormal Pap smear, impotence

Other: breast tenderness, enlargement, or secretion; gynecomastia; increased risk of breast cancer; changes in libido

NURSING CONSIDERATIONS

• Rapid treatment of dysfunctional uterine bleeding or reduction of surgical bleeding usually requires delivery by IV or IM route.

• Stop therapy at least 1 month before procedures that prolong immobilization, such as knee or hip surgery.

• Don't confuse Premarin with Primaxin, Provera, or Remeron.

PATIENT TEACHING

• Emphasize importance of regular physical exams.

• Warn patient to immediately report abdominal pain; pain, numbness, or stiffness in legs or buttocks; pressure or pain in chest; shortness of breath; severe headaches; visual disturbances, such as blind spots, flashing lights, or blurriness; vaginal bleeding or discharge; breast lumps; swelling of hands or feet; yellow skin or sclera; dark urine; and light-colored stools.

• Encourage patient to stop smoking or reduce number of cigarettes smoked because of the risk of CV complications.

Expectorants

guaifenesin

INDICATIONS
➤ Expectorant

ACTION
Increases production of respiratory tract fluids to help liquefy and reduce the thickness, surface tension, and adhesiveness of secretions, resulting in a more productive cough to clear the airway. It also provides a soothing effect on mucous membranes and the respiratory tract.

ADVERSE REACTIONS
Dizziness, drowsiness, headache, nausea, and vomiting

CONTRAINDICATIONS AND CAUTIONS
• Contraindicated in patients hypersensitive to drug or its components.
• In pregnant and breast-feeding women, safety hasn't been established; use cautiously. Don't administer to children younger than age 6. Elderly patients are more sensitive to adverse effects.

guaifenesin (glyceryl guaiacolate)

gwye-FEN-e-sin

Allfen Jr, Altarussin, Diabetic Tussin, Ganidin NR, Guiatuss, Humibid Liquibid, Mucinex, Mucinex Mini-Melts, Naldecon Senior EX, Organidin NR, Robitussin, Scot-Tussin Expectorant, Siltussin

Pharmacologic class: Propanediol derivative

INDICATIONS
➤ Expectorant

ACTION
Increases production of respiratory tract fluids to help liquefy and reduce the viscosity of tenacious secretions.

ADVERSE REACTIONS
CNS: dizziness, headache
GI: vomiting, nausea
Skin: rash

NURSING CONSIDERATIONS
• Some liquid formulations contain alcohol.
• Drug is used to liquefy thick, tenacious sputum.
• Monitor cough type and frequency.
• Stop use 48 hours before 5-hydroxyindoleacetic acid and vanillylmandelic tests.
• Don't confuse guaifenesin with guanfacine.

PATIENT TEACHING
• Tell patient to contact his health care provider if cough lasts longer than 1 week, recurs frequently, or is accompanied by high fever, rash, or severe headache.
• Inform patient that drug shouldn't be used for chronic or persistent cough, such as with smoking, asthma, chronic bronchitis, or emphysema.
• Advise patient to take each dose with one glass of water; increasing fluid intake may prove beneficial.
• Tell patient to empty entire contents of granule packet onto the tongue and to swallow without chewing for best taste.
• Encourage deep-breathing exercises.

Fluoroquinolones

ciprofloxacin
levofloxacin

INDICATIONS
➤ Bone and joint infection, bacterial bronchitis, endocervical and urethral chlamydial infection, bacterial gastroenteritis, endocervical and urethral gonorrhea, intra-abdominal infection, empiric therapy for febrile neutropenia, pelvic inflammatory disease, bacterial pneumonia, bacterial prostatitis, acute sinusitis, skin and soft-tissue infection, typhoid fever, bacterial UTI (prevention and treatment), chancroid, meningococcal carriers, and bacterial septicemia caused by susceptible organisms

ACTION
Fluoroquinolones produce a bactericidal effect by inhibiting intracellular DNA topoisomerase II (DNA gyrase), which prevents DNA replication. These enzymes are essential catalysts in the duplication, transcription, and repair of bacterial DNA.

ADVERSE REACTIONS
Adverse reactions that are rare but need medical attention include CNS stimulation (acute psychosis, agitation, hallucinations, tremors), hepatotoxicity, hypersensitivity reactions, interstitial nephritis, phlebitis, pseudomembranous colitis, and tendinitis or tendon rupture.

CONTRAINDICATIONS AND CAUTIONS
• Contraindicated in patients hypersensitive to fluoroquinolones because serious, possibly fatal reactions can occur.
• Use cautiously in patients with known or suspected CNS disorders that predispose them to seizures or lower seizure threshold, cerebral ischemia, severe hepatic dysfunction, or renal insufficiency.
• In pregnant women, these drugs cross the placenta and may cause arthropathies. Breast-feeding isn't recommended because these drugs may cause arthropathies in newborns and infants, although it isn't known if all fluoroquinolones appear in breast milk. In children, fluoroquinolones aren't recommended because they can cause joint problems. In elderly patients, reduce dosage, if needed, because these patients are more likely to have reduced renal function.

ciprofloxacin

si-proe-FLOX-a-sin

Cipro, Cipro I.V., Cipro XR, Proquin XR
Pharmacologic class: Fluoroquinolone

INDICATIONS
➤ Intra-abdominal infection, bone or joint infection, severe respiratory tract infection, skin or skin-structure infection, UTI, infectious diarrhea, typhoid fever, pyelonephritis, nosocomial pneumonia, chronic bacterial prostatitis, acute sinusitis, inhalation anthrax (postexposure)

ACTION
Inhibits bacterial DNA synthesis, mainly by blocking DNA gyrase; bactericidal.

ADVERSE REACTIONS
CNS: seizures, confusion, headache, restlessness
GI: pseudomembranous colitis, diarrhea, nausea, vomiting
GU: crystalluria, interstitial nephritis
Hematologic: leukopenia, neutropenia, thrombocytopenia
Musculoskeletal: tendon rupture
Skin: rash, Stevens–Johnson syndrome, toxic epidermal necrolysis
Other: hypersensitivity reactions

NURSING CONSIDERATIONS
• Monitor patient's intake and output and observe patient for signs of crystalluria.

PATIENT TEACHING
• Advise patient to drink plenty of fluids to reduce risk of urine crystals.
• Instruct patient to avoid caffeine while taking drug because of potential for increased caffeine effects.
• Advise patient that hypersensitivity reactions may occur even after first dose. If a rash or other allergic reaction occurs, tell him to stop drug immediately and notify prescriber.
• Tell patient that tendon rupture can occur with drug and to notify prescriber if he experiences pain or inflammation.
• Tell patient to avoid excessive sunlight or artificial ultraviolet light during therapy.

levofloxacin
lee-voe-FLOX-a-sin

Levaquin
Pharmacologic class: Fluoroquinolone

INDICATIONS
➤ Acute bacterial sinusitis, skin and skin-structure infections, chronic bronchitis, pneumonia, chronic bacterial prostatitis, UTI, acute pyelonephritis
➤ To prevent inhalation anthrax after confirmed or suspected exposure to *Bacillus anthracis*

ACTION
Inhibits bacterial DNA gyrase and prevents DNA replication, transcription, repair, and recombination in susceptible bacteria.

ADVERSE REACTIONS
CNS: encephalopathy, seizures, dizziness, headache, insomnia
GI: pseudomembranous colitis, nausea, vomiting
Hematologic: lymphopenia, eosinophilia, hemolytic anemia
Metabolic: hypoglycemia
Musculoskeletal: back pain, tendon rupture
Skin: erythema multiforme, Stevens–Johnson syndrome, photosensitivity, pruritus, rash
Other: anaphylaxis, multisystem organ failure, hypersensitivity reactions

NURSING CONSIDERATIONS
• If patient experiences symptoms of excessive CNS stimulation, stop drug and notify prescriber. Begin seizure precautions.
• Monitor glucose level and results of renal, hepatic, and blood counts.

PATIENT TEACHING
• Advise patient to take drug with plenty of fluids and to space antacids, sucralfate, and products containing iron or zinc.
• Tell patient to take oral solution 1 hour before or 2 hours after eating.
• Instruct patient to stop drug and notify prescriber if rash or other signs or symptoms of hypersensitivity develop.
• Tell patient that tendon rupture may occur with drug and to notify prescriber if he experiences pain or inflammation.
• Instruct patient to notify prescriber of loose stools or diarrhea.

Histamine-2 (H$_2$) receptor antagonists

cimetidine
famotidine
ranitidine hydrochloride

INDICATIONS
➤Acute duodenal or gastric ulcer, Zollinger–Ellison syndrome, gastroesophageal reflux

ACTION
All H$_2$-receptor antagonists inhibit the action of H$_2$ receptors in gastric parietal cells, reducing gastric acid output and concentration, regardless of stimulants, such as histamine, food, insulin, and caffeine, or basal conditions.

ADVERSE REACTIONS
H$_2$-receptor antagonists rarely cause adverse reactions. Cardiac arrhythmias, dizziness, fatigue, gynecomastia, headache, mild and transient diarrhea, and thrombocytopenia are possible.

CONTRAINDICATIONS AND CAUTIONS
• Contraindicated in patients hypersensitive to these drugs.
• Use cautiously in patients with impaired renal or hepatic function.
• In pregnant women, use cautiously. In breast-feeding women, H$_2$-receptor antagonists are contraindicated because they may appear in breast milk. In children, safety and effectiveness haven't been established.
• Elderly patients have increased risk of adverse reactions, particularly those affecting the CNS; use cautiously.

cimetidine
sye-MET-i-deen

Acid Reducer 200, Tagamet, Tagamet HB Tagamet
Pharmacologic class: H_2-receptor antagonist

INDICATIONS
➤ Duodenal ulcer; active benign gastric ulceration; gastroesophageal reflux disease with erosive esophagitis; heartburn
➤ Pathologic hypersecretory conditions

ACTION
Competitively inhibits action of histamine on the H_2-receptor sites of parietal cells, decreasing gastric acid secretion.

ADVERSE REACTIONS
CNS: confusion, dizziness, headache, peripheral neuropathy
GI: mild and transient diarrhea
GU: impotence
Musculoskeletal: arthralgia, muscle pain
Other: mild gynecomastia, hypersensitivity reactions

NURSING CONSIDERATIONS
• Assess patient for abdominal pain. Note blood in emesis, stool, or gastric aspirate.
• Wait at least 15 minutes after giving tablet before drawing sample for Hemoccult or Gastroccult test, and follow test manufacturer's instructions closely.
• Don't confuse cimetidine with simethicone.

PATIENT TEACHING
• Remind patient taking drug once daily to take it at bedtime and to take multiple daily doses with meals.
• Urge patient to avoid cigarette smoking because it may increase gastric acid secretion and worsen disease.
• Advise patient to report abdominal pain, blood in stools or emesis, black tarry stools, and coffee-ground emesis.

famotidine
fa-MOE-ti-deen

Pepcid, Pepcid AC
Pharmacologic class: H_2-receptor antagonist

INDICATIONS
➤ Duodenal ulcer, benign gastric ulcer, gastroesophageal reflux disease, heartburn
➤ Pathologic hypersecretory conditions

ACTION
Competitively inhibits action of histamine on the H_2-receptor sites of parietal cells, decreasing gastric acid secretion.

ADVERSE REACTIONS
CNS: headache, dizziness, fever, malaise, paresthesia, vertigo
CV: flushing, palpitations
EENT: orbital edema, tinnitus
GI: anorexia, constipation, diarrhea, dry mouth, taste perversion
Musculoskeletal: bone and muscle pain
Skin: acne, dry skin
Other: transient irritation at I.V. site

NURSING CONSIDERATIONS
• Assess patient for abdominal pain.
• Look for blood in emesis, stool, or gastric aspirate.

PATIENT TEACHING
• Warn patient with phenylketonuria that Pepcid AC chewable tablets contain phenylalanine.
• Tell patient to take prescription drug with a snack, if desired.
• Urge patient to avoid cigarette smoking because it may increase gastric acid secretion and worsen disease.
• Advise patient to report abdominal pain, blood in stools or vomit, black tarry stools, or coffee-ground emesis.

ranitidine hydrochloride
ra-NYE-te-deen

Zantac, Zantac 75, Zantac 150, Zantac 300
Pharmacologic class: H$_2$-receptor antagonist

INDICATIONS
➤ Active duodenal and gastric ulcer, gastroesophageal reflux disease, erosive esophagitis, heartburn
➤ Pathologic hypersecretory conditions

ACTION
Competitively inhibits action of histamine on the H$_2$-receptor sites of parietal cells, decreasing gastric acid secretion.

ADVERSE REACTIONS
CNS: headache, malaise, vertigo
EENT: blurred vision
Hepatic: jaundice
Other: anaphylaxis, angioedema, burning and itching at injection site

NURSING CONSIDERATIONS
• Assess patient for abdominal pain. Note presence of blood in emesis, stool, or gastric aspirate.
• Drug may be added to total parenteral nutrition solutions.
• Don't confuse ranitidine with rimantadine; don't confuse Zantac with Xanax or Zyrtec.

PATIENT TEACHING
• Instruct patient to take without regard to meals because absorption isn't affected by food.
• Urge patient to avoid cigarette smoking because this may increase gastric acid secretion and worsen disease.
• Advise patient to report abdominal pain, blood in stool or emesis, black tarry stools, or coffee-ground emesis.

Hypnotics

eszopiclone
temazepam
zalepion
zolpidem tartrate

INDICATIONS
➤ Insomnia

ACTION
Probably interacts with GABA receptors at binding sites close or connected to benzodiazepine receptors. Probably acts on the limbic system, thalamus, and hypothalamus of the CNS to produce hypnotic effects (temazepam). Exhibits hypnotic activity and minimal muscle relaxant and anticonvulsive properties (zolpidem tartrate).

ADVERSE REACTIONS
Headache, somnolence, unpleasant taste (eszopiclone); respiratory tract infection (eszopiclone)

CONTRAINDICATIONS AND CAUTIONS
• Use cautiously in elderly and debilitated patients, and in patients with diseases or conditions that may affect metabolism or hemodynamic responses (eszopiclone), or breast-feeding women (zalepion).
• Use cautiously in patients with compromised respiratory function or severe hepatic impairment.
• Use cautiously in patients with signs and symptoms of depression (eszopiclone and temazepam).
• Contraindicated in pregnant patients and those hypersensitive to drug or other benzodiazepines (temazepam).
• Strongly consider discontinuing drug if the patient reports events such as "sleep driving" (driving when not fully awake with subsequent event amnesia) (zolpidem tartrate).

eszopiclone
ess-ZOP-ah-klone

Lunesta

Pharmacologic class: Pyrrolopyrazine derivative

INDICATIONS
➤ Insomnia

ACTION
Probably interacts with GABA receptors at binding sites close or connected to benzodiazepine receptors.

ADVERSE REACTIONS
CNS: abnormal dreams, anxiety, complex sleep-related behavior, confusion, decreased libido, depression, dizziness, headache, nervousness, pain, somnolence, neuralgia
EENT: unpleasant taste
GI: diarrhea, dry mouth, dyspepsia, nausea, vomiting
Respiratory: respiratory tract infection
Skin: pruritus, rash
Other: anaphylaxis, angioedema, accidental injury

NURSING CONSIDERATIONS
• Anaphylaxis and angioedema may occur as early as the first dose; monitor the patient closely.
• Give drug immediately before patient goes to bed or after patient has gone to bed and has trouble falling asleep.
• Use only for short periods (for example, 7 to 10 days).
• Monitor patient for changes in behavior, including those that suggest depression or suicidal thinking.

PATIENT TEACHING
• Warn patient that drug may cause allergic reactions, facial swelling, and complex sleep-related behaviors, such as driving, eating, and making phone calls while asleep. Advise patient to report these adverse effects.
• Urge patient to take drug immediately before going to bed and not to take drug unless he can get a full night's sleep.
• Advise patient to avoid taking drug after a high-fat meal.
• Advise patient to avoid alcohol while taking drug.
• Urge patient to immediately report changes in behavior and thinking.
• Warn patient not to stop drug abruptly or change dose without consulting the prescriber.

temazepam

te-MAZ-e-pam

Restoril

Pharmacologic class: Benzodiazepine

INDICATIONS
➤ Short-term treatment (7 to 10 days) of insomnia

ACTION
Probably acts on the limbic system, thalamus, and hypothalamus of the CNS to produce hypnotic effects.

ADVERSE REACTIONS
CNS: complex sleep-related behaviors, drowsiness, dizziness, lethargy, disturbed coordination, daytime sedation, confusion, nightmares, vertigo, euphoria, weakness, headache, fatigue, nervousness, anxiety, depression
EENT: blurred vision
GI: diarrhea, nausea, dry mouth
Other: anaphylaxis, angioedema, physical and psychological dependence

NURSING CONSIDERATIONS
• Monitor patient closely. Anaphylaxis and angioedema may occur as early as the first dose.
• Don't stop drug abruptly as this may cause withdrawal symptoms (cramps, seizures, tremor, and sweating). To discontinue drug, follow a gradual dosage-tapering schedule.
• Don't confuse Restoril with Vistaril.

PATIENT TEACHING
• Warn patient that drug may cause allergic reactions, facial swelling, and complex sleep-related behaviors, such as driving, eating, and making phone calls while asleep. Advise patient to report these adverse effects.
• Tell patient to avoid alcohol during therapy.
• Caution patient to avoid performing activities that require mental alertness or physical coordination.
• Warn patient not to stop drug abruptly if taken for 1 month or longer.
• Tell patient that onset of drug's effects may take as long as 2 to 2¼ hours.

zalepion
ZAL-ah-pion

Sonata
Pharmacologic class: Pyrazolopyrimidine

INDICATIONS
➤ Short-term treatment (7 to 10 days) of insomnia

ACTION
A hypnotic with chemical structure unrelated to benzodiazepines that interacts with the GABA-benzodiazepine receptor complex in the CNS. Modulation of this complex is thought to be responsible for sedative, anxiolytic, muscle relaxant, and anticonvulsant effects of benzodiazepines.

ADVERSE REACTIONS
CNS: complex sleep-related behaviors, headache, amnesia, anxiety, depression, difficulty concentrating, dizziness, malaise, nervousness, paresthesia, somnolence, tremor, vertigo
CV: chest pain, peripheral edema
EENT: abnormal vision, conjunctivitis, ear discomfort, epistaxis, eye discomfort, hyperacusis, smell alteration
GI: abdominal pain, constipation, dry mouth, dyspepsia, nausea.
Other: anaphylaxis, angioedema.

NURSING CONSIDERATIONS
• Monitor patient closely. Anaphylaxis and angioedema may occur as early as the first dose.
• Give immediately before bedtime or after patient has gone to bed and has had difficulty falling asleep.

PATIENT TEACHING
• Warn patient that drug may cause allergic reactions, facial swelling, and complex sleep-related behaviors, such as driving, eating, and making phone calls while asleep. Advise patient to report these adverse effects.
• Advise patient to take the drug immediately before bedtime or after he has gone to bed and has had trouble falling asleep.
• Advise patient to take drug only if he will be able to sleep for at least 4 undisturbed hours.
• Advise patient to avoid performing activities that require mental alertness until CNS adverse reactions are known.
• Advise patient to avoid alcohol use while taking drug.
• Tell patient not to take drug after a high-fat or heavy meal.

zolpidem tartrate

ZOL-pih-dem

Ambien, Ambien CR, Edluar, Zolpimist
Pharmacologic class: Imidazopyridine

INDICATIONS
➤ Short-term management of insomnia

ACTION
Although drug interacts with one of three identified GABA-benzodiazepine receptor complexes, it isn't a benzodiazepine. It exhibits hypnotic activity and minimal muscle relaxant and anticonvulsant properties.

ADVERSE REACTIONS
CNS: headache, amnesia, change in dreams, complex sleep-related behaviors, daytime drowsiness, depression, dizziness, hangover, nervousness, sleep disorder
GI: dry mouth, dyspepsia, nausea, vomiting
Other: anaphylaxis, angioedema, back or chest pain, flulike syndrome, hypersensitivity reactions

NURSING CONSIDERATIONS
• Anaphylaxis and angioedema may occur as early as the first dose. Monitor patient closely.
• Use drug only for short-term management of insomnia, usually 7 to 10 days.
• Don't confuse Ambien with Amen.

PATIENT TEACHING
• Warn patient that drug may cause allergic reactions, facial swelling, and complex sleep-related behaviors, such as driving, eating, and making phone calls while asleep. Advise patient to report these adverse effects.
• Instruct patient to take drug immediately before going to bed.
• Tell patient to avoid alcohol use while taking drug.
• Tell patient to place the S.L. tablet under the tongue and allow the tablet to disintegrate. Tell the patient not to swallow, chew, break, or split the tablet, or take the tablet with water.
• Tell patient to aim the spray directly over the tongue and press down fully to make sure the full dose is delivered.
• Caution patient to avoid performing activities that require mental alertness or physical coordination during therapy.

Inotropics

digoxin

INDICATIONS
➤ Heart failure and supraventricular arrhythmias, including supraventricular tachycardia, atrial fibrillation, and atrial flutter

ACTION
Inotropics help move calcium into the cells, which increases cardiac output by strengthening contractility. Digoxin also acts on the central nervous system to slow heart rate.

ADVERSE REACTIONS
Inotropics may cause arrhythmias, nausea, vomiting, diarrhea, headache, fever, mental disturbances, visual changes, and chest pain.

CONTRAINDICATIONS AND CAUTIONS
• Contraindicated in patients hypersensitive to any of the drug components.
• Digoxin is contraindicated in ventricular fibrillation.
• Use digoxin cautiously in patients with renal insufficiency because of the potential for digoxin toxicity. Use digoxin cautiously in patients with sinus node disease or AV block because of the potential for advanced heart block.

digoxin
di-JOX-in

Lanoxicaps, Lanoxin
Pharmacologic class: Cardiac glycoside

INDICATIONS
➤ Heart failure, paroxysmal supraventricular tachycardia, atrial fibrillation and flutter

ACTION
Inhibits sodium potassium–activated ADT, promoting movement of calcium from extracellular to intracellular cytoplasm and strengthening myocardial contraction. Enhances vagal tone, slowing conduction through the SA and AV nodes.

ADVERSE REACTIONS
CNS: agitation, fatigue, generalized muscle weakness, hallucinations, dizziness, headache, stupor, vertigo
CV: arrhythmias, heart block
EENT: blurred vision, diplopia, light flashes, photophobia, yellow-green halos around visual images
GI: anorexia, nausea, diarrhea, vomiting

NURSING CONSIDERATIONS
• Monitor digoxin level. Therapeutic level ranges from 0.8 to 2 nanogram/ml. Obtain blood at least 6 to 8 hours after last oral dose, preferably just before next scheduled dose.
• In children, cardiac arrhythmias, including sinus bradycardia, are usually early signs of toxicity.
• Toxic effects on the heart may be life-threatening and require immediate attention.
• Excessively slow pulse rate (60 beats/minute or less) may be a sign of digitalis toxicity. Withhold drug and notify prescriber.
• Monitor potassium level carefully.

PATIENT TEACHING
• Tell patient to report pulse less than 60 beats/minute or more than 110 beats/minute, or skipped beats or other rhythm changes.
• Instruct patient to report adverse reactions promptly. Nausea, vomiting, diarrhea, appetite loss, and visual disturbances may be indicators of toxicity.
• Encourage patient to eat a consistent amount of potassium-rich foods.

Laxatives

bisacodyl
docusate calcium/docusate sodium
lactulose

INDICATIONS
➤ Constipation, irritable bowel syndrome, diverticulosis

ACTION
Laxatives promote movement of intestinal contents through the colon and rectum in several ways: bulk-forming, emollient, hyperosmolar, and stimulant.

ADVERSE REACTIONS
All laxatives may cause flatulence, diarrhea, and abdominal disturbances. Bulk-forming laxatives may cause intestinal obstruction, impaction, or (rarely) esophageal obstruction.

Emollient laxatives may irritate the throat. Hyperosmolar laxatives may cause fluid and electrolyte imbalances. Stimulant laxatives may cause urine discoloration, malabsorption, and weight loss.

CONTRAINDICATIONS AND CAUTIONS
• Contraindicated in patients with GI obstruction or perforation, toxic colitis, megacolon, nausea and vomiting, or acute surgical abdomen.
• Use cautiously in patients with rectal or anal conditions, such as rectal bleeding or large hemorrhoids.
• For pregnant women and breast-feeding women, recommendations vary for individual drugs. Infants and children have an increased risk of fluid and electrolyte disturbances; use cautiously. In elderly patients, dependence is more likely to develop because of age-related changes in GI function. Monitor these patients closely.

bisacodyl
bye-suh-KOH-dil

Bisac-Evac, Bisa-Lax, Correctol, Dulcolax, Ex-Lax Ultra, Feen-a-Mint, Fleet Bisacodyl, Fleet Bisacodyl Enema, Fleet Laxative

Pharmacologic class: Diphenylmethane derivative

INDICATIONS
➤ Chronic constipation; preparation for childbirth, surgery, or rectal or bowel examination

ACTION
Unknown. Stimulant laxative that increases peristalsis, probably by direct effect on smooth muscle of the intestine, by irritating the muscle or stimulating the colonic intramural plexus. Drug also promotes fluid accumulation in colon and small intestine.

ADVERSE REACTIONS
CNS: dizziness, faintness, muscle weakness with excessive use
GI: abdominal cramps, burning sensation in rectum with suppositories, nausea, vomiting, diarrhea with high doses
Metabolic: fluid and electrolyte imbalance, hypokalemia

NURSING CONSIDERATIONS
• Give drug at times that don't interfere with scheduled activities or sleep. Soft, formed stools are usually produced 15 to 60 minutes after rectal use.
• Before giving for constipation, determine whether patient has adequate fluid intake, exercise, and diet.
• Tablets and suppositories are used together to clean the colon before and after surgery and before barium enema.

PATIENT TEACHING
• Advise patient to swallow enteric-coated tablet whole to avoid GI irritation. Instruct him not to take within 1 hour of milk or antacid.
• Teach patient about dietary sources of bulk, including bran and other cereals, fresh fruit, and vegetables.
• Tell patient to take drug with a full glass of water or juice.

docusate calcium/docusate sodium

DOK-yoo-sayt

DC Softgels, Surfak/Colace, Dulcolax Stool Softener, Ex-Lax Stool Softener Caplets, Phillips' Liqui-Gels, Regulax SS

Pharmacologic class: Surfactant

INDICATIONS

➤ Stool softener

ACTION

Stool softener that reduces surface tension of interfacing liquid contents of the bowel. This detergent activity promotes incorporation of additional liquid into stools, thus forming a softer mass.

ADVERSE REACTIONS

GI: bitter taste, mild abdominal cramping, diarrhea
Other: laxative dependence with long-term or excessive use

NURSING CONSIDERATIONS

• Drug isn't used to treat existing constipation but prevents constipation from developing.
• Give liquid (not syrups) in milk, fruit juice, or infant formula to mask bitter taste.
• Before giving drug, determine whether patient has adequate fluid intake, exercise, and diet.
• Drug is laxative of choice for patients who shouldn't strain during defecation, including patients recovering from MI or rectal surgery, those with rectal or anal disease that makes passage of firm stools difficult, and those with postpartum constipation.

PATIENT TEACHING

• Teach patient about dietary sources of fiber, including bran and other cereals, fresh fruit, and vegetables.
• Instruct patient to use drug only occasionally and not for longer than 1 week without prescriber's knowledge.
• Tell patient to stop drug and notify prescriber if severe cramping occurs.
• Notify patient that it may take from 1 to 3 days to soften stools.

lactulose
LAK-tyoo-lose

Cephulac, Constulose, Enulose, Kristalose
Pharmacologic class: Disaccharide

INDICATIONS
➤ Constipation
➤ To prevent and treat hepatic encephalopathy, including hepatic precoma and coma in patients with severe hepatic disease

ACTION
Produces an osmotic effect in colon; resulting distention promotes peristalsis. Also decreases ammonia, probably as a result of bacterial degradation, which lowers the pH of colon contents.

ADVERSE REACTIONS
GI: abdominal cramps, belching, diarrhea, flatulence, gaseous distention, nausea, vomiting

NURSING CONSIDERATIONS
• To minimize sweet taste, dilute with water or fruit juice or give with food.
• Prepare enema (not commercially available) by adding 200 g (300 ml) to 700 ml of water or normal saline solution. The diluted solution is given as retention enema for 30 to 60 minutes. Use a rectal balloon. If enema isn't retained for at least 30 minutes, repeat dose.
• Monitor sodium level for hypernatremia, especially when giving in higher doses to treat hepatic encephalopathy.
• Monitor mental status and potassium levels when giving to patients with hepatic encephalopathy.
• Replace fluid loss.
• Don't confuse lactulose with lactose.

PATIENT TEACHING
• Show home care patient how to mix and use drug.
• Inform patient about adverse reactions and tell him to notify prescriber if reactions become bothersome or if diarrhea occurs.
• Instruct patient not to take other laxatives during lactulose therapy.

Macrolide anti-infectives

azithromycin
clarithromycin
erythromycin/erythromycin ethylsuccinate/erythromycin lactobionate/erythromycin stearate

INDICATIONS
➤ Various common infections

ACTION
Inhibit RNA-dependent protein synthesis by acting on a small portion of the 50S ribosomal unit.

ADVERSE REACTIONS
These drugs may cause nausea, vomiting, diarrhea, abdominal pain, palpitations, chest pain, vaginal candidiasis, nephritis, dizziness, headache, vertigo, somnolence, rash, and photosensitivity.

CONTRAINDICATIONS AND CAUTIONS
• Contraindicated in patients hypersensitive to any of the drug components.
• Contraindicated in patients with concomitant use of terfenadine, astemizole, or cisapride due to the potential for cardiac arrhythmias. These drugs also have the potential to cause many other drug interactions when given with other drugs; screen carefully.

azithromycin
ay-zi-thro-MY-sin

Zithromax, Zmax
Pharmacologic class: Macrolide

INDICATIONS
➤ Skin and skin-structure infections, community-acquired pneumonia, acute bacterial sinusitis, chancroid, nongonococcal urethritis or cervicitis, pelvic inflammatory disease, otitis media, pharyngitis, tonsillitis

ACTION
Binds to the 50S subunit of bacterial ribosomes, blocking protein synthesis; bacteriostatic or bactericidal, depending on concentration.

ADVERSE REACTIONS
CNS: fatigue, headache, somnolence
CV: chest pain, palpitations
GI: abdominal pain, anorexia, diarrhea, nausea, vomiting, pseudomembranous colitis, dyspepsia, flatulence, melena
GU: candidiasis, nephritis, vaginitis
Hepatic: cholestatic jaundice
Skin: photosensitivity reactions, rash, pain at injection site, pruritus
Other: angioedema

NURSING CONSIDERATIONS
• Obtain specimen for culture and sensitivity tests before giving first dose. Begin therapy while awaiting results.
• Give Zmax 1 hour before or 2 hours after a meal. Don't give with antacids.
• Monitor patient for superinfection.
• If patient vomits within 60 minutes of taking Zmax, notify prescriber; additional or different therapy may be needed.

PATIENT TEACHING
• Advise patient to avoid excessive sunlight and to wear protective clothing and use sunscreen when outside.
• Tell patient to report adverse reactions promptly.

clarithromycin

klar-ITH-ro-my-sin

Biaxin, Biaxin XL

Pharmacologic class: Macrolide

INDICATIONS

➤ Pharyngitis or tonsillitis; acute maxillary sinusitis; acute worsening of chronic bronchitis; community-acquired pneumonia; uncomplicated skin and skin-structure infections; acute otitis media

➤ *Helicobacter pylori*, to reduce risk of duodenal ulcer recurrence

ACTION

Binds to the 50S subunit of bacterial ribosomes, blocking protein synthesis; bacteriostatic or bactericidal, depending on concentration.

ADVERSE REACTIONS

CNS: headache

GI: pseudomembranous colitis, abdominal pain or discomfort, diarrhea, nausea, taste perversion, vomiting (in children)

Hematologic: coagulation abnormalities

Skin: rash (in children)

NURSING CONSIDERATIONS

• Obtain specimen for culture and sensitivity tests before giving. Begin therapy while awaiting results.

• Grapefruit juice may inhibit metabolism, increasing adverse effects. Don't take with grapefruit juice.

• Use cautiously in patients with hepatic or renal impairment.

• Monitor patient for superinfection.

• Giving clarithromycin with a drug metabolized by CYP3A may increase drug levels and prolong therapeutic and adverse effects.

PATIENT TEACHING

• Advise patient to report persistent adverse reactions.

• Inform patient that drug may be taken with or without food.

erythromycin/erythromycin ethylsuccinate/ erythromycin lactobionate/erythromycin stearate

er-ith-roe-MYE-sin

E-Mycin, Eryc, Ery-Tab/E.E.S., EryPed/Erythrocin Lactobionate/ Erythrocin Stearate

Pharmacologic class: Macrolide

INDICATIONS

➤ Acute pelvic inflammatory disease; intestinal amebiasis; respiratory tract, skin, or soft-tissue infection; nongonococcal urethritis; Legionnaires' disease; uncomplicated urethral, endocervical, or rectal infection; pertussis; primary syphilis

ACTION

Inhibits bacterial protein synthesis by binding to the 50S subunit of the ribosome; bacteriostatic or bactericidal, depending on concentration.

ADVERSE REACTIONS

CNS: fever
CV: vein irritation or thrombophlebitis after I.V. injection, ventricular arrhythmias
GI: pseudomembranous colitis, abdominal pain and cramping, diarrhea, nausea, vomiting
Hepatic: hepatocellular or cholestatic hepatitis
Skin: eczema, rash, urticaria
Other: anaphylaxis, overgrowth of nonsusceptible bacteria or fungi

NURSING CONSIDERATIONS

• Obtain specimen for culture and sensitivity tests before giving. Begin therapy while awaiting results.
• For I.V. administration, dilute each 250 mg in at least 100 ml of normal saline solution. Infuse over 1 hour.
• Monitor patient for superinfection. Drug may cause overgrowth of nonsusceptible bacteria or fungi.
• Monitor hepatic function. Drug may cause hepatotoxicity.

PATIENT TEACHING

• Instruct patient to take oral form of drug with full glass of water 2 hours before or 2 hours after meals for best absorption.
• Drug may be taken with food if GI upset occurs. Tell patient not to take drug with fruit juice or to swallow the chewable tablets whole.

Nitrates

isosorbide dinitrate/isosorbide mononitrate
nitroglycerin

INDICATIONS
➤ To prevent or minimize anginal attacks; hypertension from surgery; heart failure after MI; angina pectoris in acute situations; to produce controlled hypotension during surgery (nitroglycerin)

ACTION
Nitrates cause the smooth muscle of veins and, to a lesser extent, the arteries to relax and dilate. When the veins dilate, less blood returns to the heart. This, in turn, reduces the amount of blood in the ventricles at the end of diastole, when the ventricles are full (preload). By reducing preload, nitrates reduce ventricular size and wall tension (the left ventricle doesn't have to stretch as much to pump blood). This, in turn, reduces the oxygen requirements of the heart. Nitrates also decrease afterload by dilating the arterioles, reducing resistance, easing the heart's workload, and easing the demand for oxygen.

ADVERSE REACTIONS
Headache is the most common adverse reaction. Hypotension may occur, accompanied by dizziness and increased heart rate.

CONTRAINDICATIONS AND CAUTIONS
• Contraindicated in patients with hypersensitivity or idiosyncrasy to nitrates and in those with severe hypotension, angle-closure glaucoma, increased intracranial pressure, shock, or acute MI with low left ventricular filling pressure.
• Use cautiously in patients with blood volume depletion (such as from diuretic therapy) or mild hypotension.
• I.V. nitroglycerin is contraindicated in patients hypersensitive to I.V. form, with cardiac tamponade, restrictive cardiomyopathy, or constrictive pericarditis.

isosorbide dinitrate/isosorbide mononitrate

eye-soe-SOR-bide

Dilatrate-SR, Isordil, Titradose/ISMO, Monoket

Pharmacologic class: Nitrate

INDICATIONS

➤ Acute anginal attacks (S.L. isosorbide dinitrate only); to prevent situations that may cause anginal attacks

ACTION

Reduces cardiac oxygen demand by decreasing preload and afterload. Increases blood flow through the coronary vessels.

ADVERSE REACTIONS

CNS: headache, dizziness, weakness
CV: orthostatic hypotension, tachycardia, palpitations, ankle edema, flushing, fainting
Skin: cutaneous vasodilation, rash

NURSING CONSIDERATIONS

• Monitor blood pressure and heart rate and intensity and duration of drug response.
• Don't confuse Isordil with Isuprel or Inderal.

PATIENT TEACHING

• Tell patient to take S.L. tablet at first sign of attack. He should wet tablet with saliva and place under his tongue until absorbed; he should sit down and rest. Dose may be repeated every 10 to 15 minutes for a maximum of three doses. If drug doesn't provide relief, tell patient to seek medical help promptly.
• Advise patient taking P.O. form of isosorbide dinitrate to take oral tablet on an empty stomach either 30 minutes before or 1 to 2 hours after meals and to swallow oral tablets whole.
• Tell patient to minimize dizziness upon standing up by changing to upright position slowly. Advise him to go up and down stairs carefully and to lie down at first sign of dizziness.
• Caution patient to avoid alcohol because it may worsen low blood pressure effects.

nitroglycerin

nye-troe-GLIH-ser-in

Nitro-Dur, NitroMist, Nitrostat

Pharmacologic class: Nitrate

INDICATIONS

➤ Acute angina pectoris

➤ Hypertension from surgery; heart failure after MI; angina pectoris in acute situations; to produce controlled hypotension during surgery (by I.V. infusion)

ACTION

Reduces cardiac oxygen demand by decreasing preload and afterload. Increases blood flow through the coronary vessels.

ADVERSE REACTIONS

CNS: headache, dizziness, syncope, weakness

CV: orthostatic hypotension, tachycardia, flushing, palpitations

Skin: cutaneous vasodilation, contact dermatitis, rash

NURSING CONSIDERATIONS

• Monitor blood pressure and intensity and duration of drug response.

• Wipe off nitroglycerin paste or remove patch before defibrillation to avoid patient burns.

• Don't confuse nitroglycerin with nitroprusside.

PATIENT TEACHING

• Tell patient to take S.L. tablet at first sign of attack. Patient should wet the tablet with saliva, place it under tongue until absorbed, and then sit down and rest. Dose may be repeated every 5 minutes for a maximum of three doses. If drug doesn't provide relief, he should obtain medical help promptly.

• Tell patient to take oral tablets on an empty stomach either 30 minutes before or 1 to 2 hours after meals, to swallow oral tablets whole, and not to chew tablets.

• Remind patient using translingual aerosol form that he shouldn't inhale the spray but should release it onto or under the tongue and wait about 10 seconds or so before swallowing.

• Advise patient to avoid alcohol.

• To minimize dizziness when standing up, tell patient to rise slowly. Advise him to go up and down stairs carefully and to lie down at the first sign of dizziness.

Nonopioid analgesics

acetaminophen
tramadol

INDICATIONS
➤ Mild pain or fever (acetaminophen), moderate to moderately severe chronic pain (tramadol)

ACTION
The pain-control effects aren't completely understood, but it's thought to produce analgesia by inhibiting prostaglandin and other substances that sensitize pain receptors (acetaminophen) or bind to opioid receptors and inhibit reuptake of norepinephrine and serotonin (tramadol). It may relieve fever through central action in the hypothalamic heat-regulating center (acetaminophen).

ADVERSE REACTIONS
Rash, hypoglycemia, neutropenia (acetaminophen), dizziness, headache, somnolence, vertigo, constipation, nausea and vomiting (tramadol)

CONTRAINDICATIONS AND CAUTIONS
• Contraindicated in patients with hypersensitivity to drug.
• Use cautiously in patients with any type of liver disease and patients with long-term alcohol use.
• Use cautiously in patients taking tranquilizers or antidepressants, or who suffer from depression or emotional disturbances (tramadol).
• Use cautiously in patients at risk for seizures or respiratory depression, or patients with increased intracranial pressure or head injury or acute abdominal conditions, or patients with physical dependence on opioids (tramadol).

acetaminophen

a-seet-a-MIN-a-fen

Aminofen, Aspirin Free Anacin, FeverAll, Tylenol, Valorin

Pharmacologic class: Para-aminophenol derivative

INDICATIONS

➤ Mild pain or fever

ACTION

Thought to produce analgesia by inhibiting prostaglandin and other substances that sensitize pain receptors. Drug may relieve fever through central action in the hypothalamic heat-regulating center.

ADVERSE REACTIONS

Hematologic: hemolytic anemia, leukopenia, neutropenia, pancytopenia

Hepatic: jaundice

Metabolic: hypoglycemia

Skin: rash, urticaria

NURSING CONSIDERATIONS

• Use liquid form for children and patients who have difficulty swallowing.
• If suppository is too soft, refrigerate for 15 minutes or run under cold water in wrapper.
• Many OTC and prescription products contain acetaminophen; be aware of this when calculating total daily dose.
• In children, don't exceed five doses in 24 hours.

PATIENT TEACHING

• Tell parents to consult prescriber before giving drug to children younger than age 2.
• Warn patient that high doses or unsupervised long-term use can cause liver damage. Excessive alcohol use may increase the risk of liver damage.
• Tell breast-feeding women that drug appears in breast milk in low levels (< 1% of dose). Drug may be used safely if therapy is short-term and doesn't exceed recommended doses.

tramadol hydrochloride
TRAM-uh-dohl

Rybix ODT, Ryzolt, Ultram, Ultram ER
Pharmacologic class: Synthetic, centrally active analgesic

INDICATIONS
➤ Moderate to moderately severe chronic pain

ACTION
Unknown. Thought to bind to opioid receptors and inhibit reuptake of norepinephrine and serotonin.

ADVERSE REACTIONS
CNS: dizziness, headache, somnolence, vertigo, seizures, CNS stimulation, confusion, coordination disturbance
EENT: visual disturbances
GI: constipation, nausea, vomiting, abdominal pain, anorexia
Respiratory: respiratory depression
Skin: diaphoresis, pruritus, rash

NURSING CONSIDERATIONS
• Reassess patient's level of pain at least 30 minutes after administration.
• Monitor CV and respiratory status. Withhold dose and notify prescriber if respirations are shallow or rate is below 12 breaths/minute.
• Monitor patients at risk for seizures. Drug may reduce seizure threshold.
• Withdrawal symptoms may occur if drug is stopped abruptly. Reduce dosage gradually.
• Don't confuse tramadol with trazodone or trandolapril.

PATIENT TEACHING
• Caution ambulatory patient to be careful when rising and walking. Warn outpatient to avoid driving and other potentially hazardous activities that require mental alertness until drug's CNS effects are known.

Nonsteroidal anti-inflammatory drugs

aspirin
celecoxib
diclofenac epolamine/diclofenac potassium/diclofenac sodium
etodolac
ibuprofen
indomethacin/indomethacin sodium trihydrate
ketoprofen
ketorolac tromethamine
nabumetone
naproxen/naproxen sodium

INDICATIONS
➤ Mild to moderate pain, inflammation, stiffness, swelling, or tenderness

ACTION
The analgesic effect of NSAIDs may result from interference with the prostaglandins involved in pain. Prostaglandins appear to sensitize pain receptors to mechanical stimulation or to other chemical mediators.

ADVERSE REACTIONS
Adverse reactions chiefly involve the GI tract, particularly erosion of the gastric mucosa. The most common symptoms are abdominal pain, epigastric distress, heartburn, and nausea.

CONTRAINDICATIONS AND CAUTIONS
• Contraindicated in patients with GI lesions or GI bleeding and in patients hypersensitive to these drugs.
• NSAIDs cause an increased risk of serious GI adverse events, including bleeding, ulceration, and perforation of the stomach or intestines, which can be fatal.
• May increase the risk of serious thrombotic events, MI, or stroke, which can be fatal. The risk may be greater with longer use or in patients with CV disease or risk factors for CV disease.
• In pregnant women, use cautiously in the first and second trimesters; don't use in the third trimester. For breast-feeding women, NSAIDs aren't recommended. In children younger than age 14, safety of long-term therapy hasn't been established. Patients older than age 60 may be more susceptible to toxic effects of NSAIDs because of decreased renal function.
• NSAIDs may mask signs and symptoms of infection because of their antipyretic and anti-inflammatory actions.

aspirin (acetylsalicylic acid, ASA)

ASS-pir-in

Bayer, Ecotrin, Empirin, Halfprin, Heartline, Norwich, St Joseph, ZORprin

Pharmacologic class: Salicylate

INDICATIONS

➤ Mild to moderate pain or fever; rheumatoid arthritis, osteoarthritis, or other polyarthritic or inflammatory conditions; suspected acute MI; to reduce risk of recurrent transient ischemic attacks and stroke or death; acute ischemic stroke

ACTION

Produces analgesia and exerts its anti-inflammatory effect by inhibiting prostaglandin and other substances that sensitize pain receptors. In low doses, also appears to interfere with clotting by keeping a platelet-aggregating substance from forming.

ADVERSE REACTIONS

EENT: tinnitus, hearing loss
GI: nausea, GI bleeding, dyspepsia, GI distress, occult bleeding
Hematologic: prolonged bleeding time, leukopenia, thrombocytopenia
Hepatic: hepatitis
Skin: rash, bruising, urticaria.
Other: angioedema, Reye syndrome, hypersensitivity reactions.

NURSING CONSIDERATIONS

• Anticoagulants may increase risk of bleeding. Use with extreme caution if must be used together.
• Use cautiously in patients with GI lesions, impaired renal function, hypoprothrombinemia, vitamin K deficiency, thrombocytopenia, thrombotic thrombocytopenic purpura, or severe hepatic impairment.
• Don't give to children or teens that have or are recovering from chickenpox or flulike symptoms because of the risk of Reye syndrome.
• Febrile, dehydrated children can develop toxicity rapidly.

PATIENT TEACHING

• Advise patient to take drug with food, milk, antacid, or large glass of water to reduce GI reactions.
• Instruct patient to discard aspirin tablets that have a strong vinegar-like odor.

celecoxib

sell-ah-COCKS-ib

Celebrex

Pharmacologic class: Cyclooxygenase-2 (COX-2) inhibitor

INDICATIONS

➤ Osteoarthritis; rheumatoid arthritis; ankylosing spondylitis; juvenile rheumatoid arthritis; acute pain and primary dysmenorrhea

ACTION

Thought to inhibit prostaglandin synthesis, impeding COX-2, to produce anti-inflammatory, analgesic, and antipyretic effects.

ADVERSE REACTIONS

CNS: headache, dizziness, insomnia
GI: abdominal pain, diarrhea, flatulence, GI reflux, nausea
Respiratory: dyspnea, upper respiratory tract infection
Skin: erythema multiforme, exfoliative dermatitis, Stevens–Johnson syndrome, toxic epidermal necrolysis, rash

NURSING CONSIDERATIONS

• Watch for signs and symptoms of overt and occult bleeding.
• Drug can cause fluid retention; monitor patient with hypertension, edema, or heart failure.
• Don't confuse Celebrex with Cerebyx or Celexa.

PATIENT TEACHING

• Tell patient to report history of allergic reactions to sulfonamides, aspirin, or other NSAIDs before therapy.
• Instruct patient to promptly report signs of GI bleeding, such as blood in vomit, urine, or stool; or black, tarry stools.
• Instruct patient to take drug with food if stomach upset occurs.
• Inform patient that it may take several days before he feels consistent pain relief.
• Advise patient that using OTC NSAIDs with celecoxib may increase the risk of GI toxicity.

diclofenac epolamine/diclofenac potassium/ diclofenac sodium

dye-KLOE-fen-ak

Flector/Apo-Diclo, Cambia, Cataflam, Voltaren, Zipsor/Voltaren, Voltaren-XR

Pharmacologic class: NSAID

INDICATIONS
➤ Ankylosing spondylitis, osteoarthritis, rheumatoid arthritis, analgesia, primary dysmenorrhea
➤ Acute pain due to minor strains, sprains, and contusions

ACTION
May inhibit prostaglandin synthesis, to produce anti-inflammatory, analgesic, and antipyretic effects.

ADVERSE REACTIONS
CNS: aseptic meningitis, anxiety, depression, dizziness
CV: heart failure, edema, fluid retention, hypertension
EENT: laryngeal edema, blurred vision, epistaxis, tinnitus
GI: bleeding, melena, nausea, peptic ulceration, taste disorder
GU: nephrotic syndrome, acute renal failure, fluid retention
Hepatic: jaundice, hepatitis, hepatotoxicity
Metabolic: hypoglycemia, hyperglycemia
Respiratory: asthma
Skin: Stevens–Johnson syndrome, rash, urticaria
Other: anaphylactoid reactions, anaphylaxis, angioedema

NURSING CONSIDERATIONS
• Monitor liver function test.
• Different formulations of oral diclofenac are not bioequivalent even if the milligram strength is the same.
• Don't confuse diclofenac with Diflucan.

PATIENT TEACHING
• Tell patient to take tablets or capsules with milk, meals, or antacids to minimize GI distress.
• Teach patient signs and symptoms of GI bleeding and tell him to notify prescriber immediately if any of these occurs.
• Advise patient to avoid drinking alcohol or taking aspirin during drug therapy.
• Advise patient that use of OTC NSAIDs and diclofenac may increase the risk of GI toxicity.

etodolac

ee-toe-DOE-lak

Pharmacologic class: NSAID

INDICATIONS

➤ Acute pain

➤ Osteoarthritis, rheumatoid arthritis, juvenile rheumatoid arthritis

ACTION

Produces anti-inflammatory, analgesic, and antipyretic effects, possibly by inhibiting prostaglandin synthesis.

ADVERSE REACTIONS

CNS: asthenia, malaise, dizziness, insomnia, syncope, fever

CV: hypertension, heart failure palpitations, fluid retention

EENT: blurred vision, tinnitus, photophobia

GI: dyspepsia, peptic ulceration with or without GI bleeding or perforation, ulcerative stomatitis, thirst, dry mouth

GU: dysuria, urinary frequency, renal failure

Hematologic: anemia, leukopenia, hemolytic anemia

Hepatic: hepatitis.

Respiratory: asthma.

Skin: pruritus, rash, Stevens–Johnson syndrome

NURSING CONSIDERATIONS

• Because NSAIDs impair the synthesis of renal prostaglandins, they can decrease renal blood flow and lead to reversible renal impairment, especially in patients with renal or heart failure or liver dysfunction, in elderly patients, and in those taking diuretics. Monitor these patients closely.

PATIENT TEACHING

• Tell patient to take drug with milk or meals to minimize GI discomfort.

• Teach patient signs and symptoms of GI bleeding and tell him to notify prescriber immediately if any of these occurs.

• Advise patient to avoid drinking alcohol or taking aspirin during drug therapy.

• Advise patient that use of OTC NSAIDs and etodolac may increase the risk of GI toxicity.

ibuprofen
eye-byoo-PROH-fen

Advil, Caldolor, Excedrin IB, Motrin IB, PediaCare Fever
Pharmacologic class: NSAID

INDICATIONS
➤ Rheumatoid arthritis, osteoarthritis, arthritis
➤ Mild to moderate pain or fever

ACTION
May inhibit prostaglandin synthesis, to produce anti-inflammatory, analgesic, and antipyretic effects.

ADVERSE REACTIONS
CNS: dizziness, headache, nervousness
CV: edema, fluid retention
GI: abdominal pain, bloating, constipation, decreased appetite, diarrhea, nausea, nonnecrotizing enterocolitis, vomiting
GU: acute renal failure, azotemia, cystitis, hematuria
Hematologic: agranulocytosis, aplastic anemia, leukopenia, neutropenia, pancytopenia, thrombocytopenia
Metabolic: hyperkalemia, hypoglycemia
Skin: pruritus, rash

NURSING CONSIDERATIONS
• Check renal and hepatic function periodically in patients on long-term therapy.
• Monitor patients for signs and symptoms of GI ulceration and bleeding.

PATIENT TEACHING
• Tell patient to take with meals or milk to reduce adverse GI reactions.
• Drug is available OTC. Instruct patient not to exceed 1.2 g daily, not to give to children younger than age 12, and not to take for extended periods (longer than 3 days for fever or longer than 10 days for pain) without consulting prescriber.
• Caution patient that use with aspirin, alcohol, or corticosteroids may increase risk of GI adverse reactions.
• Teach patient to watch for and report to prescriber immediately signs and symptoms of GI bleeding.

indomethacin/indomethacin sodium trihydrate
in-doe-METH-a-sin

Indocin, Indocin SR/Indocin I.V.
Pharmacologic class: NSAID

INDICATIONS
➤ Rheumatoid arthritis, osteoarthritis, ankylosing spondylitis, acute gouty arthritis

ACTION
May inhibit prostaglandin synthesis, to produce anti-inflammatory, analgesic, and antipyretic effects.

ADVERSE REACTIONS
CNS: headache, dizziness, depression, fatigue, somnolence, syncope, vertigo
CV: edema, hypertension
EENT: hearing loss, tinnitus
GI: pancreatitis, abdominal pain, anorexia, constipation, diarrhea, dyspepsia, GI bleeding, nausea, peptic ulceration
Other: hypersensitivity reactions

NURSING CONSIDERATIONS
• Because of the high risk of adverse effects from long-term use, drug shouldn't be used routinely as an analgesic or antipyretic.
• Watch for bleeding in patients receiving anticoagulants, patients with coagulation defects, and neonates.
• Drug causes sodium retention; watch for weight gain (especially in elderly patients) and increased blood pressure in patients with hypertension.
• Monitor patient on long-term oral therapy for toxicity.

PATIENT TEACHING
• Tell patient to take oral dose with food, milk, or antacid to prevent GI upset.
• Alert patient that using oral form with aspirin, alcohol, other NSAIDs, or corticosteroids may increase risk of adverse GI reactions.
• Teach patient signs and symptoms of GI bleeding and tell him to notify prescriber immediately if any of these occurs.
• Tell patient to immediately report signs or symptoms of cardiac events, such as chest pain, shortness of breath, weakness, and slurred speech.

ketoprofen
kee-toe-PROE-fen

Pharmacologic class: NSAID

INDICATIONS
➤ Rheumatoid arthritis, osteoarthritis
➤ Mild to moderate pain, dysmenorrhea

ACTION
Produces anti-inflammatory, analgesic, and antipyretic effects, possibly by inhibiting prostaglandin synthesis.

ADVERSE REACTIONS
CNS: headache, dizziness, CNS excitation or CNS depression
CV: peripheral edema
EENT: tinnitus, visual disturbances
GI: dyspepsia, abdominal pain, nausea, stomatitis, vomiting
GU: nephrotoxicity, UTI signs and symptoms
Skin: photosensitivity reactions, rash

NURSING CONSIDERATIONS
• Don't use sustained-release form for patients in acute pain.
• Check renal and hepatic function every 6 months or as indicated.
• Drug decreases platelet adhesion and aggregation and can prolong bleeding time about 3 to 4 minutes from baseline.

PATIENT TEACHING
• Instruct patient not to exceed 75 mg daily.
• Tell patient to take drug 30 minutes before or 2 hours after meals with a full glass of water. If adverse GI reactions occur, patient may take drug with milk or meals.
• Teach patient signs and symptoms of GI bleeding and tell him to notify prescriber immediately if any of these occurs.
• Alert patient that using with aspirin, alcohol, other NSAIDs, or corticosteroids may increase risk of adverse GI reactions.
• Instruct patient to report problems with vision or hearing immediately.
• Tell patient to protect drug from direct light and excessive heat and humidity.

ketorolac tromethamine

KEE-toe-role-ak

Sprix
Pharmacologic class: NSAID

INDICATIONS
➤ Moderately severe, acute pain

ACTION
May inhibit prostaglandin synthesis, to produce anti-inflammatory, analgesic, and antipyretic effects.

ADVERSE REACTIONS
CNS: headache, dizziness, drowsiness, sedation
CV: arrhythmias, edema, hypertension, palpitations
EENT: (nasal spray only) nasal discomfort, rhinalgia, rhinitis
GI: dyspepsia, GI pain, nausea, constipation, vomiting
GU: renal failure
Skin: diaphoresis, pruritus, rash

NURSING CONSIDERATIONS
• Correct hypovolemia before giving. Oral therapy is only indicated as a continuation of I.V./I.M. therapy. Maximum combined duration of parenteral, nasal, and oral therapy is 5 days.
• Carefully observe patients with coagulopathies and those taking anticoagulants. Drug can prolong bleeding time.

PATIENT TEACHING
• Tell patient to discard nasal spray within 24 hours of the first dose, even if medication remains in the bottle.
• Warn patient using nasal spray that he may experience transient, mild to moderate nasal irritation that lasts for a few minutes and won't worsen with next dose.
• Advise patient to take a sip of water after using nasal spray to decrease throat sensation.
• Warn patient not to take ketorolac with other NSAIDs.
• Advise patient to maintain adequate fluid intake.
• Advise patient to be alert for signs and symptoms of CV events and to seek medical attention immediately if they occur.
• Teach patient signs and symptoms of GI bleeding and tell him to notify prescriber immediately if any of these occurs.

nabumetone
nah-BYOO-meh-tone
Pharmacologic class: NSAID

INDICATIONS
➤ Rheumatoid arthritis, osteoarthritis

ACTION
Produces anti-inflammatory, analgesic, and antipyretic effects, possibly by inhibiting prostaglandin synthesis.

ADVERSE REACTIONS
CNS: dizziness, fatigue, headache, insomnia, nervousness
CV: edema, vasculitis
EENT: tinnitus
GI: abdominal pain, diarrhea, dyspepsia, bleeding, anorexia, constipation, dry mouth, nausea, ulceration, vomiting
Skin: increased diaphoresis, pruritus, rash

NURSING CONSIDERATIONS
• During long-term therapy, periodically monitor renal and liver function, CBC, and hematocrit; assess patients for signs and symptoms of GI bleeding.

PATIENT TEACHING
• Instruct patient to take drug with food, milk, or antacids. Drug is absorbed more rapidly when taken with food or milk.
• Advise patient to limit alcohol intake because using drug with alcohol increases the risk of GI problems.
• Teach patient signs and symptoms of GI bleeding and tell him to notify prescriber immediately if any of these occurs.
• Advise patient that use of OTC NSAIDs in combination with nabumetone may increase the risk of GI toxicity.

naproxen/naproxen sodium
na-PROX-en

EC-Naprosyn, Naprosyn/Aleve, Anaprox, Anaprox DS
Pharmacologic class: NSAID

INDICATIONS
➤ Rheumatoid arthritis, osteoarthritis, juvenile arthritis, ankylosing spondylitis, pain, dysmenorrhea, tendinitis, bursitis, acute gout
➤ Mild to moderate pain, primary dysmenorrhea

ACTION
May inhibit prostaglandin synthesis to produce anti-inflammatory, analgesic, and antipyretic effects.

ADVERSE REACTIONS
CNS: dizziness, drowsiness, headache, vertigo
CV: edema, palpitations
EENT: tinnitus, auditory disturbances, visual disturbances
GI: abdominal pain, constipation, diarrhea, dyspepsia, epigastric pain, heartburn, nausea, occult blood loss, peptic ulceration, stomatitis, thirst
GU: renal failure
Hematologic: ecchymoses, increased bleeding time
Metabolic: hyperkalemia
Respiratory: dyspnea
Skin: diaphoresis, pruritus, purpura, rash, urticaria

NURSING CONSIDERATIONS
• Monitor CBC and renal and hepatic function every 4 to 6 months during long-term therapy.

PATIENT TEACHING
• Tell patient not to take more than 600 mg in 24 hours. Dosage in patient older than age 65 shouldn't exceed 400 mg daily.
• Advise patient to take drug with food or milk to minimize GI upset. Tell him to drink a full glass of water or other liquid with each dose.
• Warn patient against taking naproxen and naproxen sodium at the same time.
• Teach patient signs and symptoms of GI bleeding and tell him to notify prescriber immediately if any of these occurs.
• Caution patient that use with aspirin, alcohol, other NSAIDs, or corticosteroids may increase risk of adverse GI reactions.

Nucleoside reverse transcriptase inhibitors

zidovudine

INDICATIONS
➤ HIV infection, AIDS, prevention of maternal–fetal HIV transmission, prevention of HIV infection after occupational exposure (as by needle stick) or nonoccupational exposure to blood, genital secretions, or other potentially infectious body fluids of an HIV-infected person when there's substantial risk of transmission

ACTION
Nucleoside reverse transcriptase inhibitors (NRTIs) suppress HIV replication by inhibiting HIV DNA polymerase. Competitive inhibition of nucleoside reverse transcriptase inhibits DNA viral replication by chain termination, competitive inhibition of reverse transcriptase, or both.

ADVERSE REACTIONS
Because of the complexity of HIV infection, it's often difficult to distinguish between disease-related symptoms and adverse drug reactions. The most frequently reported adverse effects of NRTIs are anemia, leukopenia, and neutropenia. Thrombocytopenia is less common. Rare adverse effects of NRTIs are hepatotoxicity, myopathy, and neurotoxicity. Any of these adverse effects requires prompt medical attention. Adverse effects that don't need medical attention unless they persist or are bothersome include headache, severe insomnia, myalgias, nausea, or hyperpigmentation of nails.

CONTRAINDICATIONS AND CAUTIONS
• Contraindicated in patients hypersensitive to these drugs.
• Use cautiously in patients with compromised bone marrow function.
• In pregnant women, use drug only if benefits outweigh risks. HIV-infected mothers shouldn't breast-feed, to reduce the risk of transmitting the virus. It isn't known if NRTIs appear in breast milk. The pharmacokinetic and safety profile of NRTIs is similar in children and adults. NRTIs may be used in children age 3 months and older, but the half-life may be prolonged in neonates. In elderly patients, elimination half-life may be prolonged.

zidovudine
zid-oh-VEW-den

Retrovir

Pharmacologic class: Nucleoside reverse transcriptase inhibitor

INDICATIONS
➤ HIV infection, with other antiretrovirals
➤ To prevent maternal–fetal transmission of HIV

ACTION
Nucleoside reverse transcriptase inhibitor that inhibits replication of HIV by blocking DNA synthesis.

ADVERSE REACTIONS
CNS: asthenia, dizziness, fever, headache, malaise, seizures
GI: anorexia, nausea, vomiting, pancreatitis, abdominal pain, constipation, diarrhea, dyspepsia, taste perversion
Hematologic: agranulocytosis, severe bone marrow suppression, thrombocytopenia, anemia
Hepatic: hepatomegaly
Metabolic: lactic acidosis
Respiratory: cough, wheezing
Skin: rash, diaphoresis

NURSING CONSIDERATIONS
• Monitor blood studies every 2 weeks to detect anemia or agranulocytosis.
• If administering by I.V., infuse drug over 1 hour at a constant rate. Avoid rapid infusion or bolus injection.
• Don't confuse Retrovir with ritonavir.

PATIENT TEACHING
• Instruct patient to take drug on an empty stomach. To avoid esophageal irritation, tell patient to take drug while sitting upright and with adequate fluids.
• Tell patient that his gums may bleed. Recommend good mouth care with a soft toothbrush.
• Advise pregnant, HIV-infected patient that drug therapy only reduces the risk of HIV transmission to her newborn. Long-term risks to infants are unknown.
• Tell patient not to keep capsules in the kitchen, bathroom, or other places that may be damp or hot. Heat and moisture may cause the drug to break down and affect the intended results.

Opioid antagonist

Naloxone hydrochloride

INDICATIONS
➤ Known or suspected opioid-induced respiratory depression, postoperative opioid depression, and opioid overdose

ACTION
Naloxone may displace opioid analgesics from the receptors. The drug has no pharmacological activity on its own.

ADVERSE REACTIONS
Edema, hypertension, palpitations, phlebitis, shortness of breath, anxiety, depression, disorientation, dizziness, nausea, vomiting, and headache.

CONTRAINDICATIONS AND CAUTIONS
➤ Contraindicated in patients with hypersensitivity to drug.
➤ Use cautiously in patients with any type of liver disease and patients with long-term alcohol use.
➤ Use cautiously in patients with cardiac irritability or opioid addiction.

naloxone hydrochloride

nal-OX-one

Pharmacologic class: Opioid antagonist

INDICATIONS
➤Known or suspected opioid-induced respiratory depression; postoperative opioid depression

ACTION
May displace opioid analgesics from their receptors (competitive antagonism).

ADVERSE REACTIONS
CNS: seizures, tremors
CV: ventricular fibrillation, tachycardia, hypertension with higher than recommended doses, hypotension
GI: nausea, vomiting
Respiratory: pulmonary edema
Skin: diaphoresis
Other: withdrawal symptoms in opioid-dependent patients with higher than recommended doses

NURSING CONSIDERATIONS
• Duration of action of the opioid may exceed that of naloxone, and patients may relapse into respiratory depression.
• Respiratory rate increases within 1 to 2 minutes.
• Drug is effective only for reversing respiratory depression caused by opioids and not for other drug-induced respiratory depression, including that caused by benzodiazepines.
• Patients who receive drug to reverse opioid-induced respiratory depression may exhibit tachypnea.
• Monitor respiratory depth and rate. Provide oxygen, ventilation, and other resuscitation measures.
• Don't confuse naloxone with naltrexone.

PATIENT TEACHING
• Reassure family that patient will be monitored closely until effects of opioid resolve.

Opioids

codeine phosphate/codeine sulfate
fentanyl citrate/fentanyl transdermal system/fentanyl transmucosal
hydrocodone bitartrate and acetaminophen
hydromorphone hydrochloride
meperidine hydrochloride
methadone hydrochloride
morphine sulfate
oxycodone hydrochloride

INDICATIONS
➤ Moderate to severe pain from acute and some chronic disorders; diarrhea; dry, nonproductive cough; management of opioid dependence; anesthesia support; sedation

ACTION
Opioids act as agonists at specific opioid receptor binding sites in the CNS and other tissues, altering perception of pain.

ADVERSE REACTIONS
Respiratory and circulatory depression are the major hazards of opioids. Other adverse CNS effects include agitation, coma, depression, dizziness, faintness, mental clouding, nervousness, restlessness, sedation, seizures, visual disturbances, and weakness. Adverse GI effects include biliary colic, constipation, nausea, and vomiting. Urine retention or hypersensitivity also may occur. Tolerance to the drug and psychological or physical dependence may follow prolonged therapy.

CONTRAINDICATIONS AND CAUTIONS
• Contraindicated in patients hypersensitive to these drugs and in those who have recently taken an MAO inhibitor. Also contraindicated in those with acute or severe bronchial asthma or respiratory depression.
• Use cautiously in patients with increased intracranial or intraocular pressure, hepatic or renal dysfunction, mental and emotional disturbances, or drug-seeking behaviors.
• In pregnant or breast-feeding women, use cautiously; codeine, meperidine, methadone, and morphine appear in breast milk. Breast-feeding infants of women taking methadone may develop physical dependence. In children, safety and effectiveness of some opioids haven't been established; use cautiously. Elderly patients may be more sensitive to opioids, and lower doses are usually given.

codeine phosphate/codeine sulfate

koe-DEEN

Pharmacologic class: Opioid

INDICATIONS

➤ Mild to moderate pain

ACTION

May bind with opioid receptors in the CNS, altering perception of and emotional response to pain. Also suppresses the cough reflex by direct action on the cough center in the medulla.

ADVERSE REACTIONS

CNS: clouded sensorium, sedation, dizziness, euphoria, light-headedness, physical dependence

CV: bradycardia, flushing, hypotension

GI: constipation, dry mouth, ileus, nausea, vomiting

GU: urine retention

Respiratory: respiratory depression

Skin: diaphoresis, pruritus

NURSING CONSIDERATIONS

• Reassess patient's level of pain at least 15 and 30 minutes after use.

• For full analgesic effect, give drug before patient has intense pain.

• Monitor respiratory and circulatory status.

• Opioids may cause constipation. Assess bowel function and need for stool softeners and stimulant laxatives.

• Codeine may delay gastric emptying, increase biliary tract pressure from contraction of the sphincter of Oddi, and interfere with hepatobiliary imaging studies.

• Don't confuse codeine with Cardene, Lodine, or Cordran.

PATIENT TEACHING

• Advise patient that GI distress caused by taking drug P.O. can be eased by taking drug with milk or meals.

• Instruct patient to ask for or to take drug before pain is intense.

• Caution ambulatory patient about getting out of bed or walking. Warn outpatient to avoid driving and other hazardous activities that require mental alertness until drug's effects on the CNS are known.

• Advise patient to avoid alcohol during therapy.

fentanyl citrate/fentanyl transdermal system/ fentanyl transmucosal

FEN-ta-nil

Onsolis, Sublimaze/Duragesic/Actiq, Fentora

Pharmacologic class: Opioid agonist

INDICATIONS

➤ Preoperative medication; adjunct to regional or general anesthetic
➤ Postoperative pain, restlessness, tachypnea, and emergence delirium; moderate to severe chronic pain

ACTION

Unknown. Binds with opioid receptors in the CNS, altering perception of and emotional response to pain.

ADVERSE REACTIONS

CNS: asthenia, clouded sensorium, confusion, euphoria, sedation, somnolence, seizures, anxiety, depression, dizziness
CV: arrhythmias, chest pain, hypertension, hypotension
GI: constipation, dyspepsia, dry mouth, ileus, nausea, vomiting
Musculoskeletal: skeletal muscle rigidity (dose-related)
Respiratory: apnea, hypoventilation, respiratory depression
Skin: diaphoresis, pruritus

NURSING CONSIDERATIONS

• For better relief, give drug before patient has intense pain.
• Monitor circulatory and respiratory status and urinary function carefully. Drug may cause respiratory depression, hypotension, or altered level of consciousness, no matter how it's given.
• Identify all daily drugs, particularly CYP3A4 inhibitors, which may increase fentanyl levels.
• Don't confuse fentanyl with alfentanil.

PATIENT TEACHING

• Tell home care patient to avoid drinking alcohol or taking other CNS-type drugs because additive effects can occur.
• Tell patient that pain relief with the patch may not occur for several hours after the patch is applied. Oral, immediate-release opioids may be needed for initial pain relief.
• Inform patient that heat from fever or environment, such as from heating pads or electric blankets, may increase transdermal delivery and cause toxicity requiring dosage adjustment.

hydrocodone bitartrate and acetaminophen
Hye-droe-COD-one
Pharmacologic class: Opioid analgesic combination

INDICATIONS
➤ Mild to moderate pain

ACTION
May bind with opioid receptors in the CNS, altering perception of and emotional response to pain.

ADVERSE REACTIONS
CNS: drowsiness, sedation, dizziness, light-headedness, physical dependence, confusion
CV: bradycardia, flushing, hypotension
GI: constipation, dry mouth, nausea, vomiting
GU: urine retention
Respiratory: respiratory depression

NURSING CONSIDERATIONS
• Reassess patient's level of pain at least 15 and 30 minutes after use.
• For full analgesic effect, give drug before patient has intense pain.
• Monitor respiratory and circulatory status.
• Opioids may cause constipation. Assess bowel function and need for stool softeners and stimulant laxatives.
• Codeine may delay gastric emptying, increase biliary tract pressure from contraction of the sphincter of Oddi, and interfere with hepatobiliary imaging studies.

PATIENT TEACHING
• Advise patient that GI distress caused by taking drug P.O. can be eased by taking drug with milk or meals.
• Instruct patient to ask for or to take drug before pain is intense.
• Caution ambulatory patient about getting out of bed or walking. Warn outpatient to avoid driving and other hazardous activities that require mental alertness until drug's effects on the CNS are known.
• Advise patient to avoid alcohol during therapy.

hydromorphone hydrochloride

Hye-droe-MOR-fone

Dilaudid, Dilaudid-HP, Exalgo

Pharmacologic class: Opioid

INDICATIONS
➤ Moderate to severe pain

ACTION
Binds with opioid receptors in the CNS, altering perception of and emotional response to pain. Also suppresses the cough reflex by direct action on the cough center in the medulla.

ADVERSE REACTIONS
CNS: sedation, somnolence, clouded sensorium, dizziness, euphoria, light-headedness, insomnia, headache, pain
CV: hypotension, flushing, bradycardia, edema
EENT: blurred vision, diplopia, nystagmus
GI: nausea, vomiting, constipation, diarrhea, ileus, dry mouth
Respiratory: respiratory depression, bronchospasm

NURSING CONSIDERATIONS
• Reassess patient's level of pain at least 15 and 30 minutes after administration.
• For better effect, give drug before patient has intense pain.
• Discontinue all other extended-release opioids before giving extended-release form of hydromorphone.
• Monitor respiratory and circulatory status and bowel function.
• Keep opioid antagonist (naloxone) available.
• Don't use extended-release form within 14 days of stopping MAO inhibitor.
• Don't confuse hydromorphone with morphine or oxymorphone or Dilaudid with Dilantin.

PATIENT TEACHING
• Instruct patient to request or take drug before pain becomes intense.
• Advise patient to take drug with food if GI upset occurs.
• Caution patient about getting out of bed or walking. Warn outpatient to avoid hazardous activities that require mental alertness until drug's CNS effects are known.
• Advise patient to avoid alcohol during therapy.

meperidine hydrochloride
me-PER-i-deen

Demerol

Pharmacologic class: Opioid

INDICATIONS
➤ Moderate to severe pain; preoperative analgesia; adjunct to anesthesia; obstetric analgesia

ACTION
Unknown. Binds with opioid receptors in the CNS, altering perception of and emotional response to pain.

ADVERSE REACTIONS
CNS: clouded sensorium, dizziness, euphoria, light-headedness, sedation, somnolence, seizures, hallucinations, headache
CV: bradycardia, cardiac arrest, shock, hypotension, tachycardia
GI: biliary tract spasms, constipation, ileus, nausea, vomiting
Respiratory: respiratory arrest, respiratory depression
Skin: diaphoresis, pruritus, urticaria

NURSING CONSIDERATIONS
• In elderly patients or in those with renal dysfunction, active metabolite may accumulate, causing increased adverse CNS reactions.
• Reassess patient's level of pain at least 15 and 30 minutes after administration.
• In neonates exposed to drug during labor, monitor respirations. Have resuscitation equipment and naloxone available.
• Monitor respiratory and CV status carefully. Don't give if respirations are below 12 breaths/minute, if respiratory rate or depth is decreased, or if change in pupils is noted.
• Monitor bowel function. Patient may need a stimulant laxative and stool softener.
• Don't confuse Demerol with Demulen.

PATIENT TEACHING
• Caution ambulatory patient about getting out of bed or walking. Warn outpatient to avoid driving and other potentially hazardous activities that require mental alertness until drug's CNS effects are known.
• Advise patient to avoid alcohol during therapy.

methadone hydrochloride
METH-a-done

Dolophine, Methadose
Pharmacologic class: Opioid agonist

INDICATIONS
➤ Severe pain; opioid withdrawal syndrome

ACTION
Unknown. Binds with opioid receptors in the CNS, altering perception of and emotional response to pain.

ADVERSE REACTIONS
CNS: clouded sensorium, hallucinations, dizziness, light-headedness, sedation, somnolence, seizures, syncope
CV: arrhythmias, bradycardia, prolonged QT interval, cardiac arrest, shock, cardiomyopathy, heart failure, flushing, edema
GI: nausea, vomiting, abdominal pain, anorexia, biliary tract spasm, constipation, dry mouth, glossitis, ileus
Metabolic: hypokalemia, hypomagnesemia, weight gain
Respiratory: respiratory arrest, respiratory depression, pulmonary edema
Skin: diaphoresis, pruritus, urticaria

NURSING CONSIDERATIONS
• Respiratory depression, QT interval prolongation, and torsades de pointes have been observed during treatment. Be vigilant during treatment initiation and dose titration.
• Reassess patient's level of pain at least 15 and 30 minutes after parenteral administration and 30 minutes after oral administration.
• Patient treated for opioid withdrawal syndrome usually needs an additional analgesic if pain control is needed.
• Monitor patient closely because drug has cumulative effect; marked sedation can occur after repeated doses.
• When used as an adjunct in the treatment of opioid addiction (maintenance), withdrawal is usually delayed and mild.

PATIENT TEACHING
• Instruct patient to increase fluid and fiber in diet, if not contraindicated, to combat constipation.
• Advise patient to avoid alcohol during therapy. Caution patients not to use CNS depressants during initiation of treatment with methadone.

morphine sulfate

MOR-feen

Astramorph PF, Avinza, DepoDur, Duramorph MS Contin, MSIR

Pharmacologic class: Opioid

INDICATIONS

➤ Moderate to severe pain

ACTION

Unknown. Binds with opioid receptors in the CNS, altering perception of and emotional response to pain.

ADVERSE REACTIONS

CNS: dizziness, euphoria, light-headedness, nightmares, sedation, somnolence, seizures, syncope

CV: bradycardia, cardiac arrest, shock, hypertension, hypotension, tachycardia

GI: constipation, nausea, vomiting, anorexia, biliary tract spasms, dry mouth, ileus

Hematologic: thrombocytopenia

Respiratory: apnea, respiratory arrest, respiratory depression

NURSING CONSIDERATIONS

• Reassess patient's level of pain at least 15 and 30 minutes after giving parenterally and 30 minutes after giving orally.

• Keep opioid antagonist (naloxone) and resuscitation equipment available.

• Monitor circulatory, respiratory, bladder, and bowel functions carefully.

• Preservative-free preparations are available for epidural and intrathecal use.

• When drug is given epidurally, monitor patient closely for respiratory depression up to 24 hours after the injection.

• Don't confuse morphine with hydromorphone or Avinza with Invanz.

PATIENT TEACHING

• Warn patient to read labels on OTC drugs carefully and not to use alcohol in any form.

• Tell patient to swallow morphine sulfate whole or to open capsule and sprinkle beads or pellets on a small amount of applesauce immediately before taking.

oxycodone hydrochloride
ox-i-KOE-done

ETH-Oxydose, M-Oxy, OxyContin, Roxicodone
Pharmacologic class: Opioid

INDICATIONS
➤ Moderate to severe pain

ACTION
Unknown. Binds with opioid receptors in the CNS, altering perception of and emotional response to pain.

ADVERSE REACTIONS
CNS: clouded sensorium, dizziness, euphoria, light-headedness, physical dependence, sedation, somnolence
CV: bradycardia, hypotension
GI: constipation, nausea, vomiting, ileus
Respiratory: respiratory depression

NURSING CONSIDERATIONS
• Reassess patient's level of pain at least 15 and 30 minutes after administration.
• For full effect, give drug before patient has intense pain.
• Monitor circulatory and respiratory status. Withhold dose and notify prescriber if respirations are shallow or if respiratory rate falls below 12 breaths/minute.
• Monitor patient's bladder and bowel patterns.
• For patients who are taking more than 60 mg daily, stop drug gradually to prevent withdrawal symptoms.
• Drug isn't intended for as-needed use or for immediate postoperative pain. Drug is indicated only for postoperative use if patient was receiving it before surgery or if pain is expected to persist for an extended time.

PATIENT TEACHING
• Instruct patient to take drug before pain is intense.
• Tell patient to take drug with milk or after eating. Tell patient to swallow extended-release tablets whole.
• Caution ambulatory patient about getting out of bed or walking. Warn outpatient to avoid driving and other hazardous activities that require mental alertness until drug's CNS effects are known.
• Advise patient to avoid alcohol use during therapy.

Ovulation stimulant

clomiPHENE citrate

INDICATIONS
➤ To induce ovulation

ACTION
Clomiphene is thought to stimulate release of follicle-stimulating hormone, luteinizing hormone, and pituitary gonadotropins, resulting in maturation of the ovarian follicle, ovulation, and development of the corpus luteum.

ADVERSE REACTIONS
Ovarian enlargement, hot flashes, abdominal or pelvic discomfort, bloating, and breast discomfort

CONTRAINDICATIONS AND CAUTIONS
• Contraindicated in patients with a known hypersensitivity or allergy to clomiphene or to any of its ingredients.
• Contraindicated in pregnant women and in those with undiagnosed abnormal genital bleeding, ovarian cyst not related to polycystic ovarian syndrome, hepatic disease or dysfunction, uncontrolled thyroid or adrenal dysfunction, or organic intracranial lesion.

clomiPHENE citrate
KLOE-mi-feen

Clomid, Serophene

Pharmacologic class: Chlorotrianisene derivative

INDICATIONS
➤ To induce ovulation

ACTION
Appears to stimulate release of follicle-stimulating hormone, luteinizing hormone, and pituitary gonadotropins, resulting in maturation of the ovarian follicle, ovulation, and development of the corpus luteum.

ADVERSE REACTIONS
CNS: headache
EENT: blurred vision, diplopia, scotoma, photophobia
GI: nausea, vomiting, bloating, distention
GU: ovarian enlargement, urinary frequency and polyuria, abnormal uterine bleeding, ovarian cyst
Metabolic: weight gain
Skin: reversible alopecia, urticaria, rash, dermatitis
Other: hot flashes, breast discomfort

NURSING CONSIDERATIONS
• Monitor patient closely because of potentially serious adverse reactions.
• Don't confuse clomiphene with clomipramine or clonidine. Don't confuse Serophene with Sarafem.

PATIENT TEACHING
• Tell patient about the risk of multiple births.
• Teach patient to take and chart basal body temperature to ascertain if ovulation has occurred.
• Advise patient to stop drug and contact prescriber immediately if pregnancy is suspected because drug may have teratogenic effect.
• Advise patient to stop drug and contact prescriber immediately if abdominal symptoms or pain occur; these symptoms may indicate ovarian enlargement or ovarian cyst. Also, tell patient to immediately notify prescriber if signs and symptoms of impending visual toxicity occur, such as blurred vision, double vision, vision defect in one part of the eye (scotoma), or sensitivity to the sun.

Penicillins

amoxicillin
ampicillin/ampicillin sodium/ampicillin trihydrate
penicillin G benzathine
penicillin G potassium
penicillin G procaine
penicillin G sodium
penicillin V potassium

INDICATIONS
➤ Streptococcal pneumonia; endocarditis; diphtheria; anthrax; meningitis; tetanus; botulism; actinomycosis; syphilis; relapsing fever; Lyme disease; pneumococcal infections; rheumatic fever; bacterial endocarditis; neonatal group B streptococcal disease; septicemia; gynecologic infections; infections of urinary, respiratory, and GI tracts; infections of skin, soft tissue, bones, and joints

ACTION
Penicillins are generally bactericidal. They inhibit synthesis of the bacterial cell wall, causing rapid cell destruction. They're most effective against fast-growing susceptible bacteria. Their sites of action are enzymes known as penicillin-binding proteins (PBPs). The affinity of certain penicillins for PBPs in various microorganisms helps explain the different activities of these drugs.

ADVERSE REACTIONS
With all penicillins, hypersensitivity reactions range from mild rash, fever, and eosinophilia to fatal anaphylaxis. Hematologic reactions include hemolytic anemia, leukopenia, thrombocytopenia, and transient neutropenia. Certain adverse reactions are more common with specific classes.

CONTRAINDICATIONS AND CAUTIONS
• Contraindicated in patients hypersensitive to these drugs.
• Use cautiously in patients with history of asthma or drug allergy, mononucleosis, renal impairment, CV diseases, hemorrhagic condition, or electrolyte imbalance.
• In pregnant women, use cautiously. For breast-feeding patients, recommendations vary depending on the drug. For children, dosage recommendations have been established for most penicillins. Elderly patients are susceptible to superinfection and renal impairment, which decreases excretion of penicillins; use cautiously and at a lower dosage.

amoxicillin

a-mox-i-SILL-in

DisperMox, Moxatag

Pharmacologic class: Aminopenicillin

INDICATIONS

➤ Infections of the ear, nose, and throat; skin and skin structure; GU tract; respiratory tract; uncomplicated gonorrhea

➤ *Helicobacter pylori* eradication

ACTION

Inhibits cell-wall synthesis during bacterial multiplication.

ADVERSE REACTIONS

CNS: seizures, lethargy, confusion, dizziness, fatigue, headache

GI: diarrhea, nausea, pseudomembranous colitis, vomiting, glossitis, stomatitis, gastritis, enterocolitis, abdominal pain, black hairy tongue

GU: interstitial nephritis, nephropathy, vaginitis

Hematologic: agranulocytosis, leukopenia, thrombocytopenia, thrombocytopenic purpura, eosinophilia, hemolytic anemia

Other: anaphylaxis, hypersensitivity reactions

NURSING CONSIDERATIONS

• If large doses are given or if therapy is prolonged, bacterial or fungal superinfection may occur.

• Clostridium difficile–associated diarrhea, ranging from mild diarrhea to fatal colitis, has been reported following use of amoxicillin. Evaluate patient if diarrhea occurs.

• Drug may decrease hormonal contraceptive effectiveness. Advise use of another form of contraception during therapy.

• Don't confuse amoxicillin with amoxapine.

PATIENT TEACHING

• Instruct patient to take extended-release tablets with a meal.

• Tell patient to notify prescriber if rash, fever, or chills develop. A rash is the most common allergic reaction, especially if allopurinol is also being taken.

• Tell parent to place drops directly on child's tongue for swallowing or add to formula, milk, fruit juice, water, ginger ale, or a cold drink for immediate and complete consumption.

ampicillin/ampicillin sodium/ampicillin trihydrate
am-pi-SILL-in

Principen
Pharmacologic class: Aminopenicillin

INDICATIONS
➤ Infections of the respiratory tract, skin and skin-structures, GI tract; UTIs; uncomplicated gonorrhea
➤ Bacterial meningitis or septicemia

ACTION
Inhibits cell-wall synthesis during bacterial multiplication.

ADVERSE REACTIONS
GI: diarrhea, nausea, pseudomembranous colitis, abdominal pain, black hairy tongue, enterocolitis, gastritis, glossitis, stomatitis, vomiting
Hematologic: leukopenia, thrombocytopenia, thrombocytopenic purpura, anemia, eosinophilia, hemolytic anemia, agranulocytosis
Other: hypersensitivity reactions, overgrowth of nonsusceptible organisms

NURSING CONSIDERATIONS
• Monitor sodium level because each gram of ampicillin contains 2.9 mEq of sodium.
• Obtain specimen for culture and sensitivity tests before giving. Begin therapy while awaiting results.
• Give drug 1 to 2 hours before or 2 to 3 hours after meals.
• Watch for signs and symptoms of hypersensitivity, such as erythematous maculopapular rash, urticaria, and anaphylaxis.
• Drug may decrease hormonal contraceptive effectiveness. Advise use of another form of contraception during therapy.

PATIENT TEACHING
• Tell patient to take entire quantity of drug exactly as prescribed, even after he feels better.
• Instruct patient to take oral form on an empty stomach 1 hour before or 2 hours after meals.
• Inform patient to notify prescriber if rash, fever, or chills develop. A rash is the most common allergic reaction, especially if allopurinol is also being taken.

penicillin G benzathine

pen-i-SILL-in

Bicillin L-A, Permapen

Pharmacologic class: Natural penicillin

INDICATIONS
➤ Syphilis
➤ Group A streptococcal upper respiratory tract infections
➤ To prevent poststreptococcal rheumatic fever and glomerulonephritis

ACTION
Inhibits cell-wall synthesis during bacterial multiplication.

ADVERSE REACTIONS
CNS: neuropathy
GI: pseudomembranous colitis, enterocolitis, nausea, vomiting
GU: interstitial nephritis, nephropathy
Hematologic: agranulocytosis, leukopenia, thrombocytopenia, anemia, eosinophilia, hemolytic anemia
Skin: exfoliative dermatitis, maculopapular rash
Other: anaphylaxis, hypersensitivity reactions, sterile abscess at injection site

NURSING CONSIDERATIONS
• Obtain specimen for culture and sensitivity tests before giving first dose. Begin therapy while awaiting results.
• Bicillin L-A is the only penicillin G benzathine product indicated for sexually transmitted infections. Don't substitute Bicillin C-R because it may not be effective.
• Inadvertent I.V. use may cause cardiac arrest and death. Never give I.V.
• Drug may decrease hormonal contraceptive effectiveness. Advise use of another form of contraception during therapy.
• Don't confuse drug with Polycillin, penicillamine, or the various types of penicillin.

PATIENT TEACHING
• Tell patient to report adverse reactions promptly.
• Warn patient that I.M. injection may be painful but that ice applied to the site may ease discomfort.

penicillin G potassium
pen-i-SILL-in

Pfizerpen

Pharmacologic class: Natural penicillin

INDICATIONS
➤ Moderate to severe systemic infection
➤ Anthrax; meningitis; neurosyphilis; syphilis
➤ Group B streptococcal infection

ACTION
Inhibits cell-wall synthesis during bacterial multiplication.

ADVERSE REACTIONS
CNS: seizures, agitation, anxiety, confusion, depression, dizziness, fatigue, hallucinations, lethargy, neuropathy
CV: thrombophlebitis, cardiac arrest, arrhythmias
GI: pseudomembranous colitis, enterocolitis, nausea, vomiting
GU: interstitial nephritis, nephropathy
Hematologic: agranulocytosis, leukopenia, thrombocytopenia, anemia, eosinophilia, hemolytic anemia
Metabolic: severe potassium poisoning
Skin: exfoliative dermatitis, maculopapular eruptions
Other: anaphylaxis, hypersensitivity reactions, overgrowth of nonsusceptible organisms

NURSING CONSIDERATIONS
• Obtain specimen for culture and sensitivity tests before giving first dose. Begin therapy while awaiting results.
• Monitor renal function closely.
• Due to increased risk of electrolyte imbalances, monitor potassium and sodium levels closely in patients receiving more than 10 million units I.V. daily.
• Drug may decrease hormonal contraceptive effectiveness. Advise use of another form of contraception during therapy.
• Don't confuse drug with Polycillin, penicillamine, or the various types of penicillin.

PATIENT TEACHING
• Tell patient to notify prescriber if rash, fever, or chills develop. A rash is the most common allergic reaction.
• Warn patient that I.M. injection may be painful but that ice applied to the site may help alleviate discomfort.

penicillin G procaine

pen-i-SILL-in

Pharmacologic class: Natural penicillin

INDICATIONS
➤ Moderate to severe systemic infection
➤ Anthrax
➤ Syphilis

ACTION
Inhibits cell-wall synthesis during bacterial multiplication.

ADVERSE REACTIONS
CNS: seizures, agitation, anxiety, confusion, depression, dizziness, fatigue, hallucinations, lethargy
GI: pseudomembranous colitis, enterocolitis, nausea, vomiting
GU: interstitial nephritis, nephropathy
Hematologic: agranulocytosis, thrombocytopenia, hemolytic anemia, leukopenia, anemia, eosinophilia
Musculoskeletal: arthralgia
Other: anaphylaxis, hypersensitivity reactions, overgrowth of nonsusceptible organisms

NURSING CONSIDERATIONS
• Obtain specimen for culture and sensitivity tests before giving first dose. Begin therapy while awaiting results.
• Monitor renal and hematopoietic function periodically.
• Inadvertent I.V. use may cause CNS toxicity and death. Toxic reaction may occur after one dose. Never give I.V.
• Drug may decrease hormonal contraceptive effectiveness. Advise use of another form of contraception during therapy.
• Don't confuse drug with Polycillin, penicillamine, or the various types of penicillin.

PATIENT TEACHING
• Tell patient to report adverse reactions promptly. A rash is the most common allergic reaction.
• Warn patient that I.M. injection may be painful but that ice applied to the site may help alleviate discomfort.

penicillin G sodium

pen-i-SILL-in

Pharmacologic class: Natural penicillin

INDICATIONS

➤ Moderate to severe systemic infection

➤ Meningitis

➤ Neurosyphilis

ACTION

Inhibits cell-wall synthesis during bacterial multiplication.

ADVERSE REACTIONS

CNS: neuropathy, seizures, agitation, anxiety, confusion, depression, dizziness, fatigue, hallucinations, lethargy

CV: heart failure, thrombophlebitis

GI: enterocolitis, ischemic colitis, nausea, vomiting, pseudomembranous colitis

GU: nephropathy, interstitial nephritis

Hematologic: hemolytic anemia, agranulocytosis, leukopenia, thrombocytopenia, anemia, eosinophilia

Musculoskeletal: arthralgia

Other: hypersensitivity reactions, anaphylaxis, overgrowth of nonsusceptible organisms, pain at injection site, vein irritation

NURSING CONSIDERATIONS

• Obtain specimen for culture and sensitivity tests before giving first dose. Begin therapy while awaiting results.

• Drug may decrease hormonal contraceptive effectiveness. Advise use of another form of contraception during therapy.

• Don't confuse drug with Polycillin, penicillamine, or the various types of penicillin.

PATIENT TEACHING

• Tell patient to report adverse reactions promptly.

• Instruct patient to report discomfort at I.V. site.

• Warn patient receiving I.M. injection that the injection may be painful but that ice applied to site may help alleviate discomfort.

penicillin V potassium
pen-i-SILL-in

Penicillin VK, Veetids

Pharmacologic class: Natural penicillin

INDICATIONS
➤ Mild to moderate systemic infections
➤ To prevent recurrent rheumatic fever
➤ To prevent inhalation anthrax after possible exposure

ACTION
Inhibits cell-wall synthesis during bacterial multiplication.

ADVERSE REACTIONS
CNS: neuropathy
GI: epigastric distress, nausea, diarrhea, black hairy tongue, vomiting
GU: nephropathy
Hematologic: leukopenia, thrombocytopenia, eosinophilia, hemolytic anemia
Other: anaphylaxis, hypersensitivity reactions, overgrowth of nonsusceptible organisms

NURSING CONSIDERATIONS
• Obtain specimen for culture and sensitivity tests before giving first dose. Begin therapy while awaiting results.
• Periodically assess renal and hematopoietic function in patients receiving long-term therapy.
• Drug may decrease hormonal contraceptive effectiveness. Advise use of another form of contraception during therapy.
• Don't confuse drug with Polycillin, penicillamine, or the various types of penicillin.

PATIENT TEACHING
• Tell patient to take drug with food if stomach upset occurs.
• Advise patient to notify prescriber if rash, fever, or chills develop. A rash is the most common allergic reaction.

Peripheral vasodilator

hydrALAZINE hydrochloride

INDICATION
➤ Hypertension

ACTION
Hydralazine is a direct-acting peripheral vasodilator that relaxes smooth muscle, causing blood vessels to dilate. This lowers the blood pressure by increasing the diameter of the blood vessels, reducing total peripheral resistance.

ADVERSE REACTIONS
Headache, angina pectoris, palpitations, tachycardia, nausea, vomiting, diarrhea, and anorexia

CONTRAINDICATIONS AND CAUTIONS
• Contraindicated in patients with a known hypersensitivity or allergy to clomiphene or to any of its ingredients.
• Contraindicated in patients with coronary artery disease or mitral valvular rheumatic heart disease.
• Use cautiously in patients with suspected cardiac disease, stroke, or severe renal impairment, and in patients taking other antihypertensives.
• Elderly patients may be more sensitive to drug's hypotensive effects.

hydrALAZINE hydrochloride
hye-DRAL-a-zeen

Pharmacologic class: Peripheral dilator

INDICATIONS
➤ Hypertension

ACTION
Unknown. A direct-acting peripheral vasodilator that relaxes arteriolar smooth muscle.

ADVERSE REACTIONS
CNS: headache, peripheral neuritis, dizziness
CV: angina pectoris, palpitations, tachycardia, orthostatic hypotension, edema, flushing
EENT: nasal congestion
GI: nausea, vomiting, diarrhea, anorexia, constipation
Hematologic: neutropenia, leukopenia, agranulocytopenia, agranulocytosis, thrombocytopenia with or without purpura
Skin: rash
Other: lupuslike syndrome

NURSING CONSIDERATIONS
• Drug is compatible with normal saline, Ringer's, lactated Ringer's, and several other common I.V. solutions.
• Monitor patient's blood pressure, pulse rate, and body weight frequently.
• Monitor patient closely for signs and symptoms of lupuslike syndrome (sore throat, fever, muscle and joint aches, rash), and notify prescriber immediately if they develop.
• Don't confuse hydralazine with hydroxyzine.

PATIENT TEACHING
• Instruct patient to take oral form with meals to increase absorption.
• Inform patient that low blood pressure and dizziness upon standing can be minimized by rising slowly and avoiding sudden position changes.
• Tell woman of childbearing age to notify prescriber if she suspects pregnancy. Drug will need to be stopped.
• Tell patient to notify prescriber of unexplained prolonged general tiredness or fever, muscle or joint aching, or chest pain.

Phenothiazines

prochlorperazine/prochlorperazine edisylate/prochlorperazine maleate
promethazine hydrochloride

INDICATIONS
➤ Agitated psychotic states, hallucinations, manic-depressive illness, excessive motor and autonomic activity, nausea and vomiting, anxiety, symptomatic rhinitis

ACTION
Phenothiazines are believed to function as dopamine antagonists by blocking postsynaptic dopamine receptors in various parts of the CNS. Their antiemetic effects result from blockage of the chemoreceptor trigger zone. They also produce varying degrees of anticholinergic effects and alpha adrenergic–receptor blocking.

ADVERSE REACTIONS
Phenothiazines may produce extrapyramidal symptoms, such as dystonic movements, torticollis, oculogyric crises, and parkinsonian symptoms. Other adverse reactions include abdominal pain, agitation, anorexia, arrhythmias, confusion, constipation, dizziness, dry mouth, hematologic disorders, nausea, photosensitivity, rash, and vomiting.

CONTRAINDICATIONS AND CAUTIONS
• Contraindicated in patients with a known hypersensitivity or allergy to phenothiazines or to any of its ingredients.
• Use cautiously in debilitated patients and in those with hepatic, renal, or CV disease; respiratory disorders; hypocalcemia; seizure disorders; suspected brain tumor or intestinal obstruction; glaucoma; and prostatic hyperplasia.
• In pregnant women, use only if clearly necessary; safety hasn't been established. Women shouldn't breast-feed during therapy because most phenothiazines appear in breast milk and directly affect prolactin levels. For children younger than age 12, phenothiazines aren't recommended unless otherwise specified; use cautiously for nausea and vomiting. Acutely ill children, such as those with chickenpox, measles, CNS infections, or dehydration, have a greatly increased risk of dystonic reactions. Elderly patients are more sensitive to therapeutic and adverse effects, especially cardiac toxicity, tardive dyskinesia, and other extrapyramidal effects; use cautiously and give reduced doses, adjusting dosage to patient response.

prochlorperazine/prochlorperazine edisylate/ prochlorperazine maleate

proe-klor-PER-a-zeen

Compro/Procomp

Pharmacologic class: Dopamine antagonist

INDICATIONS
➤ Nausea and vomiting
➤ Psychotic disorders; nonpsychotic anxiety

ACTION
Acts on the chemoreceptor trigger zone to inhibit nausea and vomiting; in larger doses, it partially depresses vomiting center.

ADVERSE REACTIONS
CNS: extrapyramidal reactions, dizziness, pseudoparkinsonism
CV: orthostatic hypotension, ECG changes, tachycardia
EENT: blurred vision, ocular changes
GI: constipation, dry mouth, increased appetite
GU: urine retention, dark urine, inhibited ejaculation
Hematologic: agranulocytosis, transient leukopenia
Skin: mild photosensitivity reactions, allergic reactions

NURSING CONSIDERATIONS
• Watch for orthostatic hypotension, especially when giving drug I.V.
• Infuse slowly; rate shouldn't exceed 5 mg/minute. Maximum parenteral dose is 40 mg daily.
• Use drug only when vomiting can't be controlled by other measures or when only a few doses are needed. If more than four doses are needed in 24 hours, notify prescriber.
• Dilute oral solution with tomato juice, fruit juice, milk, coffee, carbonated beverage, tea, water, or soup. Or, mix with pudding.

PATIENT TEACHING
• Advise patient to wear protective clothing when exposed to sunlight.
• Tell patient to call prescriber if more than four doses are needed within 24 hours.

promethazine hydrochloride
proe-METH-a-zeen

Phenadoz, Promethegan

Pharmacologic class: Phenothiazine

INDICATIONS
➤ Motion sickness
➤ Nausea and vomiting
➤ Rhinitis, allergy symptoms
➤ Nighttime sedation
➤ Adjunct to analgesics for routine preoperative or postoperative sedation

ACTION
Phenothiazine derivative that competes with histamine for H_1-receptor sites on effector cells. Prevents, but doesn't reverse, histamine-mediated responses. At high doses, drug also has local anesthetic effects.

ADVERSE REACTIONS
CNS: drowsiness, sedation, confusion, sleepiness, dizziness, disorientation, extrapyramidal symptoms
EENT: dry mouth, blurred vision
GI: nausea, vomiting
GU: urine retention
Hematologic: leukopenia, agranulocytosis, thrombocytopenia
Metabolic: hyperglycemia
Respiratory: respiratory depression, apnea
Skin: photosensitivity, rash

NURSING CONSIDERATIONS
• Monitor patient for neuroleptic malignant syndrome.
• In patients scheduled for a myelogram, stop drug 48 hours before procedure. Don't resume drug until 24 hours after procedure because of the risk of seizures.

PATIENT TEACHING
• Tell patient to take oral form with food or milk.
• When treating motion sickness, tell patient to take first dose 30 to 60 minutes before travel.
• Warn patient to avoid alcohol and hazardous activities that require alertness until CNS effects of drug are known.
• Warn patient about possible photosensitivity reactions. Advise use of a sunblock.

Potassium supplements

potassium chloride
potassium gluconate

INDICATIONS
➤ To prevent or treat hypokalemia

ACTION
Potassium moves quickly into ICF to restore depleted potassium levels and reestablish balance. It is an essential element in determining cell membrane potential and excitability.

Potassium is necessary for proper functioning of all nerve and muscle cells and for nerve impulse transmission. It's also essential for tissue growth and repair and for maintenance of acid–base balance.

ADVERSE REACTIONS
Most adverse reactions to potassium are related to the method of administration. Oral potassium sometimes causes nausea, vomiting, abdominal pain, and diarrhea. Enteric-coated tablets may cause small-bowel ulcerations, stenosis, hemorrhage, and obstruction. An I.V. infusion can cause pain at the injection site and phlebitis and, if given rapidly, cardiac arrest. Infusion of potassium in patients with decreased urine production also increases the risk of hyperkalemia.

CONTRAINDICATIONS AND CAUTIONS
• Contraindicated in patients with severe renal impairment with oliguria, anuria, or azotemia; with untreated Addison's disease; or with acute dehydration, heat cramps, hyperkalemia, hyperkalemic form of familial periodic paralysis, or other conditions linked to extensive tissue breakdown.
• Use cautiously in patients with cardiac disease or renal impairment.
• Use cautiously in elderly patients because they have an increased risk of GI lesions.

potassium chloride

Kaon-C, Kay Ciel, K-Dur 10, K-Dur 20, K-Lor, Klor-Con, Klotrix, K-Lyte/Cl, K-Tab, K-Vescent, Micro-K

Pharmacologic class: Potassium salt

INDICATIONS

➤ To prevent or treat hypokalemia

ACTION

Replaces potassium and maintains potassium level.

ADVERSE REACTIONS

CNS: paresthesia of limbs, listlessness, confusion, weakness or heaviness of limbs, flaccid paralysis

CV: postinfusion phlebitis, arrhythmias, heart block, cardiac arrest, ECG changes, hypotension

GI: nausea, vomiting, abdominal pain, diarrhea

Metabolic: hyperkalemia

Respiratory: respiratory paralysis

NURSING CONSIDERATIONS

• ACE inhibitors, digoxin, and potassium-sparing diuretics may cause hyperkalemia. Use together with extreme caution. Monitor potassium level.

• Monitor ECG and electrolyte levels during therapy. Monitor renal function.

• When administering I.V., dilute the preparation before infusion and give the diluted drug slowly. Never give as an I.V. bolus or I.M. injection.

• Potassium preparations aren't interchangeable; verify preparation before use and don't switch products.

PATIENT TEACHING

• Teach patient how to prepare powders and how to take drug. Tell patient to take with or after meals with full glass of water or fruit juice to lessen GI distress.

• Teach patient signs and symptoms of hyperkalemia, and tell patient to notify prescriber if they occur.

• Tell patient to report discomfort at I.V. insertion site.

• Warn patient not to use salt substitutes concurrently, except with prescriber's permission.

potassium gluconate

Kaon, Kaylixir

Pharmacologic class: Potassium salt

INDICATIONS
• To prevent or treat hypokalemia

ACTION
Replaces potassium and maintains intracellular and extracellular potassium levels.

ADVERSE REACTIONS
CNS: paresthesia of limbs, listlessness, confusion, weakness or heaviness of legs, flaccid paralysis

CV: arrhythmias, ECG changes

GI: nausea, vomiting, abdominal pain, diarrhea

NURSING CONSIDERATIONS
• ACE inhibitors, digoxin, and potassium-sparing diuretics may cause hyperkalemia. Use together with extreme caution. Monitor potassium level.

• Give oral potassium supplements with caution because different forms deliver varying amounts of potassium. Never switch products without prescriber's order.

• Monitor ECG, fluid intake and output, and BUN, potassium, and creatinine levels.

PATIENT TEACHING
• Advise patient to sip liquid potassium slowly to minimize GI irritation. Also tell him to take drug with meals, with a full glass of water or fruit juice.

• Warn patient not to use potassium gluconate with a salt substitute, except with prescriber's permission.

• Teach patient signs and symptoms of hyperkalemia, and tell him to notify prescriber if they occur.

Progestins

medroxyPROGESTERone acetate
norethindrone/norethindrone acetate

INDICATIONS
➤Abnormal uterine bleeding, amenorrhea, contraception, endometriosis (medroxyprogesterone acetate and norethindrone/norethindrone acetate), endometrial hyperplasia, endometrial or renal cancer (medroxyprogesterone acetate)

ACTION
Medroxyprogesterone acetate suppresses ovulation, possibly by inhibiting pituitary gonadotropin secretion (medroxyprogesterone acetate and norethindrone/norethindrone acetate), preventing follicular maturation and causing endometrial thinning (medroxyprogesterone acetate), and forming a thick cervical mucus (norethindrone/norethindrone acetate).

ADVERSE REACTIONS
Bloating, abdominal pain, breakthrough bleeding, amenorrhea

CONTRAINDICATIONS AND CAUTIONS
• Contraindicated in patients with a known hypersensitivity or patients with active thromboembolic disorders or a history of thromboembolic disorders, cerebrovascular disease, apoplexy, undiagnosed abnormal vaginal bleeding, missed abortion, or hepatic.
• Contraindicated during pregnancy.
• Use cautiously in patients with diabetes, seizures, migraine, cardiac or renal disease, asthma, or depression.
• Contraindicated for use in women with breast cancer or a history of breast cancer. Use cautiously in women with a strong family history of breast cancer or who have breast nodules.

medroxyPROGESTERone acetate
me-DROX-ee-proe-JESS-te-rone

Depo-Provera, Depo-subQ, Provera 104, Provera
Pharmacologic class: Progestin

INDICATIONS
➤ Abnormal uterine bleeding; secondary amenorrhea
➤ Endometrial hyperplasia; endometrial or renal cancer; endometriosis
➤ Contraception

ACTION
Suppresses ovulation, possibly by inhibiting pituitary gonadotropin secretion, thus preventing follicular maturation and causing endometrial thinning.

ADVERSE REACTIONS
CNS: depression, stroke, pain, dizziness
CV: thrombophlebitis, pulmonary embolism, edema, thromboembolism, syncope
GI: bloating, abdominal pain
GU: breakthrough bleeding, dysmenorrhea, amenorrhea
Metabolic: weight changes
Musculoskeletal: loss of bone mineral density
Other: breast tenderness, enlargement, or secretion; hot flashes

NURSING CONSIDERATIONS
• Give by deep I.M. injection in the gluteal or deltoid muscle.

PATIENT TEACHING
• Advise patient to take medication with food if GI upset occurs.
• Tell patient to report unusual symptoms immediately and to stop drug and notify prescriber about visual disturbances or migraine.
• Advise patient to immediately report to prescriber any breast abnormalities, vaginal bleeding, swelling, yellowed skin or eyes, dark urine, clay-colored stools, shortness of breath, chest pain, or pregnancy.
• Advise patient that injection must be given every 3 months to maintain adequate contraceptive effects.

norethindrone/norethindrone acetate
nor-ETH-in-drone

Camila, Errin, Micronor, Nor-QD/Aygestin

Pharmacologic class: Progestin

INDICATIONS
➤ Amenorrhea, abnormal uterine bleeding, endometriosis
➤ Contraception

ACTION
Suppresses ovulation, possibly by inhibiting pituitary gonadotropin secretion, and forms thick cervical mucus.

ADVERSE REACTIONS
CNS: depression, stroke, headache, mood swings
CV: thrombophlebitis, pulmonary embolism, edema, thromboembolism
GI: bloating, abdominal pain or cramping
GU: breakthrough bleeding, dysmenorrhea, amenorrhea, cervical erosion, abnormal secretions
Metabolic: weight changes
Other: breast tenderness, enlargement, or secretion, premenstrual-like syndrome, anaphylactic reactions

NURSING CONSIDERATIONS
• Norethindrone acetate is twice as potent as norethindrone. Norethindrone acetate shouldn't be used for contraception.
• Watch patient closely for signs of edema.
• Don't confuse Micronor with Micro-K or Micronase.

PATIENT TEACHING
• Tell patient to take drug at the same time every day when used as a contraceptive. If she's more than 3 hours late taking the pill or if she has missed a pill, she should take the pill as soon as she remembers and then continue the normal schedule. Also tell her to use a backup method of contraception for the next 48 hours.
• Tell patient to report unusual symptoms immediately and to stop drug and notify prescriber about visual disturbances or migraine, or pain or numbness in her arms or legs.
• Encourage patient to stop or reduce smoking because of the risk of CV complications.
• Tell patient that drug does not protect against HIV or other sexually transmitted diseases.

Protease inhibitors

indinavir sulfate
lopinavir and ritonavir
nelfinavir mesylate

INDICATIONS
➤ HIV infection and AIDS

ACTION
Protease inhibitors bind to the protease active site and inhibit HIV protease activity. This enzyme is required for the proteolysis of viral polyprotein precursors into individual functional proteins found in infectious HIV. The net effect is formation of noninfectious, immature viral particles.

ADVERSE REACTIONS
The most common adverse effects, which require immediate medical attention, include kidney stones, pancreatitis, diabetes or hyperglycemia, ketoacidosis, and paresthesia. Common adverse effects that don't need medical attention unless they persist or are bothersome include generalized weakness, GI disturbances, headache, insomnia, and taste disturbance. Less common adverse effects include dizziness and somnolence.

CONTRAINDICATIONS AND CAUTIONS
• Contraindicated in patients hypersensitive to these drugs or their components and patients taking a drug highly dependent on CYP3A4 for metabolism.
• Use cautiously in patients with impaired hepatic or renal function and those with diabetes mellitus or hemophilia.
• In pregnant women, use drug only if benefits outweigh risks.
• HIV-infected mothers shouldn't breast-feed, to reduce the risk of transmitting HIV to the infant.

indinavir sulfate

in-DIN-ah-ver

Crixivan

Pharmacologic class: Protease inhibitor

INDICATIONS

➤ HIV infection, with other antiretrovirals, when antiretrovirals are warranted

ACTION

Inhibits HIV protease by binding to the protease-active site and inhibiting activity of the enzyme, preventing cleavage of the viral polyproteins and forming immature noninfectious viral particles.

ADVERSE REACTIONS

CNS: asthenia, dizziness, fatigue, headache, insomnia, malaise
GI: nausea, abdominal pain, acid regurgitation, anorexia, diarrhea, dry mouth, taste perversion, vomiting
Hematologic: neutropenia, thrombocytopenia, anemia
Metabolic: hyperbilirubinemia, hyperglycemia

NURSING CONSIDERATIONS

• Drug must be taken at 8-hour intervals.
• To prevent nephrolithiasis, patient should maintain adequate hydration (at least 48 oz or 1.5 L of fluids every 24 hours while taking indinavir).

PATIENT TEACHING

• Tell patient that drug doesn't cure HIV infection and that he or she may continue to develop opportunistic infections and other complications of HIV infection.
• Advise patient to use barrier protection during sexual intercourse.
• Caution patient not to adjust dosage or stop therapy without first consulting prescriber.
• Advise patient that if a dose is missed, he or she should take the next dose at the regularly scheduled time and shouldn't double the dose.
• Instruct patient to take drug on an empty stomach with water 1 hour before or 2 hours after a meal. Or, patient may take it with other liquids (such as skim milk, juice, coffee, or tea) or a light meal.

lopinavir and ritonavir
low-PIN-ah-ver

Kaletra

Pharmacologic class: Protease inhibitor

INDICATIONS
➤ HIV infection

ACTION
Lopinavir is an HIV protease inhibitor, which produces immature, noninfectious viral particles. Ritonavir, also an HIV protease inhibitor, slows lopinavir metabolism, thereby increasing lopinavir level.

ADVERSE REACTIONS
CNS: encephalopathy, abnormal dreams, abnormal thinking, depression, dizziness, fever, headache, hypertonia, tremors
CV: chest pain, deep vein thrombosis, edema, hypertension, palpitations, thrombophlebitis, vasculitis
GI: hemorrhagic colitis, pancreatitis, diarrhea, nausea
Hematologic: leukopenia, neutropenia, thrombocytopenia in children, anemia
Metabolic: Cushing's syndrome, dehydration, weight loss
Skin: acne, alopecia, pruritus, rash, skin discoloration, sweating
Other: chills, facial edema, flu syndrome, viral infection

NURSING CONSIDERATIONS
• Many drug interactions are possible. Review all drugs patient is taking.
• Monitor patient for signs of fat redistribution.
• Monitor total cholesterol and triglycerides before starting therapy and periodically thereafter.
• Monitor patient for signs and symptoms of pancreatitis.
• Don't confuse Kaletra with Keppra.

PATIENT TEACHING
• Tell patient to take oral solution with food. Tablets must be swallowed whole; don't crush, divide, or chew.
• Tell patient to immediately report severe nausea, vomiting, or abdominal pain.
• Inform patient that drug doesn't cure HIV infection, that opportunistic infections and other complications of HIV infection may still occur, and that transmission of HIV to others remains possible.

nelfinavir mesylate
nell-FIN-ah-veer

Viracept
Pharmacologic class: Protease inhibitor

INDICATIONS
➤ HIV infection
➤ To prevent infection after exposure to HIV

ACTION
An HIV-1 protease inhibitor, which prevents cleavage of the viral polyprotein, resulting in the production of immature, noninfectious virus.

ADVERSE REACTIONS
CNS: seizures, suicidal ideation
GI: diarrhea, pancreatitis, flatulence, nausea
Hematologic: leukopenia, thrombocytopenia
Hepatic: hepatitis
Metabolic: hypoglycemia, dehydration, diabetes mellitus, hyperlipidemia, hyperuricemia
Skin: rash
Other: redistribution or accumulation of body fat

NURSING CONSIDERATIONS
• Drug dosage is the same whether drug is used alone or with other antiretrovirals.
• Don't confuse nelfinavir with nevirapine.

PATIENT TEACHING
• Advise patient to take drug with food.
• Inform patient that drug doesn't cure HIV infection.
• If patient misses a dose, tell him or her to take it as soon as possible and then return to his normal schedule. Advise patient not to double the dose.
• Tell patient that diarrhea is the most common adverse effect and that it can be controlled with loperamide, if needed.
• Advise patient to report use of other prescribed or OTC drugs because of possible drug interactions.

Proton pump inhibitors

esomeprazole magnesium/esomeprazole sodium
lansoprazole
omeprazole/omeprazole magnesium
pantoprazole sodium
rabeprazole sodium

INDICATIONS
➤ Duodenal ulcers, gastric ulcers, erosive esophagitis, and GERD; hypersecretory conditions (Zollinger-Ellison syndrome) (lansoprazole, omeprazole, pantoprazole, rabeprazole)

ACTION
The drugs reduce stomach acid production by combining with hydrogen, potassium, and adenosine triphosphate in parietal cells of the stomach to block the last step in gastric acid secretion.

ADVERSE REACTIONS
Proton pump inhibitors (PPIs) may cause abdominal pain, diarrhea, constipation, flatulence, nausea, dry mouth, headache, asthenia, cough, abnormal liver function test results, and hyperglycemia.

CONTRAINDICATIONS AND CAUTIONS
• Contraindicated in patients hypersensitive to the drug components.
• Prolonged use of PPIs may cause low magnesium levels that require magnesium supplementation and possible discontinuation of the drug. Monitor magnesium levels before treatment and periodically during treatment. Monitor patients for signs and symptoms of low magnesium, such as abnormal heart rate or rhythm, palpitations, muscle spasms, tremors, or convulsions. In children, abnormal heart rates may present as fatigue, upset stomach, dizziness, and lightheadedness.

esomeprazole magnesium/esomeprazole sodium

ess-oh-ME-pray-zol

Nexium/Nexium I.V.

Pharmacologic class: Proton pump inhibitor

INDICATIONS
➤ GERD; erosive esophagitis; gastric ulcer prophylaxis in patients receiving continuous NSAID therapy; pathological hypersecretory conditions; *Helicobacter pylori* elimination

ACTION
Reduces gastric acid secretion and decreases gastric acidity.

ADVERSE REACTIONS
CNS: headache, dizziness
GI: abdominal pain, constipation, diarrhea, dry mouth, flatulence, nausea, vomiting
Respiratory: sinusitis, respiratory infection
Skin: pruritus

NURSING CONSIDERATIONS
• Monitor patient for rash or signs and symptoms of hypersensitivity. Monitor GI symptoms for improvement or worsening. Monitor liver function tests, especially in patients with preexisting hepatic disease.
• Drug may increase the risk for fractures of the hip, wrist, and spine.
• Long-term therapy may cause atrophic gastritis.
• Don't confuse Nexium with Nexavar.

PATIENT TEACHING
• Tell patient to take drug at least 1 hour before a meal.
• Advise patient that antacids can be used while taking drug unless otherwise directed by prescriber.
• Warn patient not to chew or crush drug pellets because this inactivates the drug.
• If patient has difficulty swallowing capsule, tell him to mix contents of capsule with 1 tablespoon of soft applesauce and swallow immediately.
• Tell patient to inform prescriber of worsening signs and symptoms or pain.
• Instruct patient to alert prescriber if rash or other signs and symptoms of allergy occur.

lansoprazole
lanz-AH-pray-zol

Prevacid, Prevacid SoluTab

Pharmacologic class: Proton pump inhibitor

INDICATIONS
➤ Duodenal ulcer, gastric ulcer, erosive esophagitis, pathological hypersecretory conditions, *Helicobacter pylori* elimination, GERD

ACTION
Inhibits proton pump activity by binding to hydrogen-potassium adenosine triphosphates, located at secretory surface of gastric parietal cells, to suppress gastric acid secretions.

ADVERSE REACTIONS
GI: abdominal pain, constipation, diarrhea, nausea

NURSING CONSIDERATIONS
• Patients with severe liver disease may need dosage adjustment, but don't adjust dosage for elderly patients or those with renal insufficiency.
• Drug may increase the risk for fractures of the hip, wrist, and spine.
• Just because symptoms respond to therapy, gastric malignancy shouldn't be ruled out.
• Don't confuse Prevacid with Pepcid, Prilosec, or Prevpac.

PATIENT TEACHING
• For best effect, instruct patient to take drug 30 to 60 minutes before eating.
• Tell patient he or she may mix the capsule's contents with a small amount (about 2 oz) of apple, cranberry, grape, orange, pineapple, prune, tomato, or vegetable juice. The patient must drink the mixture within 30 minutes. To ensure complete delivery of the dose, the patient should fill the glass two or more times with juice and swallow the contents immediately.
• Contents of capsule can be mixed with 1 tablespoon of applesauce, Ensure, pudding, cottage cheese, yogurt, or strained pears and swallowed immediately. The capsule and granules shouldn't be chewed or crushed.
• Tell patient taking ODTs to allow tablet to dissolve on tongue until all particles can be swallowed.

omeprazole/omeprazole magnesium
oh-ME-pray-zole

Prilosec/Prilosec OTC
Pharmacologic class: Proton pump inhibitor

INDICATIONS
➤ Duodenal ulcer, gastric ulcer, erosive esophagitis, pathological hypersecretory conditions, *Helicobacter pylori* elimination, GERD

ACTION
Inhibits proton pump activity by binding to hydrogen-potassium adenosine triphosphatase, located at secretory surface of gastric parietal cells, to suppress gastric acid secretion.

ADVERSE REACTIONS
CNS: asthenia, dizziness, headache
GI: abdominal pain, constipation, diarrhea, flatulence, nausea, vomiting
Musculoskeletal: back pain
Respiratory: cough, upper respiratory tract infection
Skin: rash

NURSING CONSIDERATIONS
• Dosage adjustments may be necessary in Asians and patients with hepatic impairment.
• There may be an increased risk of hip, wrist, and spine fractures associated with proton pump inhibitors.
• Use cautiously in patients with Bartter syndrome, hypokalemia, and respiratory alkalosis and in patients on a low-sodium diet.
• Don't confuse Prilosec with Prozac, Prilocaine, or Prinivil.

PATIENT TEACHING
• Tell patient to swallow tablets whole and not to open, crush, or chew them.
• Instruct patient to take drug at least 1 hour before meals.
• Advise patient that Prilosec OTC isn't intended to treat infrequent heartburn (one episode of heartburn a week or less), or for those who want immediate relief of heartburn.
• Inform patient that Prilosec OTC may take 1 to 4 days for full effect, although some patients may get complete relief of symptoms within 24 hours.

pantoprazole sodium
pan-TOE-pray-zol

Protonix, Protonix I.V.
Pharmacologic class: Proton pump inhibitor

INDICATIONS
➤ Erosive esophagitis, pathological hypersecretory conditions, GERD

ACTION
Inhibits proton pump activity by binding to hydrogen-potassium adenosine triphosphatase, located at secretory surface of gastric parietal cells, to suppress gastric acid secretion.

ADVERSE REACTIONS
CNS: anxiety, asthenia, dizziness, headache, insomnia, migraine
GI: abdominal pain, constipation, diarrhea, dyspepsia, eructation, flatulence, gastroenteritis, GI disorder, nausea, rectal disorder, vomiting
Metabolic: hyperglycemia, hyperlipemia
Skin: rash
Other: flulike syndrome, infection, injection-site reaction

NURSING CONSIDERATIONS
• Don't confuse Protonix with Prilosec, Prozac, or Prevacid.
• Drug may increase the risk for fractures of the hip, wrist, and spine.

PATIENT TEACHING
• Advise patient that drug can be taken without regard to meals.
• Tell patient to swallow tablet whole and not to crush, split, or chew it.
• Tell patient that antacids don't affect drug absorption.

rabeprazole sodium
rah-BEH-pray-zol

Aciphex

Pharmacologic class: Proton pump inhibitor

INDICATIONS
➤ Duodenal ulcer, erosive esophagitis, pathological hypersecretory conditions, *Helicobacter pylori* elimination, GERD

ACTION
Blocks proton pump activity and gastric acid secretion by inhibiting gastric hydrogen-potassium adenosine triphosphatase (an enzyme) at secretory surface of gastric parietal cells.

ADVERSE REACTIONS
CNS: headache, pain, dizziness
CV: edema
EENT: pharyngitis, dry mouth
GI: abdominal pain, constipation, diarrhea, flatulence
Hepatic: elevated liver enzyme levels, hepatitis, hepatic encephalopathy
Musculoskeletal: arthralgia, myalgia
Other: infection

NURSING CONSIDERATIONS
• Drug may increase the risk of fractures of the hip, wrist, and spine.
• If *H. pylori* eradication is unsuccessful, do susceptibility testing. If patient is resistant to clarithromycin or susceptibility testing isn't possible, expect to start therapy using a different antimicrobial.
• Patients treated for *H. pylori* eradication have developed pseudomembranous colitis with nearly all antibiotics, including clarithromycin and amoxicillin. Monitor patient closely.

PATIENT TEACHING
• Advise patient to swallow delayed-release tablet whole and not to crush, chew, or split.
• Inform patient that drug may be taken without regard to meals.

Skeletal muscle relaxants

baclofen
carisoprodol
cyclobenzaprine hydrochloride

INDICATIONS
➤ Painful musculoskeletal disorders; spasticity caused by multiple sclerosis

ACTION
Baclofen may reduce impulse transmission from the spinal cord to skeletal muscle. Carisoprodol's and cyclobenzaprine's mechanism of action is unclear.

ADVERSE REACTIONS
Skeletal muscle relaxants may cause ataxia, confusion, depressed mood, dizziness, drowsiness, dry mouth, hallucinations, headache, hypotension, nervousness, tachycardia, tremor, and vertigo. Baclofen also may cause seizures.

CONTRAINDICATIONS AND CAUTIONS
• Contraindicated in patients hypersensitive to these drugs.
• Use cautiously in patients with impaired renal or hepatic function.
• In pregnant women and breast-feeding women, use only when potential benefits to the patient outweigh risks to the fetus or infant. In children, recommendations vary. Elderly patients have an increased risk of adverse reactions; monitor them carefully.

baclofen
BAK-loe-fen

Lioresal Intrathecal
Pharmacologic class: GABA derivative

INDICATIONS
➤ Spasticity in multiple sclerosis; spinal cord injury

ACTION
Hyperpolarizes fibers to reduce impulse transmission. Appears to reduce transmission of impulses from the spinal cord to skeletal muscle, thus decreasing the frequency and amplitude of muscle spasms in patients with spinal cord lesions.

ADVERSE REACTIONS
CNS: drowsiness, dizziness, headache, weakness, hypotonia, confusion, insomnia, seizures with intrathecal use
CV: hypotension
GI: nausea, constipation
Musculoskeletal: muscle rigidity or spasticity, rhabdomyolysis
Respiratory: dyspnea
Skin: rash, pruritus, excessive sweating
Other: multiple organ-system failure

NURSING CONSIDERATIONS
• Watch for sensitivity reactions, such as fever, skin eruptions, and respiratory distress.
• Expect an increased risk of seizures in patients with seizure disorder.
• Don't withdraw drug abruptly after long-term use unless severe adverse reactions demand it; doing so may precipitate seizures, hallucinations, or rebound spasticity.
• Don't confuse baclofen with Bactroban.

PATIENT TEACHING
• Instruct patient to take oral form with meals or milk.
• Tell patient to avoid activities that require alertness until CNS effects of drug are known. Drowsiness usually is transient.
• Tell patient to avoid alcohol and OTC antihistamines while taking drug.

carisoprodol
kar-eye-soe-PROE-dol

Soma

Pharmacologic class: Carbamate derivative

INDICATIONS
➤ Adjunctive treatment for acute, painful musculoskeletal conditions

ACTION
May modify central perception of pain without modifying pain reflexes. Muscle relaxant effects may be related to sedative properties.

ADVERSE REACTIONS
CNS: drowsiness, dizziness, vertigo, ataxia, tremor, agitation, irritability, headache, depressive reactions, fever, insomnia, syncope
CV: orthostatic hypotension, tachycardia, facial flushing
GI: nausea, vomiting, epigastric distress, hiccups
Respiratory: asthmatic episodes, hiccups
Skin: erythema multiforme, pruritus, rash
Other: angioedema, anaphylaxis

NURSING CONSIDERATIONS
• Watch for idiosyncratic reactions after first to fourth doses (weakness, ataxia, visual and speech difficulties, fever, skin eruptions, and mental changes) and for severe reactions, including bronchospasm, hypotension, and anaphylactic shock. After unusual reactions, withhold dose and notify prescriber immediately.
• Don't stop drug abruptly, which may cause mild withdrawal effects, such as insomnia, headache, nausea, or abdominal cramps.

PATIENT TEACHING
• Warn patient to avoid activities that require alertness until CNS effects of drug are known. Drowsiness is transient.
• Advise patient to avoid combining drug with alcohol or other CNS depressants.
• Advise patient to avoid sudden changes in posture if dizziness occurs.
• Tell patient to take drug with food or milk if GI upset occurs.

cyclobenzaprine hydrochloride

sye-kloe-BEN-za-preen

Amrix, Flexeril

Pharmacologic class: Tricyclic antidepressant derivative

INDICATIONS
➤ Adjunct to rest and physical therapy to relieve muscle spasm from acute, painful musculoskeletal conditions

ACTION
Unknown. Relieves skeletal muscle spasms of local origin without disrupting muscle function.

ADVERSE REACTIONS
CNS: dizziness, drowsiness, seizures, headache, tremor, insomnia, fatigue, asthenia, nervousness, confusion, paresthesia, depression, attention disturbances, dysarthria, ataxia, syncope
CV: arrhythmias, palpitations, hypotension, tachycardia
EENT: visual disturbances, blurred vision
GI: dry mouth, dyspepsia, abnormal taste, constipation, nausea
Skin: rash, pruritus, acne

NURSING CONSIDERATIONS
• Monitor patient for nausea, headache, and malaise, which may occur if drug is stopped abruptly after long-term use.
• Notify prescriber immediately of signs and symptoms of overdose, including cardiac toxicity.
• Don't confuse Flexeril with Floxin.

PATIENT TEACHING
• Advise patient to report urinary hesitancy or urine retention. If constipation is a problem, suggest that patient increase fluid intake and use a stool softener.
• Warn patient to avoid activities that require alertness until CNS effects of drug are known.
• Warn patient not to combine with alcohol or other CNS depressants, including OTC cold or allergy remedies.

Sulfonamides

sulFADIAZINE
sulfamethoxazole and trimethoprim

INDICATIONS
➤ Bacterial infections, nocardiosis, toxoplasmosis, chloroquine-resistant *Plasmodium falciparum* malaria

ACTION
Sulfonamides are bacteriostatic. They inhibit biosynthesis of tetrahydrofolic acid, which is needed for bacterial cell growth. They're active against some strains of staphylococci, streptococci, *Nocardia asteroides* and *N. brasiliensis*, *Clostridium tetani* and *C. perfringens*, *Bacillus anthracis*, *Escherichia coli*, and *Neisseria gonorrhoeae* and *N. meningitidis*. Sulfonamides are also active against organisms that cause UTIs, such as *E. coli*, *Proteus mirabilis* and *P. vulgaris*, *Klebsiella*, *Enterobacter*, and *Staphylococcus aureus*, and genital lesions caused by *Haemophilus ducreyi* (chancroid).

ADVERSE REACTIONS
Many adverse reactions stem from hypersensitivity, including bronchospasm, conjunctivitis, erythema multiforme, erythema nodosum, exfoliative dermatitis, fever, joint pain, pruritus, leukopenia, Lyell syndrome, photosensitivity, rash, Stevens-Johnson syndrome, and toxic epidermal necrolysis. GI reactions include anorexia, diarrhea, folic acid malabsorption, nausea, pancreatitis, stomatitis, and vomiting. Hematologic reactions include agranulocytosis, granulocytopenia, thrombocytopenia, and, in G6PD deficiency, hemolytic anemia. Renal effects usually result from crystalluria caused by precipitation of sulfonamide in renal system.

CONTRAINDICATIONS AND CAUTIONS
• Contraindicated in patients hypersensitive to these drugs.
• Use cautiously in patients with renal or hepatic impairment, bronchial asthma, severe allergy, or G6PD deficiency.
• In pregnant women at term and in breast-feeding women, use is contraindicated; sulfonamides appear in breast milk. In infants younger than age 2 months, sulfonamides are contraindicated unless there's no therapeutic alternative. In children with fragile X chromosome and mental retardation, use cautiously. Elderly patients are susceptible to bacterial and fungal superinfection and have an increased risk of folate deficiency anemia and adverse renal and hematologic effects.

sulfADIAZINE
sul-fa-DYE-a-zeen
Pharmacologic class: Sulfonamide

INDICATIONS
➤ Asymptomatic meningococcal carrier
➤ To prevent rheumatic fever, as an alternative to penicillin
➤ Adjunctive treatment for toxoplasmosis
➤ Nocardiosis

ACTION
Inhibits formation of dihydrofolic acid from PABA, decreasing bacterial folic acid synthesis; bacteriostatic.

ADVERSE REACTIONS
CNS: seizures, depression, hallucinations, headache
GI: diarrhea, nausea, vomiting, abdominal pain
GU: toxic nephrosis with oliguria and anuria, crystalluria
Hematologic: agranulocytosis, aplastic anemia, leukopenia, thrombocytopenia, hemolytic anemia, megaloblastic anemia
Skin: generalized skin eruption, erythema multiforme, Stevens-Johnson syndrome, toxic epidermal necrolysis, exfoliative dermatitis, photosensitivity reactions, pruritus, urticaria
Other: anaphylaxis, drug fever, hypersensitivity reactions

NURSING CONSIDERATIONS
• Promptly report rash, sore throat, fever, cough, mouth sores, or iris lesions—early signs and symptoms of erythema multiforme, which may progress to life-threatening Stevens-Johnson syndrome, or of blood dyscrasias.
• Watch for signs and symptoms of superinfection, such as fever, chills, and increased pulse.
• Folic or folinic acid may be used during rest periods in toxoplasmosis therapy to reverse hematopoietic depression or anemia caused by pyrimethamine and sulfadiazine.
• Monitor fluid intake and output. Maintain intake between 3,000 and 4,000 ml daily for adults to produce output of 1,500 ml daily. Monitor urine pH daily.
• Don't confuse sulfadiazine with sulfasalazine.

PATIENT TEACHING
• Urge patient to drink a glass of water with each dose, plus plenty of water each day to prevent urine crystals.
• Warn patient to avoid prolonged sun exposure, wear protective clothing, and use sunscreen.

sulfamethoxazole and trimethoprim
sul-fa-meth-OX-a-zole and tri-meth-O-prim

Bactrim, Bactrim DS, Septra, Septra DS, Sulfatrim
Pharmacologic class: Sulfonamide and folate antagonist

INDICATIONS
➤ Shigellosis, UTIs, otitis media, traveler's diarrhea
➤ Chronic bronchitis, upper respiratory tract infections
➤ To prevent or treat *Pneumocystis jiroveci* (*carinii*) pneumonia

ACTION
Sulfamethoxazole inhibits formation of dihydrofolic acid from PABA; trimethoprim inhibits dihydrofolate reductase formation. Both decrease bacterial folic acid synthesis and are bactericidal.

ADVERSE REACTIONS
CNS: seizures, aseptic meningitis, ataxia, fatigue, hallucinations, headache, insomnia, nervousness, tinnitus, vertigo
GI: pancreatitis, pseudomembranous colitis, diarrhea, nausea, vomiting, abdominal pain, anorexia, stomatitis
GU: toxic nephrosis with oliguria and anuria, crystalluria, hematuria, interstitial nephritis
Hematologic: agranulocytosis, aplastic anemia, leukopenia, thrombocytopenia, hemolytic anemia, megaloblastic anemia.
Hepatic: hepatic necrosis, jaundice
Skin: generalized skin eruption, erythema multiforme, Stevens-Johnson syndrome, toxic epidermal necrolysis
Other: anaphylaxis, drug fever, hypersensitivity reactions

NURSING CONSIDERATIONS
• Promptly report rash, sore throat, fever, cough, mouth sores, or iris lesions—early signs and symptoms of erythema multiforme, which may progress to life-threatening Stevens-Johnson syndrome, or of blood dyscrasias.
• Watch for signs and symptoms of superinfection, such as fever, chills, and increased pulse.

PATIENT TEACHING
• Encourage patient to drink plenty of fluids to prevent crystalluria and kidney stone formation. Instruct patient to take oral form with 8 oz of water on an empty stomach.
• Advise patient to avoid prolonged sun exposure, wear protective clothing, and use sunscreen.

Tetracyclines

doxycycline/doxycycline calcium/doxycycline hyclate/doxycycline
  monohydrate
tetracycline hydrochloride

INDICATIONS
➤ Bacterial, protozoal, rickettsial, and fungal infections

ACTION
Tetracyclines are bacteriostatic but may be bactericidal against certain organisms. They bind reversibly to 30S and 50S ribosomal subunits, which inhibits bacterial protein synthesis. Susceptible gram-positive organisms include *Bacillus anthracis*, *Actinomyces israelii*, *Clostridium perfringens* and *C. tetani*, *Listeria monocytogenes*, and *Nocardia*. Susceptible gram-negative organisms include *Neisseria meningitidis*, *Pasteurella multocida*, *Legionella pneumophila*, *Brucella*, *Vibrio cholerae*, *Yersinia enterocolitica*, *Yersinia pestis*, *Bordetella pertussis*, *Haemophilus influenzae*, *H. ducreyi*, *Campylobacter fetus*, *Shigella*, and many other common pathogens. Other susceptible organisms include *Rickettsia akari*, *R. typhi*, *R. prowazekii*, and *R. tsutsugamushi*; *Coxiella burnetii*; *Chlamydia trachomatis* and *C. psittaci*; *Mycoplasma pneumoniae* and *M. hominis*; *Leptospira*; *Treponema pallidum* and *T. pertenue*; and *Borrelia recurrentis*.

ADVERSE REACTIONS
The most common adverse effects involve the GI tract and are dose related; they include abdominal discomfort; anorexia; bulky, loose stools; epigastric burning; flatulence; nausea; and vomiting. Superinfections also are common. Photosensitivity reactions may be severe. Permanent discoloration of teeth occurs if drug is given during tooth formation in children younger than age 8.

CONTRAINDICATIONS AND CAUTIONS
• Contraindicated in patients hypersensitive to these drugs.
• Use cautiously in patients with renal or hepatic impairment.
• In pregnant or breast-feeding women, use is contraindicated; tetracyclines appear in breast milk. Children younger than age 8 shouldn't take tetracyclines; these drugs can cause permanent tooth discoloration, enamel hypoplasia, and a reversible decrease in bone calcification. Elderly patients may have decreased esophageal motility; use these drugs cautiously. Elderly patients also are more susceptible to superinfection.

doxycycline/doxycycline calcium/doxycycline hyclate/doxycycline monohydrate

dox-i-SYE-kleen

Oracea/Vibramycin/Atridox, Doryx, Oraxyl, Vibramycin/Monodox, Vibramycin

Pharmacologic class: Tetracycline

INDICATIONS

➤ Gonorrhea; syphilis; uncomplicated urethral, endocervical, or rectal infections; pelvic inflammatory disease; anthrax; periodontitis; rosacea
➤ Malaria prophylaxis

ACTION

May exert bacteriostatic effect by binding to the 30S and possibly 50S ribosomal subunits of microorganisms and inhibiting protein synthesis. May also alter the cytoplasmic membrane of susceptible microorganisms.

ADVERSE REACTIONS

CNS: intracranial hypertension
GI: diarrhea, epigastric distress, nausea, oral candidiasis
Hematologic: neutropenia, thrombocytopenia, eosinophilia
Skin: maculopapular and erythematous rashes, photosensitivity reactions, increased pigmentation, urticaria
Other: anaphylaxis, hypersensitivity reactions, superinfection, permanent discoloration of teeth, enamel defects

NURSING CONSIDERATIONS

• Watch for signs and symptoms of superinfection.
• Check patient's tongue for signs of fungal infection.
• Don't confuse doxycycline, doxylamine, and dicyclomine.
• Photosensitivity reactions may occur within a few minutes to several hours after sun exposure. Photosensitivity lasts after therapy ends.

PATIENT TEACHING

• Advise patient to take oral form of drug with food or milk if stomach upset occurs.
• Advise patient to increase fluid intake and not to take oral tablets or capsules within 1 hour of bedtime because of possible esophageal irritation or ulceration.
• Warn patient to avoid direct sunlight and ultraviolet light, wear protective clothing, and use sunscreen.

tetracycline hydrochloride
tet-ra-SYE-kleen

Sumycin
Pharmacologic class: Tetracycline

INDICATIONS
➤ Uncomplicated urethral, endocervical, or rectal infections caused by *Chlamydia trachomatis*
➤ Brucellosis, gonorrhea, syphilis, acne, *Helicobacter pylori* infection

ACTION
May exert bacteriostatic effect by binding to the 30S and possibly 50S ribosomal subunits of microorganisms, thus inhibiting protein synthesis. May also alter the cytoplasmic membrane of susceptible microorganisms.

ADVERSE REACTIONS
CNS: intracranial hypertension, dizziness, headache
GI: diarrhea, epigastric distress, nausea, oral candidiasis
Hematologic: neutropenia, thrombocytopenia, eosinophilia
Skin: candidal superinfection, increased pigmentation, maculopapular and erythematous rash, photosensitivity reactions, urticaria
Other: enamel defects, hypersensitivity reactions, permanent discoloration of teeth

NURSING CONSIDERATIONS
• Using outdated or deteriorated drug has been linked to severe reversible nephrotoxicity (Fanconi syndrome).
• Watch for signs and symptoms of superinfection.
• Check patient's tongue for signs of candidal infection.
• Photosensitivity reactions may occur within a few minutes to several hours after sun exposure. Photosensitivity lasts after therapy ends.

PATIENT TEACHING
• Explain to patient that effectiveness is reduced when drug is taken with milk or other dairy products, antacids, or iron products. Also tell patient to take it at least 1 hour before bedtime to prevent esophageal irritation or ulceration.
• Warn patient to avoid direct sunlight and ultraviolet light, wear protective clothing, and use sunscreen.

Thyroid hormone replacement drugs

levothyroxine sodium (T_4)
liothyronine sodium (T_3)

INDICATIONS
➤ Thyroid hormone deficiency

ACTION
Thyroid hormones affect protein and carbohydrate metabolism and stimulate protein synthesis. They promote glucogenesis and increase the use of glycogen stores. In addition, thyroid hormones increase heart rate and cardiac output. They may even increase the heart's sensitivity to catecholamines and increase the number of beta-adrenergic receptors in the heart. Thyroid hormones may increase blood flow to the kidneys and increase the glomerular filtration rate in patients with hypothyroidism, producing diuresis.

ADVERSE REACTIONS
Most adverse reactions to thyroid drugs result from toxicity. Adverse reactions in the GI system include diarrhea, abdominal cramps, weight loss, and increased appetite. Adverse reactions in the cardiovascular system include palpitations, sweating, rapid heart rate, increased blood pressure, angina, and arrhythmias.

CONTRAINDICATIONS AND CAUTIONS
• Contraindicated in patients hypersensitive to drug and in those with acute MI uncomplicated by hypothyroidism, untreated thyrotoxicosis, or uncorrected adrenal insufficiency.
• Use cautiously in elderly patients and in those with angina pectoris, hypertension, other CV disorders, renal insufficiency, or ischemia.
• Use cautiously in patients with diabetes mellitus, diabetes insipidus, or myxedema and during rapid replacement in those with arteriosclerosis.

levothyroxine sodium (T$_4$)

lee-voe-thye-ROX-een

Levo-T, Levothroid, Levoxyl, Synthroid, Unithroid
Pharmacologic class: Thyroid hormone

INDICATIONS

➤ Thyroid hormone replacement, hypothyroidism, myxedema coma

ACTION

Not completely defined. Stimulates metabolism of all body tissues by accelerating rate of cellular oxidation.

ADVERSE REACTIONS

CNS: nervousness, insomnia, tremor, headache, fever, fatigue
CV: tachycardia, arrhythmias, angina pectoris, cardiac arrest
GI: diarrhea, vomiting
Metabolic: weight loss, increased appetite
Musculoskeletal: decreased bone density, muscle weakness
Skin: allergic skin reactions, diaphoresis, hair loss
Other: heat intolerance, impaired fertility

NURSING CONSIDERATIONS

• Patients with diabetes mellitus may need increased antidiabetic doses when starting thyroid hormone replacement.
• Watch for angina, coronary occlusion, or stroke in patients with arteriosclerosis who are receiving rapid replacement.
• Patients taking anticoagulants may need their dosage modified and require careful monitoring of coagulation status.
• Dosage may need to be increased in pregnant patients.
• Don't confuse levothyroxine with liothyronine!

PATIENT TEACHING

• Teach patient the importance of compliance. Tell him or her to take drug at same time each day, preferably ½ to 1 hour before breakfast, to maintain constant hormone levels and help prevent insomnia.
• Make sure patient understands that replacement therapy is usually for life. The drug should never be stopped unless directed by prescriber.
• Advise patient who has achieved stable response not to change brands.

liothyronine sodium (T$_3$)

lye-oh-THYE-roe-neen

Cytomel, Triostat

Pharmacologic class: Thyroid hormone

INDICATIONS
➤ Thyroid hormone replacement, hypothyroidism, myxedema coma, premyxedema coma, simple (nontoxic) goiter

ACTION
Unclear. Enhances oxygen consumption by most tissues of the body; increases the basal metabolic rate and the metabolism of carbohydrates, lipids, and proteins.

ADVERSE REACTIONS
CNS: nervousness, insomnia, tremor, headache, fever
CV: tachycardia, arrhythmias, angina, cardiac decompensation and collapse, MI
GI: diarrhea, vomiting
Metabolic: weight loss
Skin: skin reactions, diaphoresis
Other: heat intolerance

NURSING CONSIDERATIONS
• Watch for angina, coronary occlusion, or stroke in patients with arteriosclerosis who are receiving rapid replacement. In patients with coronary artery disease who must receive thyroid hormones, watch for possible coronary insufficiency.
• Monitor pulse and blood pressure.
• In pregnant patients, dosage may need to be increased.
• Don't confuse levothyroxine with liothyronine or liotrix. Don't confuse Cytomel with Cytotec.

PATIENT TEACHING
• Teach patient importance of compliance. Tell him or her to take thyroid hormones at same time each day, preferably before breakfast, to maintain constant hormone levels and help prevent insomnia.
• Make sure patient understands that replacement therapy is usually for life. Drug should never be stopped unless directed by prescriber.
• Advise patient who has achieved a stable response not to change brands.

Urinary analgesic

phenazopyridine hydrochloride

INDICATIONS
➤ Pain with urinary tract irritation or infection

ACTION
Phenazopyridine exerts local anesthetic action on urinary mucosa.

ADVERSE REACTIONS
Headache, nausea, vomiting, rash, pruritus, anaphylactoid reactions

CONTRAINDICATIONS AND CAUTIONS
• Contraindicated in patients hypersensitive to drug and in those with glomerulonephritis, severe hepatitis, uremia, renal insufficiency, or pyelonephritis during pregnancy.

phenazopyridine hydrochloride

fen-az-oh-PEER-i-deen

Azo-Gesic, Azo-Standard, Baridium, Pyridium, Urogesic, UTI-Relief

Pharmacologic class: Urinary analgesic

INDICATIONS

➤ Pain with urinary tract irritation or infection

ACTION

Unknown; exerts local anesthetic action on urinary mucosa.

ADVERSE REACTIONS

CNS: headache
EENT: staining of contact lenses
GI: nausea, GI disturbances
Hematologic: hemolytic anemia, methemoglobinemia
Skin: rash, pruritus
Other: anaphylactoid reactions

NURSING CONSIDERATIONS

• When drug is used with an antibacterial, therapy shouldn't extend beyond 2 days.
• Patients with red blood cell G6PD deficiency may be predisposed to hemolysis.
• Don't confuse Pyridium with pyridoxine.

PATIENT TEACHING

• Advise patient that taking drug with meals may minimize GI distress.
• Caution patient to stop drug and notify prescriber immediately if skin or sclera becomes yellow-tinged, which may indicate drug accumulation from impaired renal excretion.
• Inform patient that drug colors urine red or orange and may stain fabrics and contact lenses.
• Advise patient that drug doesn't treat the infection and to notify prescriber if urinary tract pain persists. Tell him or her that drug shouldn't be used for long-term treatment.

Urinary tract antispasmodics

oxybutynin chloride
tolterodine tartrate
trospium chloride

INDICATIONS
➤ Overactive bladder; uninhibited or reflex neurogenic bladder (oxybutynin)

ACTION
Urinary tract antispasmodics relieve smooth-muscle spasms by inhibiting parasympathetic activity, which causes the detrusor and urinary muscles to relax. Oxybutynin also exhibits many anticholinergic effects.

ADVERSE REACTIONS
Blurred vision, headache, somnolence, urinary retention, dry mouth, dyspepsia, constipation, nausea, vomiting.

CONTRAINDICATIONS AND CAUTIONS
• Contraindicated in patients hypersensitive to drug or its components and in those with myasthenia gravis, GI obstruction, untreated angle-closure glaucoma, megacolon, adynamic ileus, severe colitis, ulcerative colitis with megacolon, urine or gastric retention, or obstructive uropathy.
• Contraindicated in elderly or debilitated patients with intestinal atony and in hemorrhaging patients with unstable CV status.
• Use cautiously in elderly, pregnant, or breast-feeding patients and in those with autonomic neuropathy, reflux esophagitis, or hepatic or renal disease.

oxybutynin chloride
ox-i-BYOO-ti-nin

Ditropan, Ditropan XL, Gelnique, Oxytrol

Pharmacologic class: Antimuscarinic

INDICATIONS
➤ Neurogenic bladder, overactive bladder

ACTION
Relaxes smooth muscle of bladder by antagonizing muscarinic receptors, relieving symptoms of overactive bladder.

ADVERSE REACTIONS
CNS: dizziness, insomnia, restlessness, fever, headache
CV: palpitations, tachycardia, vasodilation
EENT: mydriasis, cycloplegia, blurred vision, dry eyes
GI: constipation, dry mouth, nausea, vomiting
GU: urinary hesitancy, urine retention, impotence
Skin: pruritus

NURSING CONSIDERATIONS
• Drug may aggravate symptoms of hyperthyroidism, coronary artery disease, heart failure, arrhythmias, tachycardia, hypertension, or prostatic hyperplasia.
• Obtain periodic cystometry as directed to evaluate response to therapy.
• Monitor patient for residual urine after voiding.
• Don't confuse Ditropan with diazepam or Dithranol, or oxybutynin with Oxycontin.

PATIENT TEACHING
• Warn patient to avoid hazardous activities, such as operating machinery or driving, until CNS effects of drug are known.
• Caution patient that using drug during very hot weather may cause fever or heatstroke because it suppresses sweating.
• Tell patient to swallow Ditropan XL whole and not to chew or crush it.
• Instruct patient using transdermal patch to change patch twice a week and to choose a new application site with each new patch to avoid the same site within 7 days. Warn patient to only wear one patch at a time.
• Advise patient using topical gel to rotate application sites.
• Advise patient to avoid alcohol while taking drug.

tolterodine tartrate
toll-TEAR-oh-deen

Detrol, Detrol LA

Pharmacologic class: Antimuscarinic

INDICATIONS
➤ Overactive bladder

ACTION
Relaxes smooth muscle of bladder by antagonizing muscarinic receptors, relieving symptoms of overactive bladder.

ADVERSE REACTIONS
CNS: headache, fatigue, paresthesia, vertigo, dizziness, nervousness, somnolence
CV: hypertension, chest pain
EENT: abnormal vision, pharyngitis, rhinitis, sinusitis
GI: dry mouth, abdominal pain, constipation, diarrhea, dyspepsia, flatulence, nausea, vomiting
GU: dysuria, micturition frequency, urine retention, UTI
Respiratory: bronchitis, coughing, URI
Skin: pruritus, rash, erythema, dry skin
Other: flulike syndrome, fungal infection, infection

NURSING CONSIDERATIONS
• Assess baseline bladder function and monitor therapeutic effects.
• Monitor patient for residual urine after voiding.

PATIENT TEACHING
• Advise patient to avoid driving or other potentially hazardous activities until visual effects of drug are known.
• Advise women to stop breast-feeding during therapy.
• Instruct patient to immediately report signs of infection, urine retention, or GI problems.
• Tell patient taking extended-release form to swallow capsule whole and take with liquids.

trospium chloride

TROZ-pee-um

Sanctura, Sanctura XR

Pharmacologic class: Antimuscarinic

INDICATIONS
➤ Overactive bladder

ACTION
Relaxes smooth muscle of bladder by antagonizing muscarinic receptors, relieving symptoms of overactive bladder.

ADVERSE REACTIONS
CNS: fatigue, headache
EENT: dry eyes
GI: constipation, dry mouth, abdominal pain, dyspepsia, flatulence
GU: urine retention

NURSING CONSIDERATIONS
• Assess patient to determine baseline bladder function, and monitor patient for therapeutic effects.
• Monitor patient for residual urine after voiding.
• If patient has bladder outflow obstruction, watch for evidence of urine retention.
• Monitor patient for decreased gastric motility and constipation.
• Elderly patients typically need a reduced dosage because they have an increased risk of anticholinergic effects.

PATIENT TEACHING
• Tell patient to take drug on an empty stomach or at least 1 hour before meals.
• Tell patient to take extended release form with water in the morning on an empty stomach, at least 1 hour before a meal.
• Tell patient that alcohol may increase drowsiness and fatigue. Urge him to avoid excessive alcohol consumption while taking trospium.
• Explain that drug may decrease sweating and increase the risk of heatstroke when used in hot environments or during strenuous activities.
• Urge patient to avoid activities that are hazardous or require mental alertness until he knows how the drug affects him.

Appendices

The eight "rights" of medication administration

Traditionally, nurses have been taught the "five rights" of medication administration. These are broadly stated goals and practices to help individual nurses administer drugs safely.

1. **The right drug:** Check the drug label and verify that the drug and form to be given is the drug that was prescribed.

2. The **right patient:** Confirm the patient's identity by checking at least two patient identifiers.

3. The **right dose:** Verify that the dose and form to be given is appropriate for the patient, and check the drug label with the prescriber's order.

4. The **right time:** Ensure that the drug is administered at the correct time and frequency.

5. The **right route:** Verify that the route by which the drug is to be given is specified by the prescriber and is appropriate for the patient.

   In addition to the traditional "five rights" of individual practice, best practice researchers have added three additional "rights":

6. The **right reason:** Verify that the drug prescribed is appropriate to treat the patient's condition.

7. The **right response:** Monitor the patient's response to the drug administered.

8. The **right documentation:** Completely and accurately document in the patient's medical record the drug administered, the monitoring of the patient, including his response, and other nursing interventions.

Avoiding common drug errors: Best practices and prevention

In addition to following your institution's administration policies, you can help prevent errors in drug administration by reviewing these common errors and ways to prevent them. The Joint Commission, the Institute for Safe Medication Practices (ISMP), and the FDA also maintain resources to help improve drug safety.

Topic	Error	Best practices and prevention
Drug orders		
Pharmacy computer system	The system may not detect all unsafe orders.	• Don't rely on the pharmacy computer system to detect all unsafe orders. • Before giving a drug, understand the correct indication, dosage, and potential adverse effects. • Consult the pharmacist if there is any question, and verify the information using a current drug reference.
Confusing drug names	Many drugs have names that look alike–sound alike and may easily be mistaken one for the other.	• Be aware of the drugs your patient takes regularly, and question any deviations from his routine. • Take your time and read the label carefully. • Consult the ISMP list of look alike–sound alike drugs. • Be aware of tall man lettering, which helps differentiate similar drug names.
Abbreviations	Using dangerous abbreviations can result in giving the wrong drug or wrong dose, by the wrong route, or at the wrong time.	• Don't abbreviate drug names. • Be aware of The Joint Commission's official "Do not use" list of drug abbreviations to avoid (see *Abbreviations to avoid*, page 388). • Consult your facility's list of approved abbreviations and the ISMP's list of "Error-prone abbreviations, symbols, and dose designations" (www.ismp.org/tools/errorproneabbreviations.pdf).
Unclear order	A drug order with incomplete or unclear information can result in giving the wrong drug or wrong dose, by the wrong route, or at the wrong time.	• Keep in mind that each order should specify the correct drug name, dosage, route, and frequency of administration. • Clarify all incomplete or unclear orders with the prescriber.
Inadvertent overdose	A prescriber may write an order for a combination drug such as acetaminophen/opioid analgesic tablets without realizing the total acetaminophen dose could be toxic (exceed 4 g).	• Note the amount of acetaminophen in each combined formulation. • Be aware of pharmacy substitutions because acetaminophen amounts may vary. • Warn patients not to take additional drugs that contain acetaminophen.

Topic	Error	Best practices and prevention

Drug orders (continued)

Anticoagulants	Lack of standardization for drug naming, labeling, and packaging can create confusion. Dosing regimens, assay methods, narrow therapeutic ranges, complex drug interactions, and drug monitoring create high potential for complications.	• Keep current with the different dosing, assay methods, drug interactions, monitoring methods, and reversal regimens for each anticoagulant given. • Be especially aware of the correct doses and indications for neonates and children. • Teach patients to manage their therapy appropriately.

Drug preparation

Crushing drugs for oral or enteral administration	Crushing certain oral or enteral drugs may • alter the drug's effects, causing overdose or other adverse reactions • result in skin irritation or other adverse reactions for the preparer • produce teratogenic effects in pregnant women.	• Use a liquid formulation instead of crushing a drug whenever possible. • Before crushing a drug, always check with the pharmacist and established references, such as the ISMP's list of "Oral dosage forms that should not be crushed" (www.ismp.org/tools/donotcrush.pdf).
Solution color change or particulate matter	Unusual appearance may indicate that • the drug has been improperly stored or manufactured • the drug has expired • the wrong drug was provided by the pharmacy.	• Closely examine all solutions before giving them and know what their appearance should be. • If you note a color change, contact the pharmacist who dispensed the solution and report it. • Don't give a drug until verifying that the drug has been correctly labeled and that it is safe to give.
Incorrect drug storage	Incorrect storage may change a drug's physical properties or result in its being inadvertently administered.	• Follow your facility's policy for storing drugs. • Always store drugs in the appropriate container, in the appropriate place, at the appropriate temperature.
Incomplete or incorrect drug labels	Incorrect or incomplete labeling can result in giving the wrong drug, formulation, or dose.	• Never give a drug whose label is incomplete or incorrect. Notify the pharmacy immediately and obtain the correctly labeled drug. • Label all medications, medication containers, and other solutions on and off the sterile field.

Topic	Error	Best practices and prevention

Drug administration

Topic	Error	Best practices and prevention
Using a parenteral syringe for oral or enteral drugs	Using a parenteral syringe with a luer-lock to prepare small amounts of oral or enteral drugs can result in misadministration because the drug could be accidentally injected into an I.V. line.	• Always use special oral syringes to give oral or enteral drugs. Their hubs won't support a needle and they don't have a luer-lock, so they can't be attached to I.V. lines.
Infusion pump safety problems	Problems with infusion pumps (used to deliver controlled fluids, drugs, and nutrients) can cause fluid overload or administration of inaccurate doses.	• Make sure you know how to safely operate an infusion pump. Consult your facility's policy on proper usage. • Before beginning an infusion, always verify that the pump is working properly. Make sure all alarms are functional and never bypass them. • Double-check all dosing.
Calculation errors	Dosage calculation errors can cause significant patient harm, especially with "high alert" medications, and in neonates and children.	• Be aware of medications that are considered high alert. • Write out the mg/kg or mg/m^2 dose and the calculated dose as a safeguard. • Whenever a prescriber provides a calculation, double-check it and document that the dose was verified in the medical record. • Use only approved abbreviations, and be aware of the placement of decimal points.
Herbal supplements	Because herbal supplements aren't subject to the same quality assurance standards as drugs, their labels may be misrepresented and their effects and interactions with drugs may not be well studied.	• Always assess and document all drugs and herbal supplements that the patient is taking in his medical record. • Monitor the patient carefully, and report unusual adverse reactions. • Consult a drug reference for known drug–herb interactions.

Abbreviations to avoid

The Joint Commission requires every health care facility to develop a list of approved abbreviations for staff use. Certain abbreviations should be avoided because they're easily misunderstood, especially when handwritten. The Joint Commission has identified a minimum list of dangerous abbreviations, acronyms, and symbols. This do-not-use list includes the following items.

Official "Do Not Use" List[1]

Do not use	Potential problem	Use instead
U (unit)	Mistaken for "0" (zero), the number "4" (four) or "cc"	Write "unit"
IU (International Unit)	Mistaken for IV (intravenous) or the number 10 (ten)	Write "International Unit"
Q.D., QD, q.d., qd (daily)	Mistaken for each other	Write "daily"
Q.O.D., QOD, q.o.d, qod (every other day)	Period after the Q mistaken for "I" and the "O" mistaken for "I"	Write "every other day"
Trailing zero (X.0 mg)* Lack of leading zero (.X mg)	Decimal point is missed	Write X mg Write 0.X mg
MS	Can mean morphine sulfate or magnesium sulfate	Write "morphine sulfate" Write "magnesium sulfate"
MSO_4 and $MgSO_4$	Confused for one another	

[1]Applies to all orders and all medication-related documentation that is handwritten (including free-text computer entry) or on pre-printed forms.

*Exception: A "trailing zero" may be used only where required to demonstrate the level of precision of the value being reported, such as for laboratory results, imaging studies that report size of lesions, or catheter/tube size. It may not be used in medication orders or other medication-related documentation.

Additional Abbreviations, Acronyms and Symbols
(For <u>possible</u> future inclusion in the Official "Do Not Use" List)

Do not use	Potential problem	Use instead
> (greater than) < (less than)	Misinterpreted as the number "7" (seven) or the letter "L" Confused for one another	Write "greater than" Write "less than"
Abbreviations for drug names	Misinterpreted due to similar abbreviations for multiple drugs	Write drug names in full
Apothecary units	Unfamiliar to many practitioners Confused with metric units	Use metric units
@	Mistaken for the number "2" (two)	Write "at"
cc	Mistaken for U (units) when poorly written	Write "mL" or "ml" or "milliliters" ("mL" is preferred)
µg	Mistaken for mg (milligrams) resulting in one thousand-fold overdose	Write "mcg" or "micrograms"

© The Joint Commission, 2010. Reprinted with permission.

Patient education guidelines

Patients and their families should be active participants in the patient's care and should understand the patient's care plan, including the purpose of newly prescribed medications. The patient and family need to be taught what to watch for, how the patient's condition will be monitored, and what signs and symptoms to report, and to report anything that doesn't seem right, including unfamiliar medications. Before administering a medication, the nurse needs to verify with the patient any medication allergies or unusual past reactions to medications.

The following general teaching guidelines will help ensure that the patient receives the maximum therapeutic benefit from his medication regimen and will help him avoid adverse reactions, accidental overdose, and harmful changes in effectiveness.

- Instruct the patient to learn the brand names, generic names, and dosages of all drugs and supplements (such as herbs and vitamins) that he's taking.

- Tell the patient to notify the pharmacist and prescriber about everything he takes, including prescription drugs, OTC drugs, and herbal or other supplements, and about any drug allergies.

- Advise the patient to always read the label before taking a drug, to take it exactly as prescribed, and never to share prescription drugs.

- Warn the patient not to change brands of a drug without consulting the prescriber, to avoid harmful changes in effectiveness. For example, certain generic preparations aren't equivalent in effect to brand-name preparations of the same drug.

- Tell the patient to check the expiration date before taking a drug.

- Show the patient how to safely discard drugs that are outdated or no longer needed.

- Caution the patient to keep all drugs safely out of the reach of children and pets.

- Advise the patient to store drugs in their original container, at the proper temperature, and in areas where they won't be exposed to sunlight or excessive heat or humidity. Sunlight, heat, and humidity can cause drug deterioration and reduce a drug's effectiveness.

- Encourage the patient to report adverse or unusual reactions to the prescriber, and teach him proper techniques to monitor his condition (for example, how to obtain a resting heart rate before taking Lanoxin).

- Suggest that the patient have all prescriptions filled at the same pharmacy so that the pharmacist can warn against potentially harmful drug interactions.

- Tell the patient to report his complete medication history to all health care providers he sees, including his dentist.

- Instruct the patient to call the prescriber, poison control center, or pharmacist immediately and to seek immediate medical attention if he or someone else has taken an overdose. Tell the patient to keep emergency numbers handy at all times.

- Advise the patient to make sure he has a sufficient supply of drugs when traveling. He should carry them with him in their original containers and not pack them in luggage. Also, recommend that he carries a letter from his prescriber authorizing the use of a drug, especially if the drug is a controlled substance.

Special pediatric drug administration considerations

Biochemically, a drug displays the same mechanisms of action in all people. But the response to a drug can be affected by a child's age and size, as well as by the maturity of the target organ. To ensure optimal drug effect and minimal toxicity, consider the following factors when giving drugs to children.

Adjusting dosages for children

When calculating children's dosages, don't use formulas that only modify adult dosages. Base pediatric dosages on either body weight (mg/kg) or body surface area (mg/m^2). A child isn't a scaled-down version of an adult. Reevaluate dosages at regular intervals to ensure needed adjustments as the child develops. Although body surface area provides a useful standard for adults and older children, use the body weight method instead in premature or full-term infants.

Giving oral drugs

Remember the following when giving oral drugs to a child:

- If the patient is an infant, give drugs in liquid form, if possible. For accuracy, measure and give the preparation by oral syringe, never a parenteral syringe. It's very important to remove the syringe cap to keep the infant from aspirating it. Be sure to instruct parents to do the same. Never use a vial or cup. Lift the patient's head to prevent aspiration of the drug, and press down on his chin to prevent choking. You may also place the drug in a nipple and allow the infant to suck the contents.

- If the patient is a toddler, explain how you're going to give him the drug. If possible, have the parents enlist the child's cooperation. Don't call the drug "candy," even if it has a pleasant taste. Let the child drink a liquid drug from a calibrated medication cup rather than a spoon. It's easier and more accurate. If the preparation is available only in tablet form, crush and mix it with an appropriate buffer, such as jelly or applesauce. (First, verify with the pharmacist that the tablet can be crushed without compromising its effectiveness.)

- If the patient is an older child who can swallow a tablet or capsule by himself, have him place the drug on the back of his tongue and swallow it with water or nonacidic fruit juice.

Giving I.V. infusions

For I.V. infusions in infants, use a peripheral vein or a scalp vein in the temporal region. The arms and legs are the most accessible insertion sites, but because patients tend to move about, take these precautions:

- Protect the insertion site to keep the catheter or needle from being dislodged.

- Use a padded arm board to reduce the risk of dislodgment. Remove the arm board during range-of-motion exercises.

- Place the clamp out of the child's reach. If extension tubing is used to allow the child greater mobility, securely tape the connection.

- During an infusion, monitor flow rates and check the child's condition and insertion site at least every hour. Infants, small children, and children with compromised cardiopulmonary status are especially vulnerable to fluid overload with I.V. drug administration. To prevent this problem and help ensure that a limited amount of fluid is infused in a controlled manner, use an infusion pump.

Giving I.M. injections

I.M. injections are preferred when a drug can't be given by other parenteral routes and rapid absorption is needed.

The vastus lateralis muscle is the preferred injection site in children younger than age 2. To select the correct needle size, consider the patient's age, muscle mass, nutritional status, and drug viscosity. Record and rotate injection sites. Explain to the patient that the injection will hurt but that the drug will help him. Restrain him during the injection, if needed, and comfort him afterward.

Giving Topical Drugs

When you give a child a topical drug, consider the following:

- Use eardrops warmed to room temperature. Cold drops can cause pain and vertigo. To give drops, turn the patient on his side, with the affected ear up. If he's younger than age 3, pull the pinna down and back; if age 3 or older, pull the pinna up and back.

- Use topical corticosteroids cautiously because prolonged use in children may delay growth. When you apply topical corticosteroids to the diaper area of infants, don't cover the area with plastic or rubber pants, which act as an occlusive dressing and may enhance systemic absorption.

Index